The Chemical Analysis of Prehistoric Bones

A paleodietary and ecoarcheological study of Bronze Age West-Friesland

L. T. Runia

BAR International Series 363
1987

B.A.R.

5, Centremead, Osney Mead, Oxford OX2 0DQ, England.

BAR -S363, 1987: 'The Chemical Analysis of Prehistoric Bones'

ISBN 9780860544715 paperback
ISBN 9781407346380 e-book
DOI https://doi.org/10.30861/9780860544715
A catalogue record for this book is available from the British Library
This book is available at www.barpublishing.com

"Denken alleen is niet voldoende",
  zegt de vos.
"De volgende keer
  moet je het zeker weten."

Waar is Piep
N. Benchley & A. Lobel
Amsterdam: Ploegsma

ACKNOWLEDGEMENTS

The present work and the analyses described and discussed in it could not have been carried out and completed without the help, assistance, cooperation, criticism and patience of a number of persons. I wish to thank them all: dr. Gerard IJzereef, dr. Clason, drs. de Haas, drs. van de Walle-van der Woude, dr. Constandse-Westerman and drs. Bergström for submitting bones and bone samples; dr. A.C. Zeven, mr. van Laar and mr. Topper for plant samples; drs. van Raaphorst, Dick Börger, Bart Broerse, Gerard Heeringa and dr. Tjip Lub for analytical facilities; dr. George Maat for physical-anthropological instructions; dr. W.G. Mook and staff of his laboratory for stable isotope analyses; dr. Margaret Schoeninger for hospitality and introducing me into bone chemistry; Fred Gijbels, Bob Donker, Bert Brouwestijn and Ab Visser for drawings and photographs; Jakob Tiesinga and Sytze Faber for many books and papers; Rik Maliepaard for cleaning and measuring bones; dr. Jan Albert Bakker, drs. Roel Brandt, drs. Jan Peter Pals, drs. Linda Therkorn and drs. Willy de Vries-Metz for discussions; Bert de Leeuw for XRD and DTA and Domela Grondstra for providing working space.

Special thanks are due to dr. Willy Groenman-van Waateringe and dr. Loes van Wijngaarden-Bakker for giving me the opportunity to carry out this study, for continuous support and for critical discussions; and to dr. Carol van Driel-Murray for correcting the English text and for stimulating ideas.

The investigations were supported by the Foundation for Archaeological Research, which is subsidised by the Netherlands Organization for the Advancement of Pure Research (ZWO). A grant from the St.Christophorileen tot Oldehove, founded in 1480, is gratefully acknowledged.

Wieke, Tessel, Jetteke, Merlijn and Elke had to endure seeing me change into an addict of bones, graphs and floppy disks- I hope to change back.

Contents

I. Chemical analysis of bone in archeology 4

II. The geographical and archeological context 23

III. Analytical procedures in bone analysis 53

IV. Analysis of bone: the macro elements calcium, phosphorus and iron 55

V. Analysis of bone: strontium 60

VI. Analysis of bone: zinc 90

VII. Analysis of bone: miscellaneous trace elements 108

VIII. Trace elements in cremations 125

IX. Analysis of soil and plant material 130

X. Stable isotopes in bone collagen 152

XI. Discussion: agricultural and dietary implications 161

References 199

Appendix 1: Catalogue of prehistoric human bone material from West-Friesland 213

Appendix 2: Abbreviations 234

I
CHEMICAL ANALYSIS OF BONE IN ARCHEOLOGY

A. INTRODUCTION

A.1 General aspects

Albert Egges van Giffen, the founder of modern Dutch archeology, was trained as a biologist. The subject of his dissertation (1913) was "Die Fauna der Wurten", and during his long and active career as an all-round archeologist he remained interested in zooarcheology and in paleoenvironmental research in general (Waterbolk 1973, Clason 1983). Reputedly, there have been occasions where he entertained little regard for human remains: upon discovery of some human burial he recorded its position, took a photograph, collected skull, pelvis and one femur and discarded the rest of the bones. Obviously, Van Giffen could not foresee the potentials of prehistoric bones in the reconstruction of 'past behaviour', though even in his time analyses of bones from Roman times were being attempted in relation to lead pollution (Nriagu 1983a). His sampling strategy resulted in the loss of material, but he saved enough to make the present study concerning the chemical analysis of human and animal bones possible: a study which was conducted at the Institute bearing his name.

Van Giffen's dissertation is an example in the long history of the morphological study of human and animal bones from archeological sites. The study of morphology, metrical characteristics, provenance and many other aspects of prehistoric human and animal bones still remains an important field of research in archeology. In the Netherlands, more or less in the line of Van Giffen's attitude towards human bones, the study of prehistoric human bones is not very well established. Archeologists leave the study of human bones from their excavations to interested physical anthropologists on a more or less ad-hoc basis. This approach might result, for instance, in the situation whereby the Neolithic and Bronze Age skeletons from the Oostwoud barrows (Van Giffen 1962), the largest complex of skeletons of that period in the Netherlands, were mislayed in a depot. The recent policy of reducing government expenses and the closing of the 'Instituut voor Anthropobiologie' in Utrecht will not cause an improvement of this situation.

In contrast to this, the study of animal bones from excavated prehistoric sites is well established in the Netherlands: the archeological institutes of Amsterdam and Groningen and the ROB all have zoological departments. The initiative for the present study of, principally, human skeletal material was taken by the zooarcheological department of the IPP. In personal contacts with Dutch physical anthropologists, it appeared that their research interests are, more or less as a consequence of their positions in faculties of medicine, mainly in research areas other than the study of skeletal material from archeological excavations. The possibilities of chemical analyses of prehistoric bone in relation to paleodietary and paleoecological problems appeared to be unfamiliar.

Though chemical analysis of bone in relation to archeological problems is not "as old as the road to Rome", the first attempts were made in the beginning of this century when Rosenblatt analysed human bones from the Roman Period (Rosenblatt 1906, Kobert 1909, cited in Gilfillan 1965 and

Nriagu 1983a). These analyses, probably with doubtful results because of the inaccurate analytical techniques, were a contribution to the discussion on lead pollution and lead poisoning in Roman times. The causal relation between lead pollution and the decline and fall of the Roman Empire is still disputed even though bone analysis remains one of the tools in the study of this problem.

This early use of bone analyses in archeological contexts is but a small foretaste of the menu of potential uses of bone chemistry in archeological, anthropological and paleoecological research. At present, the focus of analyses of prehistoric bones is on dietary reconstruction by means of analysis of trace element (strontium, zinc and others) concentrations in bone mineral and determination of stable isotope (carbon, nitrogen) ratios in bone collagen. Price (1986) states that 'the study of archaeological bone chemistry is at a turning point, in transition from an experimental procedure to a major research technique'. Though this statement may be optimistic in the light of the problems still present in the interpretation of bone trace element levels in terms of dietary composition, we may agree with Price in that 'there is justification for enthusiasm about the potential of this methodology to provide greater resolution for our views of the past', but (Price et al. 1985b:429) 'trace element analysis, along with isotopic studies, as a tool in the study of the past is in its infancy'.

Bone chemistry studies rely on data gathered by researchers with medical and physiological interests. However, little was done in the field of bone chemistry, e.g. on trace element concentrations, before the 1960's. The interest in the incorporation in bone of radioactive strontium deriving from atmospheric nuclear testing is an exception to this general picture (Comar et al. 1957). In one of the first reports on bone trace element concentrations, Alexander & Nusbaum (1962) give zinc concentrations in 25 human rib samples. These rib samples had originally been collected for strontium analysis. Many papers on trace elements in fresh human and animal tissues do not contain information on concentrations in bone mineral (for instance, Schroeder & Balassa 1966, Schroeder et al. 1966).

The paper by Becker et al. (1968) may be the first to contain reliable data on trace element concentrations in prehistoric human bones. Besides fresh bone samples, prehistoric Peruvian and Pennsylvanian bones were analysed in order to compare recent and prehistoric levels of trace elements. No dietary extrapolations were made.

The study of the chemistry of prehistoric bones aims to add new, independent information and to broaden and refine the picture of prehistoric human diets that has been produced by the established archeological and ecoarcheological research methods. 'Traditional' phyto- and zooarcheological research is carried out as a matter of routine (or, at least, it should be) in many archeological projects. Besides giving clues on the past environment and, for instance, seasonality of sites, one of the aims of the ecoarcheologist is to provide insight in the range of available food resources, animal and vegetable, marine and terrestrial (Wing & Brown 1979, Mann 1981, Gilbert & Mielke 1985). The characteristics of the remains of plants and animals and of taphonomic processes inevitably result in a qualitatively and quantitatively incomplete and biased picture of the foods that were consumed (Jones 1983). Usually, the methods used in ecoarcheological studies do not allow for distinguishing differences in the composition of diets of various individuals and groups of individuals. Even differences between sites may not be quantifiable by the traditional methods.

The chemical composition of human and animal bone, and especially the concentrations of trace elements and the ratios of the stable isotopes of carbon and nitrogen, in principle reflects the dietary regime of the individuals concerned. Thus, theoretically, by extracting the information on diet that is hidden in the composition of the bones, it is possible to reconstruct individual diets. After filtering out biases due to a number of factors, such as diagenetic alteration of the bone composition, physiological effects of age, sex and disease, and geographical variations, the diets of various individuals, or rather groups of individuals, can be compared. Obviously, this is a clear advantage of the bone analysis method compared to the 'traditional' ecoarcheological methods. The need for this kind of data on prehistoric diets, and especially on the amount of meat therein, may be most urgently felt by researchers of hominids and early humans (Harding & Teleki 1981, Sillen 1981, compare also Schoeninger 1982) where archeological and ecoarcheological 'Begleitfunde' next to the fossil hominid bones are relatively scarce. Unfortunately, in the fossilized bones of hominids and early humans diagenetic changes of trace element levels may be considerable. Still another problem is posed by the wide range of food resources which were probably exploited by our ancestors (Mann 1981) the trace element concentrations of which are incompletely known (section V.A, IX.E). Basic research in this field is urgently needed.

Prehistoric bone tissue may be used for other purposes. For instance, paleoserological studies (Borgognini Tarli et al. 1986). However, the reliability of these studies are questioned by some anthropologists (compare Piepenbrink 1986)

A number of reviews of uses and potentials of 'bone chemistry and past behaviour' were published recently (Parker & Toots 1980, Sillen & Kavanagh 1982, Price et al. 1985b, Gilbert 1985), to which another contribution is added here (section I. B.).

A.2. The present study

The present study was initiated and carried out at the Albert Egges van Giffen Instituut voor Prae- en Protohistorie (IPP) in Amsterdam. The IPP was founded in 1951, and a tradition of close cooperation of archeologists and ecoarcheological researchers was established in the period after 1960. Ecoarcheological information is considered essential in the description and reconstruction of prehistoric human behaviour.

When the potentials and first results of the chemical study of prehistoric bones in America became known in Europe, it was recognized that the complexes of human and animal bones from a number of Bronze Age sites in West-Friesland were potentially suitable for chemical analysis in relation to dietary reconstruction. A crucial role in the process of recognition of the potentials of bone chemistry was played by dr. C.S. Peebles, who had just finished a paper on strontium in human bones (Schoeninger & Peebles 1981), and who was at that time a guest professor at the IPP. In the same period, G.F. IJzereef was working on his dissertation, which contains a model for the agricultural exploitation of a part of West-Friesland (Brandt & IJzereef 1980, IJzereef 1981, 1983), and R.W. Brandt wrote a paper on a comparable subject (Brandt 1980). The Assendelver Polder Project, with important contributions by ecoarcheologists, was planned and carried out (Brandt et al. 1985). Thus, there was, and still is, a wide interest in the reconstruction of the paleoenvironment and of the activities of humans living in that environment. Chemical analysis of the human and animal bones from West-Friesland was potentially capable of adding another and new dimension to archeological research. The present work should show whether or not the attempt to add this dimension was succesful.

A grant for the analysis of West-Frisian bones was requested by dr. L.H. van Wijngaarden- Bakker and prof. dr. W. Groenman- van Waateringe, and was awarded by the Foundation for Archaeological Research, which is a subsidiary of the Netherlands Organization for the Advancement of Pure Research (grant 123-21-022). On March 1st, 1984, the actual work commenced.
Chemical analyses were carried out at the Netherlands Energy Research Foundation (ECN) in Petten (N-H), and stable isotope assesment was done at the Laboratium voor Isotopenfysica in Groningen.

B. CHEMICAL ANALYSIS OF PREHISTORIC BONE

Ideally, excavated, non-fossilized prehistoric bone consists of two fractions: organic and inorganic. In vivo, the inorganic fraction of bone is hydroxyapatite, which is present in bone as small crystals, whereas the organic fraction of bone is made up of collagen: long, helical chains of aminoacids. The two bone fractions have their own potentials and problems in chemical analysis and in resistence to diagenetic influences. Hydroxyapatite is studied for its trace element concentrations. In collagen, the in vivo stable isotope ratios may be preserved more or less unaltered. The natural bipartition demands for separate treatises on the 'state of the art' of analyses of the fraction involved.

B.1. Trace elements

B.1.1. Trace elements in paleodietary research

The potential of prehistoric bones for dietary analysis were first exploited with the analysis of strontium concentrations in animal bones some twenty years ago (Toots & Voorhies 1965). Strontium was the first element to be used in bone analysis for dietary reconstruction, and it is still the most important trace element in paleodietary research. Other elements of interest are zinc, copper and barium. Some basic physical characteristics of the most important elements in chemical analysis of prehistoric bone are assembled in table I.1.

Table I.1. Physical characteristics of some macro- and trace elements (Weast 1974).

element	symbol	---atomic--- no.	weight	ionic(+2) radius nm	abundance in lithosphere absolute ppm	rel.to Ca mg / g Ca
phosphorus	P	15	30.98		1180	32.51
calcium	Ca	20	40.08	0.099	36300	1000
iron	Fe	26	55.85	0.074	50000	1377
copper	Cu	29	63.54	0.072	70	1.93
zinc	Zn	30	65.37	0.074	132	3.63
arsenic	As	33	74.92		5	0.14
strontium	Sr	38	87.62	0.112	300	8.26
barium	Ba	56	137.34	0.134	250	6.89
lead	Pb	82	207.19	0.120	16	0.44

* in lithosphere

The early use of strontium and its important place in bone analyses is a consequence of a number of factors. Before dealing with strontium in more detail, it is useful to review the requirements of trace elements in bone analyses.

To be of potential use in palaeodietary studies, the ante-mortem, in vivo behaviour, and the post-mortem, in soil, behaviour of a trace element has to be understood qualitatively and, above all, also quantitatively. The in vivo behaviour of the trace element comprises the relationships between dietary composition, intake and uptake of the element, disease and stress, and the ultimate concentration of the element in the bone mineral. A prerequisite is that the provenance of the trace element in various food items, in relation to the concentrations of other elements, such as calcium, and the energy value has to be known. Ideally, the distribution of a trace element in the range of food items should be correlated with different origins of food items: vegetable, animal, terrestrial or marine. An element with a well-known relationship between dietary levels and bone concentrations, but with a uniform distribution over the food-stuffs, is of little use in paleodietary studies. However, such an element might be useful in other aspects, for instance, the study of diseases.

The second aspect in the behaviour of potentially usable trace elements comprises the post-mortem behaviour of the element concentrations in bone. Bones from an archeological context have generally been enveloped in a soil matrix between death and the moment of analysis. The main taphonomic process is the influence of the soil solution on elemental concentrations in the bone mineral. Obviously, for elements to be used, this diagenetic influence should be absent or small: we are interested in the ante-mortem concentrations of the element. In general, elements that closely resemble Ca (table I.1) will be the least affected by diagenetic processes.

Strontium is an element that answers well to the above-mentioned requirements. Strontium and calcium turnover in the food chain are relatively well-known as a result of much research in the 1950's and 1960's (for instance, Comar et al. 1957, Russell 1966a,b). The interest in Sr was a result of the concern over the dangerous consequences of radioactive fallout, especially of Sr-90, that resulted from atmospheric nuclear tests and, potentially, from nuclear war. After the banning of atmospheric testing in 1963, the interest in Sr in the food chain faded away. Stable Sr is not an essential nor a toxic element (Underwood 1977). In the 1970's and 1980's, the interest in the role of trace elements, toxic and/or essential, in human and animal metabolism in health and disease increased. Little new work on Sr was done by nutritionists. However, the amount of data collected on Sr turnover (section V.A) enabled anthropologists to use Sr in paleodietary research. A synopsis of the knowledge on Sr and Ca turnover in food chains is visualized in figure 2 of Price et al. (1985b), however, the figures in this scheme are arithmetically inconsistent (compare Van Wijngaarden-Bakker 1986).

The danger of radioactive Sr-90 for human health is connected with the affinity of Sr for bone. Like Ca, which resembles Sr in chemical characteristics, the major part of body Sr is present in the skeleton. Thus, radioactive Sr, once in the body, would be incorporated in the bone mineral matrix as an ion substituting for a Ca ion. The Sr-90, incorparated in bone, becomes a semi-permanent source of radiation in the body, which may cause radiation diseases such as bone marrow cancer.

The properties of Sr, which in its radioactive form make it dangerous for human and animal health, on the other hand make it a suitable element for paleodietary studies. The insensitivity of bone Sr concentrations to influences of the soil solution is a consequence of the location of Sr ions as substitutes for Ca in the hydroxyapatite crystal lattice (Posner 1969). Thus, the ratio of Sr and Ca in the body, which is of interest because of its dependency on dietary Sr and Ca concentrations, is fixed in the bone mineral matrix.

A further requirement for a trace element to be used in paleodietary analyses is that it should exhibit a non-uniform distribution in the range of available food items. In the case of Sr, the discrimination against Sr in favour of Ca in the intestinal tract of animals causes distinct differences between Sr/Ca ratios in vegetable and animal tissues. Thus, Sr concentrations in bones of humans and animals reflect the relative importance of animal and vegetable foods in the diets of the involved individuals. The bipartition: animal versus vegetable food items is a relevant one in many archeological and anthropological contexts (Harding & Teleki 1981, Jones 1983). Besides, there is a difference in Sr concentrations in terrestrial and marine habitats, a distinction which may also have archeological relevance. Strontium and calcium relationships in various steps of the food chain will be dealt with in more detail in sections V.A and IX.C.

B.1.2. Strontium in paleodietary studies

Toots & Voorhies (1965) analysed Sr concentrations in fossil bones of Pliocene animals in order to be able to compare their feeding habits with dental morphology. Though their methodology is sound and uptil now the basis for dietary reconstruction, the material used was probably not suitable for their purposes, and thus the validity of their conclusions may be questioned (Sillen & Kavanagh 1982). In my view, the virtual absence of any difference between the mean Sr concentrations in various skeletal elements of Merycodus and the low coefficients of variation in the samples of Toots and Voorhies may be seen as indicators for diagenetic alterations of Sr concentrations. In table I.2, the data of Toots and Voorhies are compared with data on fresh bone Sr concentrations. Compared with these data, the Merycodus values appear unrealisticcally uniform.

Table I.2. Comparison between data of Toots & Voorhies (1965) and other data on bone Sr concentrations (Schoeninger 1979) and bone Sr/1000 Ca ratios (Price et al. 1985a, Tanaka et al. 1981)

sample		n	mean	SD	CV(%)
Merycodus	mandibles	10	523	27	5.1
	mature metacarpals	10	526	34	6.5
	immature metacarpals	10	529	28	5.3
fresh mink bones		35	270	52	19.3
fresh white tailed deer foreleg,	males	26	0.385	0.125	32.5
	females	12	0.273	0.091	33.3
	fawns	15	0.301	0.082	27.2
fresh human bones, Japan:	age 8 year	7	0.334	0.024	7.2
	13 year	10	0.484	0.175	36.2
	20-25 year	15	0.506	0.081	16.0

Toots & Voorhies (1965) sought to differentiate between grazing and browsing animals. However, their assumptions on Sr contents in food of grazers versus that in food of browsers, i.e. relatively high Sr concentrations in succulents and herbs that are consumed by browsing animals, are not relevant if Ca concentrations are not taken into account. Interestingly, Toots and Voorhies's assumptions on differences in Sr concentrations in the vegetation are not reflected in later Sr studies where equal Sr/Ca ratios in the vegetation are equally assumed. The problems encountered here, i.e. differences between grazers and browsers and variations in Sr/Ca ratios in a vegetation remain of interest (sections V.A, IX.D).

Bone analysis can be applied in two partly overlapping fields of research: the first concerns diachronic problems, the other with problems within narrower time and space limits may be terme 'isochronous'.
In diachronic applications, the focus is on shifts in dietary habits in the course of time. Changes in diet in time will usually be a reflection of changes in the exploitation of the environmental resources. Such changes may be forced upon the people as a consequence of environmental factors, for instance climatic changes. In coastal areas in general, and in our study area West-Friesland in particular, marine regression and transgression influence the availability of areas of land suitable for food procurement, which in turn affects the hunting/gathering and agricultural potential. Technical improvements, cultural evolution and population pressure may be other causes for changing strategies in the exploitation of environmental capacities.

In diachronic studies, the differences between individuals or groups of individuals within sites receive less attention. Bone chemistry-based dietary reconstruction appears to be more successful in the diachronic field than in the isochronic field. In the light of the greater differences in dietary composition and in Sr concentrations that occur in time and in space than that within a given site, this would appear to be obvious.

In the isochronous research field, few papers have been published in which a reflection of the archeologically determined status differences on the bone Sr levels was found. In the classic paper of Schoeninger (1979) on status differences in Chalcatzingo, no control on physiological factors (e.g., sex and age) as a cause for the observed status differences in Sr levels was performed (Sillen & Kavanagh 1982). However, this paper remains one of the few in which a correlation between archeologically determined status and bone Sr levels is described. The diachronic aspects of the Chalcatzingo site remain unclear due to the limited number of bones.

Lambert and co-workers used bones from two North-American Woodland sites primarily for methodological studies on trace element levels in bones. They produced useful data on diagenetic influences on the concentrations of various trace elements (Lambert et al. 1979, 1982, 1984, 1985). Isochronic aspects of trace element levels are limited to differences between males and females (Lambert et al. 1982) and between age groups (Lambert et al. 1979). The diachronic aspect of these sites consists of the differences between hunter/gatherers of the Gibson site and maize cultivating people of the Ledders site. These differences appear to be rather small.

Special cases of isochronic studies are those in which weaning ages of infants are determined (Sillen & Smith 1984, Grupe 1986b). Possibilities for such studies are limited because in most excavated complexes of human bones the very young children are underrepresented or absent.

In the diachronic research field, Sr analysis may yield information on the change from hunting/gathering to agriculture. Schoeninger (1981, 1982) and Sillen (1981) studied this problem using bones from Middle-Eastern sites. Sillen (1981) in his methodological study did not venture any conclusions on Natufian dietary composition. Though the bones he used were to a certain extent affected by diagenesis, the difference between herbivorous and carnivorous animal bone Sr concentrations corroborates theoretical considerations. Humans are intermediate between carnivores and herbivores.

Schoeninger (1981, 1982) in a number of Middle-Eastern sites compared Sr/Ca ratios in human and herbivorous animal bones. The number of animal bones was small and no carnivores were studied. X-ray diffraction patterns suggest recristallization of at least part of the hydroxyapatite. Schoeninger states that this will affect Sr levels in all species equally so that the relative levels are not affected. There is, however, no check for this statement. There appear to be clear differences between sites. Some of the hunter/gatherers groups more closely resemble settled groups (i.e. agriculturalists) than other hunter/gatherer groups. According to Schoeninger, this is a consequence of the environment: on the one hand, some of the hunter/gatherers probably relied heavily on abundantly growing wild cereals for their subsistence, while others relied more on animal food; on the other hand some settled groups kept herds for a living rather than growing cereals.

On the North-American continent, the introduction of agriculture (i.e. maize cultivation) is in many instances better traceable by using carbon isotope analysis than by trace element analysis (section I.B.2). Beck (1985) used Zn and Sr concentrations in an attempt to trace agricultural activities. Diachronic studies in Europe will, in many cases, not deal with the introduction of agriculture, but will rather be carried out in order to detect changes in the exploitation of vegetable and animal food resources within agricultural systems.

Consumption of seafood will result in high Sr concentrations in bone (Kyle 1986). Thus, Sr levels may be used to compare diets of coastal and inland sites. Connor & Slaughter (1984) used Sr and other trace element levels in bones from mummified Inuit to compare diets from Alaskan coastal sites. Strontium levels in these people were, however, not high compared to Sr levels in bones from a small island on the Papua New Guinean coast (Kyle 1986)

B.1.3. Practical problems and research needs in strontium studies

The results of previous analyses of bones have emphasised that much fundamental research remains to be done in order to be able to filter out the background noise resulting from various factors and which obscures the dietary or ecological meaning of bone trace element concentrations. This is the case for Sr, but even more for other trace elements, such as zinc, which play essential roles in plant and animal metabolism. Some experimental work has been carried out already. Schoeninger (1979) studied mink for data on the variation in Sr levels in animals raised on the same diet. Price et al. (1985a) measured Sr concentrations in fresh white-tailed deer, a species they propose using as a baseline species. Runia (1987b) analysed various grain species and varieties for their Sr/Ca ratios.

Few data on concentrations of stable Sr in fresh human bones have been published. The paper by Tanaka et al. (1981) is often cited for the data on the differences in Sr/Ca ratios within individuals (table I.3). Relatively high Sr/Ca ratios are found in the skull, probably in part due to high Sr contents in the teeth which may take up Sr and Ca directly from the food (compare data in Comar et al. 1961). Bones with a relatively large amount of trabecular bone, e.g. ribs and vertebrae, show relatively low Sr/Ca ratios. Differences are small within long bones. Schoeninger (in manuscript) found no strong linear relationship between Sr concentrations in femora and vertebrae of 17th century Dutch whalers from Spitsbergen.

The rate of replacement of bone mineral is higher in vertebrae than in long bones (Bryant & Loutit 1964). Consequently, Sr levels in vertebrae will sooner be in balance with new dietary Sr levels than femoral Sr levels. This implies that marked differences between vertebra and femur Sr levels may indicate a shift in diet shortly before death.

Tanaka et al. (1981) supply data on the age dependency of human Sr/Ca ratios, and implicitely, on the variation of Sr/Ca ratios in humans (table I.2). After a rapid increase in the earliest phase of life, Sr/Ca ratios in human bones show a slight increase with age (compare also Bryant et al. 1958). This is a reflection of the age dependency of the discrimination against Sr in the uptake processes in the intestinal tract (section V.A).

Table I.3. Relative Sr/Ca ratios in the Japanese adult male. After Tanaka et al. (1981).

bone	Sr/Ca ratio relative to femur
femur	1.00
skull (including mandible and teeth)	1.13
vertebral column	0.63
chest cage (scapula, clavicula, rib and sternum)	0.72
sacrum	0.66
innominates	0.69
humerus	0.88
radius	0.88
ulna	0.88
hands	0.81
tibia	0.88
fibula	0.88
feet	0.81

To rule out regional differences in levels of Sr and other elements, the possibilities of using animal bones as reference material for trace element levels is stressed by various authors (Sillen & Kavanagh 1982, Price et al. 1985a, Runia 1985). Sillen (1981) advises the use of bones from both herbivorous and carnivorous animals. However, in many sites few or no bones of carnivorous animals are present. If only a few bones are present, it is never certain whether they stem from specimens that lived in or near the investigated site (compare Price 1985). Thus, caution in the use of these bones is necessary. Species used as baseline species are white-tailed deer (Price et al. 1985a, Price 1985), cattle and sheep/goat (Runia 1985, 1987a) as well as other herbivores (Schoeninger 1981, 1982, Sillen 1981).

Few studies exist in which Sr concentrations in bones of herbivorous, omnivorous and carnivorous animal species are given. Sillen (1981) analysed bones of various carnivorous and herbivorous species from Hayonim Cave (Israel); in this site, relative Sr concentrations in the animal species are consistant with theoretical considerations, i.e. high Sr concentrations in the herbivores, low Sr concentrations in the carnivores, with humans having intermediate Sr levels. Connor & Slaughter (1984) report on trace element concentrations in some caribou and polar bear bones but the origin of these bones remains unclear; besides, polar bear has high Sr levels due to consumption of marine food. Price (1985) gives Sr concentrations in some lynx bones besides Sr levels in deer.

The need for a baseline species in order to minimalize bias due to regional differences in soil Sr levels is apparent from various studies. Schoeninger (1985) found no consistent trophic level effect in Sr concentrations in animals from a wide geographic range. However, in a set of samples from a limited region there is a discrimination between herbivores and carnivores. Runia (1987a) has shown that in certain regions relatively large variations in soil Sr/Ca ratios may occur within short distances.

A wide range in mean Sr levels in human bones from various sites is apparent from many studies. In inland sites, Sr concentrations of a few hundred ppm in prehistoric human bones appear to be normal. In a coastal site, a mean Sr level of 1790 ppm in bone ash was found (Kyle 1986). This high level is probably largely due to consumption of shell fish. In another site near the coast, Het Valkje, a mean concentration of c. 1000 mg Sr /kg bone ash was found (Runia 1987a, compare section V.D). In this case, high Sr levels are the result of high soil Sr/Ca ratios (Runia 1987a). Sea water has a high Sr/Ca ratio (Rosenthal et al. 1970). Consequently, seafood will also have high Sr/Ca ratios, and marine sediments, such as are present in West-Friesland and in the western part of the Netherlands in general, will also be characterized by high Sr/Ca ratios.

When using a baseline species it must be certain that the animals lived in the same site or region as the humans (Pate & Brown 1985, compare also Runia 1987a). Bohman et al. (1966) found that Sr levels in cattle bones reflected the Sr levels of a new environment approximately two years after transferring the animals.

In an earlier paper, another reason for exercising caution in the selection of a baseline species was mentioned, namely the differences that may occur in Sr/Ca ratios in the various plants and plant parts that are consumed by herbivores and by man (Runia 1987b). This aspect will be discussed further in sections IX.C and IX.D.

As stated above, a number of reviews of 'the state of the art' of bone analyses have been published recently (Sillen & Kavanagh 1982, Price et al. 1985, Gilbert 1985). From these papers it becomes clear that the field of bone analysis was established and is still dominated by North-American researchers. Some of the first users of the Sr technique were paleontologists rather than archeologists. The need for information on the amount of meat in diets was initially especially felt in relation to the discussion on evolution and meat consumption, i.e. scavenging versus hunting of early humans (Harding & Teleki 1981, Mann 1981, compare also the introduction in Schoeninger 1979). Though bones from various continents were examined (North America, Gilbert 1975, 1977 (cited in Gilbert 1985), Lambert et al. 1979, 1982; Central America, Schoeninger 1979; Asia, Schoeninger 1981, 1982, Sillen 1981), the North-American, anthropological rather than archeological background of researchers may have caused a skew towards hunter/gatherers and the transition from hunting/gathering to agriculture.

In Europe, agriculture started several millennia BC and a large part of European archeological research is focussed on agricultural cultures. Unlike the situation in pre-contact America, in the Old World numerous domestic animal and plant species were developed and exploited. In America, the main food crop was maize, the importance of which in the diet is more easily detected by stable carbon isotope analysis than by trace element analysis. However, other cultures in the Americas and in tropical regions in general may have thrived on the cultivation of root crops (cassave, manihoc, yam, Hawkes 1969). In studying such cultures, the high Sr contents of roots should be remembered (Russell & Newbould 1966, Runia 1987b).

As a consequence of the dominance of agriculture in Europe since the Neolithic, paleodietary research here is faced by different problems than in America. For instance, diverging Sr and Ca ratios in various cultivated plants and parts thereof may bias the reconstruction of diets (section IX.C). Of greater importance, probably, is the production of milk by domestic animals and its consumption by humans. Milk has a relatively high Ca concentration and a low Sr/Ca ratio; milk in the diet will have a marked effect on the Sr/Ca ratio of the total diet (Runia 1987a). This aspect of milk has been recognized previously (Sillen & Kavanagh 1982), and has to some extent been used in studies on weaning ages of children (Sillen & Smith 1984, Grupe 1986b), but only one preliminary report (Runia 1987a) has yet been published on analyses of bones from potential milk-consumers. Grupe (1986a) in her extensive survey of trace elements in medieval skeletons from Northern Germany concludes that a large portion of the diet of the people concerned consisted of meat. However, she did not take milk and cheese into consideration.

As stated above, diachronic paleodietary studies in Europe in many instances will deal with changes within agricultural systems. For instance, the introduction of dairying, the exploitation of domesticated animals for their milk rather than their meat, may be detected by using trace element analyses. Another problem to which bone analyses might give clues is the change of diet which might result from the reaction of pre-or protohistoric farmers to a change in climate, such as, for example, occurred in North-Western Europe in the 10th century (Heidinga 1984).

The study of hunter/gatherer diets, the problem of the differences in the Sr/Ca ratios in animals and plants also plays a role. Modern hunter/gatherers make use of a wide variety of plants and animals for their subsistence (Hayden 1981). Besides mammals, other vertebrates and invertebrates such as birds, snails and insects are consumed. Even clay may be consumed in some cultures (Hayden 1981). Our knowledge on Sr/Ca ratios in animals other than mammals is limited (section V.A). This leaves us with a range of uncertainty on the Sr/Ca ratios of hunter/gatherer diets. Even small amounts of foods with high Ca concentrations and aberrant Sr/Ca ratios may seriously affect Sr/Ca ratios of the total diet (Runia 1987a).

In general, no exact information on the diets of prehistoric people as revealed by bone chemistry is available. Paleobotanists and zooarcheologists, by studying plant and animal remains may provide a range of food items potentially consumed by the people who are the subject of bone chemical research. The relative importance of the foods in the diets, however, remains obscure (Van Wijngaarden-Bakker 1986). Though bone analysis is executed to overcome this inherent shortcoming of traditional ecoarcheological research, it also implies that there is no independent check on the results of bone analysis in dietary reconstruction.

In at least one case, however, there is independent information on the diet of humans who were interred some 300-400 years ago: Dutch whalers, buried on Spitsbergen in the 17th-18th century and excavated in 1980 were studied by M.J. Schoeninger (in manuscript). The diet of the whalers is fairly accurately known from the Journals and 'victualing lists' (Van Wijngaarden-Bakker 1986) of the whaling ships. The reconstruction of diet based on bone chemistry was compared with historical data. A reasonably good agreement between the two reconstructions was found, though the consumption of cheese by the whalers is a complicating factor (Van Wijngaarden-Bakker 1986).

In this case, diagenetic influences on trace element concentrations are probably minor as a consequence of the relatively short period of burial in a cold environment.

B.1.4. Zinc

In the wake of the application of Sr analyses, anthropologists have searched for other elements to be used complementarily. Due to the large number of variables in the past diet, analyses of only one element, e.g. Sr, often cannot give unequivocal results on paleodietary questions (Runia 1987a). In the light of the above mentioned prerequisites for suitable trace elements for paleodietary research, only a few elements would appear to be potentially useful. Concentrations of most elements suffer from diagenetic influences (Lambert et al. 1979, 1982).

One of the potentially most promising elements is zinc. The functioning and metabolism of Zn in organisms and its distribution in both geosphere and biosphere has been the subject of much recent research (Prasad 1976). The element concentration in bone is considered to be reasonably insensitive to diagenetic influences (Lambert et al. 1979, 1982). Gilbert (1975, cited in Price et al. 1985b) was the first to use Zn concentrations. In his study, correlations between Zn concentrations and, in females, body length and, in males, incidence of diseases were recorded. More recently, bivariate plots, in which Sr and Zn concentrations are plotted, were used. However, the use of Zn is somewhat problematical due to the lack of a firm relationship between dietary Zn levels and bone Zn concentrations (Lambert et al. 1982), and the lack of detailed data on the effects of Zn shortage in diet and Zn stress in cases of pregnancy and disease on the bone Zn levels.

An example for the use of bivariate plots is the study by Beck (1985). This paper may be used to illustrate the potentials and the dangers of bivariate analyses. Using human bone samples from three North American sites, Beck tested a hypothesis on the way the transition of hunting/gathering to agriculture would be visible in human bone Sr and Zn levels. Though his results appear to be plausible enough, the large variation in the bone Zn concentrations and the lack of a control on background levels of Sr and Zn in the sites involved, in the form of analyses of animal bones from the same sites, make the interpretation less reliable. Besides, Beck (1985) is somewhat optimistic when stating that 'a firm relationship between dietary and skeletal concentrations has been demonstrated recently': the paper by Rheingold et al. (1983) to which he refers merely supplies a table with ranges of Zn concentrations in bones in three groups of animals, without any information on diet, origin or other details of the analysed specimens. This information is certainly necessary before declaring that these data provide a firm base for the interpretation of bone Zn levels. In the same paragraph, Beck stresses the regional variation in Zn levels.

B.1.5. Other trace elements

In consequence of the lack of insight in the relationship between levels in food and the concentrations in human and animal bones, identical problems to those encountered in the interpretation of zinc concentrations in bones arise for the other trace elements. Besides, concentrations in bone of many elements appear susceptible to diagenetic changes (Lambert et al. 1981). Thus, only a limited number of elements appear to answer the prerequisites for trace elements in paleodietary studies as outlined in section I.B.1.1. A multi-element approach to paleodietary or paleoenvironmental problems is advocated by several authors (Price et al. 1985b, Grupe 1986a). It would seem to be advisable to test for diagenetic influences on the concentrations of trace elements in a subsample of the complex of bones that it is intended to analyse. Such a test would also give an insight into the concentration ranges that are present in the bone samples. Analysing large numbers of bones for a wide range of trace elements may prove to be a waste of time and energy when specific answers to specific questions are being sought; on the other hand, a basic amount of reference data on naturally occurring ranges of trace element concentrations in human bones should be present though it is still lacking for a number of elements. Therefore, studies such as the one by Grupe (1986a), which list concentrations of numerous elements in a complex of medieval inhumations (11th-12th century) may prove useful as reference material in the interpretation of trace element concentrations in prehistoric human bones.

Hatch & Geidel (1985) also used a multi-element approach. Their paper contains well defined relationships between trace element levels and variables in potential paleodiets with vegetable foods, meat and nuts. Besides Sr and Zn, concentrations of Mn, Cu and V were determined. Combined trace element data suggest some status difference in two New World cultures. Vanadium levels suggest that low status groups supplemented their diet with nuts. However, diagenetic effects on V levels in bone have not been studied in detail. Besides this, there may be some doubt on the validity of assumptions of high trace element levels in nuts. When viewed in relation to energy contents, nuts appear to have not excessively high concentrations of trace elements (Runia 1987b, section VI.A)

Below Sr in the Periodic Table of the elements is barium. Possibly, discrimination against this element in favour of Ca, and probably also Sr, in digestive tracts of animals resembles the situation for Sr and Ca, but with stronger discrimination because of the greater differences between Ca and Ba than between Sr and Ca respectively (table I.1). If so, this would also make Ba suitable for paleodietary studies, provided that no post-mortem alterations of bone Ba levels occur in the soil. Unfortunately, Ba seems to be rather susceptible to diagenetic influences (Lambert et al. 1984); and there are no studies on Ba turnover relative to Ca turnover in food chains. Reports on the analysis of Ba in prehistoric human and animal bones are scarce.

B.1.6. Trace elements in cremations

As in many recent societies, the burning of the bodies of the dead formed part of the funeral ritual in numerous prehistoric cultures. Ashes of the deceased may be handled in various ways, for instance scattered over land or water. Only those prehistoric cremations that were interred have a chance of being found in excavations.

Because cremation of the dead was a predominant funeral ritual in a number of prehistoric cultures, in many instances cremated remains rather than bones are available for physical- anthropological and chemo-archeological studies. Physical- anthropological study of cremated human bone is now relatively well established (Herrmann 1972, Wahl 1982), but so far no data on trace element levels in cremated bones have been published. Some experimental work on the effects of various boiling and heating treatments on the macro and micro structure of bones has been carried out (Shipman et al. 1984).

Upon heating, bone will be altered in various ways. The organic fraction in fresh, defleshed bone, fats and collagen, will burn at temperatures of some 360 - 525 ^{o}C (Shipman et al. 1984). The organic fraction of prehistoric bones reacts with oxygen at about 300-400 ^{o}C (DTA tests by B. de Leeuw, pers.comm.). Heating to such temperatures results in charred bone, which is composed essentially of only slightly altered hydroxyapatite crystals. At higher temperatures, the crystal structure of the bones is altered. The microscopic crystals of hydroxyapatite present in fresh bone recrystallize to larger crystals of hydroxyapatite which produce sharp peaks in X-ray diffraction patterns (Shipman et al. 1984).

Considering the fact that in many instances cremations are the only human remains available for study, the potentials of this kind of material for trace element analysis should be further investigated.

B.2. Stable isotopes of carbon and nitrogen

B.2.1. Introduction

The organic fraction of bone, collagen, appears to be relatively unsusceptible to the diagenetic influences of the soil. Microbiological processes may have caused the splitting up of long chains of aminoacids into smaller units, but in many instances a large fraction of the collagen aminoacids will still be present. The carbon and nitrogen isotopic composition of the collagen appears to be relatively stable in the soil and can therefore be studied in prehistoric bones.

B.2.2. Theoretical background

Introduction

Isotopes of an element have identical atomic numbers and electron configuration, but different atomic weights due to different numbers of neutrons in the nuclei. Most elements possess stable isotopes. In many of the elements, one of the isotopes is by far the most abundant. Though chemically equal, isotopes will react at slightly different rates in consequence of the differences in mass. This effect is most pronounced in elements with a low atomic number, because their mass differences are comparatively large. The isotopes of interest in paleodietary studies are the stable isotopes of carbon and nitrogen.

Bone collagen consists of long chains of amino acids and is rich in C and N. The amino acids needed for the synthesis of collagen in the human body are mainly derived from proteins in the diet, because a number of amino acids can not be synthesised by humans (Den Hartog et al. 1978, Wing & Brown 1979). In consequence, the isotopic composition of bone collagen depends on the isotope ratios in the dietary proteins. Bone collagen C and N ratios therefore contain information in the relative importance of various protein sources in human diets (Chisholm et al. 1983a, Hobson & Schwarcz 1986, Johansen et al. 1986).

In comparison to C, N has seldom been used in paleodietary studies (Price et al. 1985b). Nitrogen isotopic ratios are not routinely measured in 14C dating laboratories as are delta 13C values (Tauber 1981, Burleigh et al. 1984).

Reference data on C and N isotopic ratios in various organic materials including bone collagen have been assembled by various authors (Schoeninger & DeNiro 1984, Schoeninger 1985, DeNiro 1985, DeNiro & Hastorf 1985, Ambrose & DeNiro 1986).

The interpretation of C and N ratios in bones is more straightforward than the interpretation of bone trace element levels. Regional differences are absent, and thus there is no need to analyse bones from a 'baseline' species as is done in trace element research (Tauber 1981, 1986). Variations in the isotopic composition in animal populations appear to be small (Hobson & Schwarcz 1986).

Terminology

The 'heavy' isotopes 13C and 15N are present in quantities that are very small when compared to the amounts of the lighter isotopes 12C and 14N. It is therefore customary to express the amounts of 13C and 15N in the form of 'delta' values relative to a standard:

delta 13C =((13C/12C sample)/(13C/12C standard) -1) * 1000 per mil

and

delta 15N =((15N/14N sample)/(15N/14N standard) -1) * 1000 per mil

The standard for C is Pee Dee Belemnite, which is relatively rich in the heavy isotope 13C and which implies that almost all delta 13C values of living tissues are negative (Van der Merwe 1982). More 13C results in less negative delta 13C values.

The standard for delta 15N is atmospheric N. Delta 15N values of organic materials are usually positive, because they contain more of the heavy isotope than air. Higher amounts of 15N results in higher delta 15N values.

Trophic level effects

In food chains, there is a general trophic level effect on C and N isotope ratios. The slightly different reaction rates of the isotopes result in a gradual change in isotopic composition.

The differences between herbivores and carnivores appear to be rather small. Schoeninger (1985) found differences of less than 2 per mil. in mean delta 13C and delta 15N values of the two and there was also an almost complete overlap in the ranges of delta 13C values. For delta 15N values, the overlap was slightly less, but still too large to be able to distinguish between trophic levels. A similar effect was also found by Schoeninger & DeNiro (1984). Within smaller areas, differences between trophic levels may, however, be somewhat less obscure.

At lower trophic levels, the isotope fractionation effects appear to be more pronounced. Differences between delta 13C and delta 15N in plants and in collagen from herbivores are about 5 per mil (Van der Merwe 1982, Schoeninger & DeNiro 1984).

Isotopic ratios in plant groups

Measurement of carbon and nitrogen isotopic ratios allows three groups of terrestrial plants to be distinguished (Bender 1968, DeNiro & Hastorf 1985, figure I.1). Legumes differ from other C4 plants in delta 15N values whereas C3 and C4 plants can be distinguished by means of their delta 13C values.

The difference between plants which utilize atmospheric N fixed by microorganisms, such as _Leguminosae_ and paddy rice, and plants which utilize N from decomposing organic matter can be seen as a result of trophic level effects. Delta 15N values in legumes are closer to zero (= delta 15N of atmospheric N) than those in other plants which utilize N from soil organic matter. Soil organic matter has delta 15N values of about +3 to +7 per mil (Letolle 1980).

The difference between C3 and C4 plants is a consequence of different photosynthetic pathways (Bender 1968, Van der Merwe 1982). C3 plants bind carbon dioxide to form a phosphoglycerate which has three C atoms while C4 plants convert carbon dioxide to a dicarboxylic acid with four C atoms (Van der Merwe 1982). The group of C3 plants encompasses almost all plants from temperate regions including major food plants such as wheat (_Triticum_ spp.) and potatoes (_Solanum tuberosum_). Plants of the C4 group occur in tropical and subtropical regions and include the important food plants _Zea mays_, millet (_Panicum_ spp.) and sugar cane (_Saccharum_ spp.).

The isotopic ratios in bone collagen of mammals reflect the isotopic ratios in their foods. Animals and man consuming predominantly either C3 or C4 plants can therefore be distinguished (Van der Merwe 1982, Ambrose & DeNiro 1986).

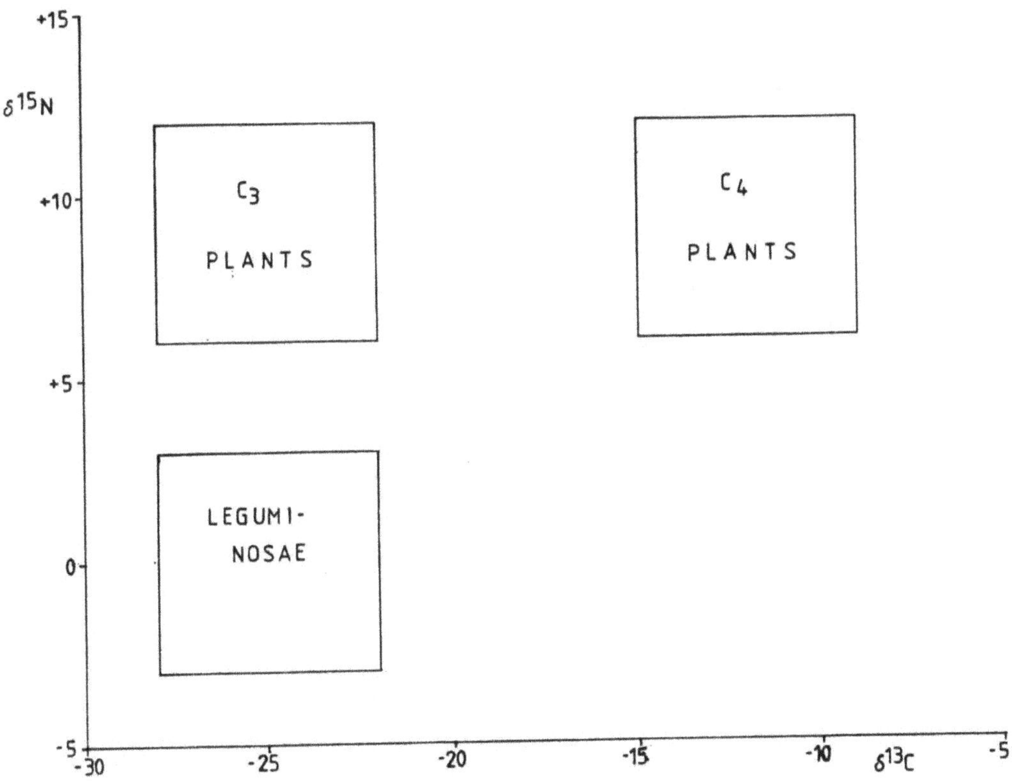

figure I.1 Groups of plants as characterized by values of delta 13C and delta 15N (adapted from DeNiro & Hastorf 1985).

Marine and terrestrial organisms

There is a clear distinction between mean C and N isotopic ratios in marine and terrestrial animals (Tauber 1981, 1983, Chisholm et al. 1983a, b, Schoeninger et al. 1983, Schoeninger & DeNiro 1984). The relative importance of marine and terrestrial protein sources can therefore be estimated on the basis of isotope ratios in human bone collagen (Tauber 1981, Chisholm et al 1983a, b, Sealy & Van der Merwe 1985, DeNiro 1985, Johansen et al. 1986).

Delta 13C values for marine mammals and fish bone collagen of about −12 to −14 per mil have been found, as compared to −19 to −23 per mil for terrestrial mammals (Tauber 1983, Schoeninger & DeNiro 1984, Hobson & Schwarcz 1986). Flesh appears to have delta 13C values that are about 4 per mil more negative: Chisholm et al. (1983a) list mean values of about −18 per mil for marine flesh and −26 per mil for terrestrial flesh.

The difference between mean delta 15N value in marine and terrestrial animals appears to be somewhat greater. Schoeninger & DeNiro found mean values of +5.3 per mil for terrestrial animals and +14.8 per mil for marine animals.

B.2.3. Stable isotope analysis in archeological studies

Isotopic studies can be used as tools in two major fields of paleodietary research. Most of the studies of stable isotope ratios in prehistoric bones have been carried out in tropical and subtropical regions or were dealing with C4 plant species in temperate regions. The point of interest in these areas is the relationship between C3 plants and C4 plants in prehistoric diets (Van der Merwe 1982). The classical example of this object of study is the spread of Zea mays cultivation on the North American continent (Van der Merwe & Vogel 1978).

Many of the problems and potentials encountered in these studies are of little relevance to studies of prehistoric cultures in temperate regions. The other paleodietary research field in which isotopic studies may be useful, i.e. the distinction of marine and terrestrial components in diets is of more interest for North-Western Europe. The potentials of C isotope analysis in this field are demonstrated by Tauber (1981, 1983) who collected a body of delta 13C values from Danish prehistoric human bones. A distinct difference in diets of Mesolithic and Neolithic peoples may be inferred from their delta 13C values, which ranged from -11 to -16 per mil and -18 to -25 per mil, respectively.

Other studies in temperate regions were carried out in North America and involved coast dwelling, salmon eating people (Chisholm et al. 1983b).

Johansen et al. (1986) found clear differences in C isotopic ratios in prehistoric and historic skeletons from a number of inland and coastal sites in Norway. These authors suggest a ranking for human diets with various amounts of marine and terrestrial proteins in relation to delta 13C values in human bone collagen.

II
THE GEOGRAPHICAL AND ARCHEOLOGICAL CONTEXT

A. INTRODUCTION

The main objective of the present study is the chemical analysis of human and animal bones from Late Neolithic and Bronze Age West-Friesland. For the interpretation of the analytical results, it is necessary to understand the archeological and ecological context from which the bone samples were taken. An overview of the archeology and paleogeography of eastern West-Friesland, the area from which bones have been analysed, is given in the present chapter, followed by a summary of the numbers and origins of the human and animal bone samples.

B. THE LANDSCAPE

The landscape of eastern West-Friesland in the Late Neolithic and Bronze Age is relatively comprehensibly described in a number of studies. The geology of the area was described by De Mulder & Bosch (1982) and by Hallewas (1981), who added archeological aspects. The vegetational history

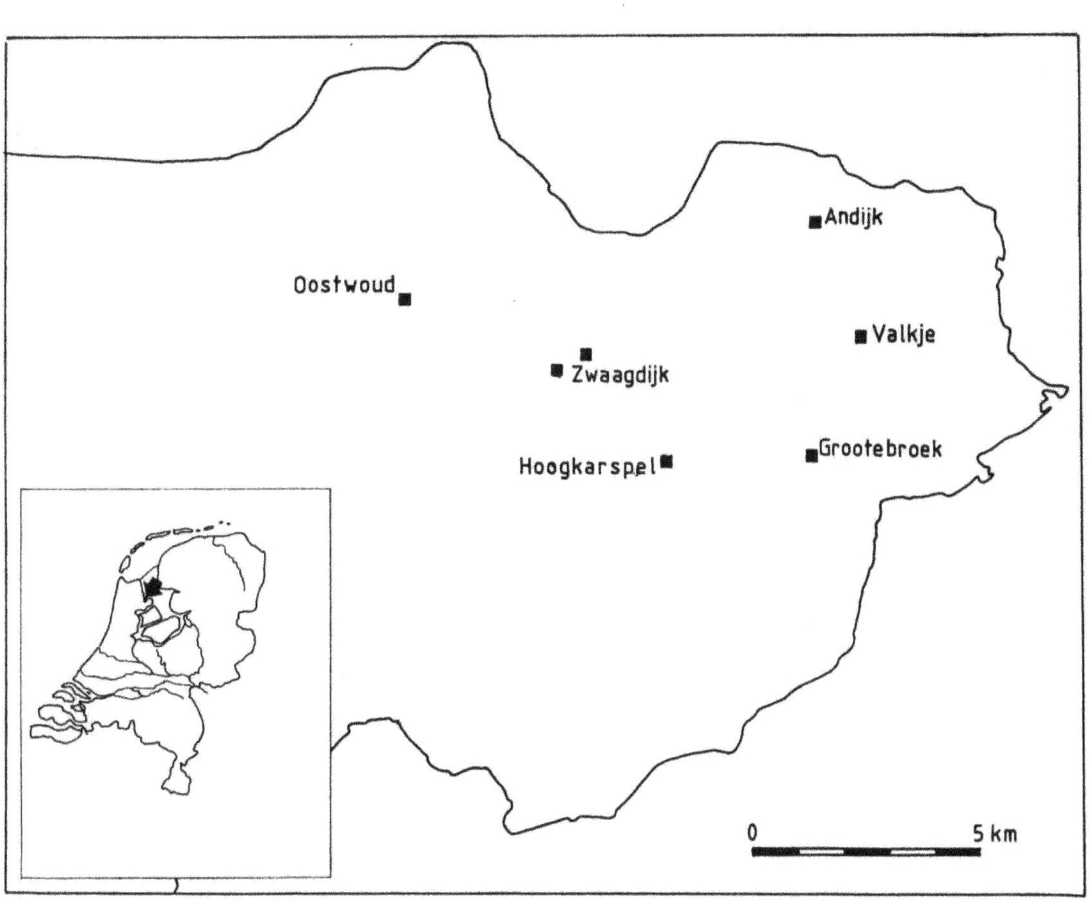

figure II.1 Location of eastern West-Friesland and some important sites mentioned in the text.

has been studied in peat sections from the Klokkeweel bog near Hoogkarspel (Pals et al. 1980) and from under the seadike near Enkhuizen (Van Geel et al. 1983).

The Late Neolithic and Bronze Age occupation traces are present on Calais IVa2-IVb deposits. The area formed the eastern end of a tidal creek system that opened to the North Sea between Bergen and Alkmaar (figure II.1, II.2).

Between c. 4300 and 3800 BP peat was formed in a large part of eastern West-Friesland. Clastic marine sediments were deposited in the Oostwoud-Hauwert region. In the following period (3800-3500 BP), all of eastern West-Friesland came under marine influence through a new branch of the tidal creek system, which ran from Hoogwoud via Wognum and Blokker to Hem, bending north in the direction of Bovenkarspel and Andijk. The sandy to sandy-loamy creek ridges and clayey basins formed in this period were the major geographic features during the subsequent Late Neolithic and Bronze Age period of occupation. The area changed into a fresh water environment after the sea had lost its influence. In the area around Westwoud-Zwaagdijk, marine sedimentation continued until c. 3000 BP.

During the occupation period c. 3300-2600 BP, the water table in the area gradually rose. As a consequence, marshes extended. Around 2600 BP, the water table had risen so much that the area became unsuitable for agriculture.

The northern part of the area was covered by a layer of so-called kiek clay.

According to Van Zeist (in Modderman 1964), the area was covered by natural grassland during the Late Neolithic and Bronze Age occupation period. This is substantiated by Bakker et al. (1977) and Van Geel et al. (1983). Trees were virtually absent. Only on the low-lying clay soils may some willow and birch have been present (Van Geel et al. 1983). Mice and vole species present in the site Het Valkje are also indicative of an almost treeless landscape with grassland, pasture and arable fields (IJzereef 1981).

C. THE SITES

C.1.1. Archeological background of eastern West-Friesland

In the last twenty years, the eastern part of West-Friesland has been extensively studied by archeologists. The large scale reallotment projects planned in these years threatened eventually to destroy much of the archeological record unless inventarization and rescue excavations could be carried out. Much of the field work and aerial survey that was done still has to be published in its definite form, though many preliminary reports and, of course the raw data, are available.

The first excavations in West-Friesland were carried out by Van Giffen in 1929, 1942 and 1949. In 1929, Neolithic settlement traces were found at Zandwerven (Van Giffen 1930, Butter 1935). Barrows near Zwaagdijk (Van Giffen 1944), Grootebroek (Van Giffen 1953) and Hoogkarspel (Bakker 1959, 1966) were mapped and some of these were excavated. Prior to these excavations, West-Friesland was archeologically almost 'terra incognita' (Woltering 1985).

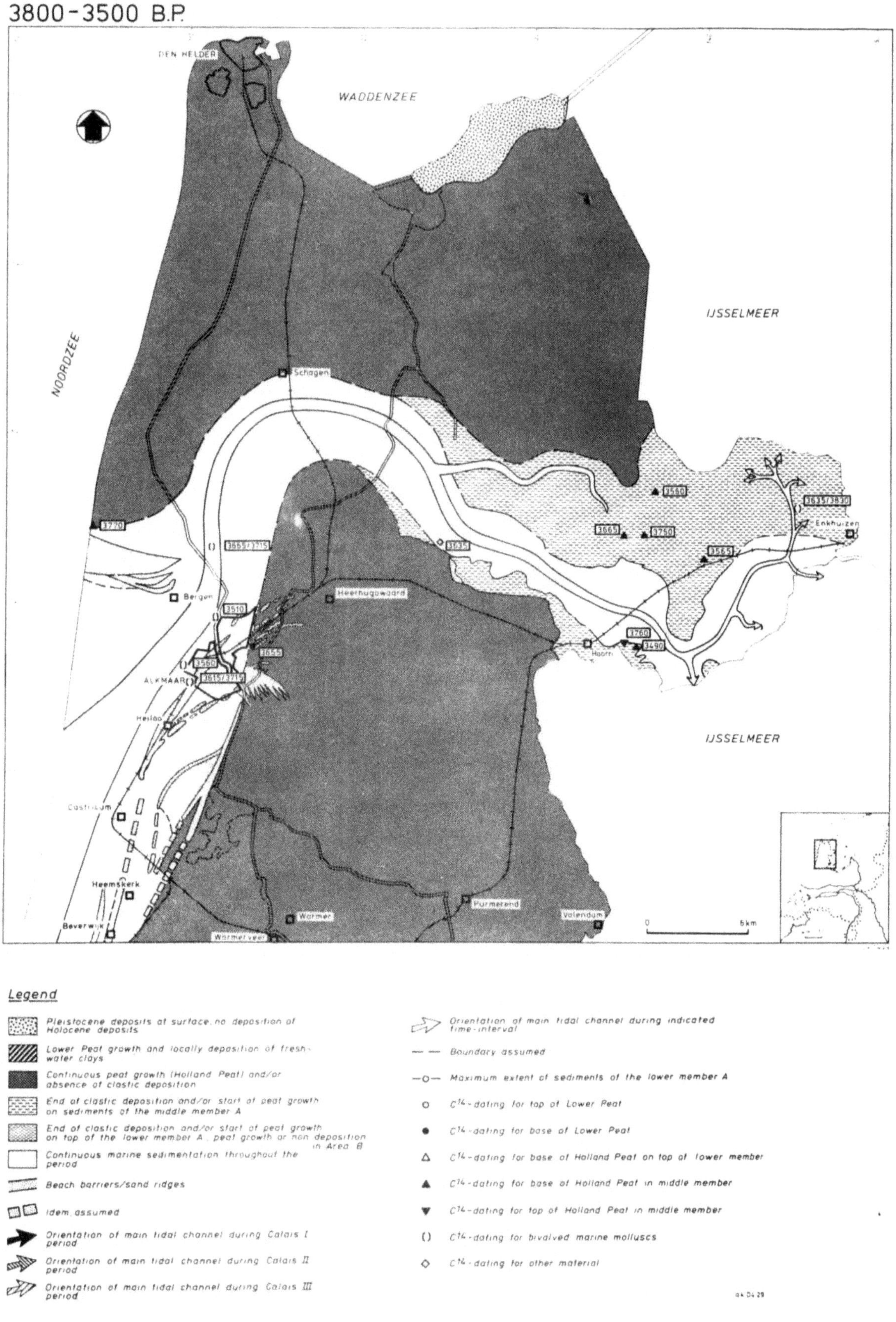

figure II.2 Paleogeographical map of the northern part of North-Holland for the period 3800-3500 BP (from De Mulder & Bosch 1982).

Various factors caused a rapid increase in interest in and knowledge of the prehistory of West-Friesland after 1950 (Woltering 1985). The mapping of part of the area by Ente (1963) resulted in a soil map on which numerous patches of 'kadetjesland', that is, land with conspicious microrelief caused by prehistoric occupation, were indicated. Parts of these settlement sites near Hoogkarspel were investigated by the IPP in a number of excavations between 1965 and 1969 (Bakker & Brandt 1966, Bakker & Metz 1967, Bakker et al. 1968, Bakker et al. 1977).

In addition to Ente's map, other soil maps of the area were made in connection with the land reallotment projects that were to be carried out in the area in the years after 1970. The reallotment schemes were a threat to practically all traces of prehistoric activity in West-Friesland. Concern in the archeological community about this situation led to large scale projects in the area. Occupation traces were mapped by systematic field walking by the ROB and air reconnaissance by the IPP (Woltering 1985). Numerous excavations were carried out.

The picture emerging from these activities is that of an area rather densely populated in the Early/Middle Bronze Age, almost uninhabited during the subsequent Iron Age and Early Middle Ages, and reclaimed again after the 10th century.

It is obvious that in an area such as West-Friesland, composed of marine sediments and with the permanent influence of a re- and transgressing sea nearby, the settlement history and the spatial characteristics of human activities cannot be separated from environmental, especially geological, variables. In the following section, some important characteristics of Bronze Age occupation of eastern West-Friesland are described.

C.1.2. The settlement traces: houses and ditches

Bronze Age farm houses are known from a number of sites in the area. Houses were three-aisled, some 6 m wide and c. 15-30 m long (Bakker et al. 1977, IJzereef 1981). The length of the houses suggests that cattle and probably other animals could be kept indoors during part of the year. Most houses were surrounded by ditches. In the later occupation phase, houses were probably built on small artificial dwelling mounds (<u>terps</u>) surrounded by ditches. Interruptions of the ditches show that the entrances of the houses were on the short sides. Plans of other buildings, such as granaries, have not been recognized.

A conspicuous feature of the Bronze Age sites in West-Friesland are the circular and figure-of-eight ditches, with diameters of c. 4 m (Modderman 1964, Bakker & Metz 1967, Buurman 1979) which are thought to have possessed a function in the agricultural system. Probably, the grain or hay harvest was temporarily stored in ricks within these circles (Bakker & Metz 1967, Bakker et al. 1977, Buurman 1979). For longer periods, the agricultural products may have been stored in the farm houses themselves.

C.1.3. The graves

The Late Neolithic and Bronze Age settlements of West-Friesland yielded a number of burial monuments, graves and isolated human bones. Only a small proportion of the known barrows have been excavated. A discussion of the grave ritual in the area is in preparation (R.W. Brandt, IPP, compare

Brandt 1980). An inventory of known barrows, based on aerial photography and fieldwork is in preparation (W.H. de Vries-Metz, IPP). A synopsis of the grave ritual, based on published data and on some new findings, is presented here.

The barrows present in the area were raised in the beginning of the Bronze Age occupation of the area. Radiocarbon dates of the tumuli fall within a timespan of c. 100 C14 years (3050-2950 BP, Lanting & Mook 1977). Only the dated skeletons from tumulus II in Oostwoud are earlier: c. 3500-3900 BP (section II.C.2.3.).

Various peripheral structures occur around the West-Frisian barrows (table II.1). The post circles that are common on the Pleistocene sands in other parts of the Netherlands in this period are virtually absent in eastern West-Friesland, possibly as a consequence of the scarcity of timber. The closely spaced posts of tumulus XIII near Zwaagdijk were removed shortly after they had been placed (Van der Waals 1961).

Most of the barrows are surrounded by a ditch which may or may not be circular. Some ditches are interrupted. In a number of cases, the ring ditches are connected to larger systems of ditches (Bakker et al. 1977).

Table II.1. Examples of peripheral structures as present in published reports on barrow excavations. Based on section C.2.

structure	barrow with structure	reference
ritual (?) ard scratches	Oostwoud II	Van Giffen 1963
ring of pits	Oostwoud I	Van Giffen 1963
double ring of posts	Zwaagdijk XIII-1,2	Van der Waals 1961
single ring of posts	Zwaagdijk IV	Van Giffen 1944
circular ditch	Zwaagdijk IV	ibid.
	Zwaagdijk XIII-3,4	Van der Waals 1961
	Hoogkarspel II	Bakker & Brandt 1966
	Grootebroek III-3	Van Giffen 1953
	Grootebroek II	ibid.
	Grootebroek I-1,2,3	ibid.
	Hoogkarspel Ia-1,2	Bakker et al. 1977
circular interrupted ditch	Grootebroek III-1,2	Van Giffen 1953
	Hoogkarspel Ia-3	Bakker et al. 1977
noncircular ditch	Zwaagdijk I-2	Van Giffen 1944
	Zwaagdijk III-2	ibid.
	Hoogkarspel III	Bakker & Brandt 1966
ditch part of field boundary	Hoogkarspel I	Bakker et al. 1977 Bakker 1959

Grave gifts from the Bronze Age are scarce in West-Friesland. The richest find, a bronze sword with a decoration of gold wire from a barrow is only known through oral tradition (Van Giffen 1944). A synopsis of grave gifts known from West-Friesland is given in table II.2. A number of these grave gifts only came to light when the storage cases containing the skeletal material were opened in the course of this study. Besides bronze objects, the grave gifts consist mainly of the bones of small wild carnivores.

Table II.2. Synopsis of grave gifts in West-Frisian Late Neolithic and Bronze Age graves. Cat. nos. refer to the catalogue (Appendix 1)

site	no.	cat.	sex	grave gift	reference
Zwaagdijk	?	-	?	bronze sword with gold wire decoration	Van Giffen 1944
Zwaagdijk	3	43	male	bronze rapier amber beads worked flint, sandstone worked (?) animal bone	Butler 1964 Runia 1986 II.C.2.1
Grootebroek	I-2	13	fem?	bronze spiral ring	Van Giffen 1953
Oostwoud	236	33	male	skull & long bones of marten (Martes sp.)	II.C.2.3
Oostwoud	533	38	male	probably: small bones of fox (Vulpes vulpes)	II.C.2.3
Hoogkarspel Ia	228	51	male?	tibia of young wild cat (Felis silvestris)	II.C.2.7

The orientation of the skeletons may be a useful parameter in the reconstruction of the grave ritual. A synopsis of the positions and orientations of the inhumations in barrows and flat graves (n=26) is given in table II.3. The crouched inhumations are, with one exception (**16**: Grootebroek, crouched on left-side looking SW) present in Oostwoud barrow II and are of Late Neolithic date. The strict correspondence between sex and the side on which the dead was interred agrees with other sites from the same period (Molenaarsgraaf: Louwe Kooymans 1974). In the group of crouched inhumations, the orientation appears to be more variable in females than in males. Interestingly, the opposite is the case for the extended individuals who date to the Bronze Age. Here, all females are interred in an E-W direction, whereas in the male group various orientations occur.

Table II.3. The position and orientation of the inhumations from West-Friesland. The orientation given is for the extended inhumations: head-feet, for the crouched individuals the direction of 'sight'. Based on data in Appendix 1.

position	orientation	---- number of individuals ---		
		males	females	sex unkown
extended on its back	S-N	3		1
	NNE-SSW			2
	E-W	2	5	
	ESE-WNW	1		1
	W-E			1
crouched on right side	facing SW		1	
	facing W		2	
	facing N		1	
crouched on left side	facing S	5		1
total		11	9	6

The way in which the Later Bronze Age inhabitants of West- Friesland treated their dead is not known. Most likely, not all the remains were interred. This follows from the absence of any cemetary or urnfield from this period. Taking the soil conservation conditions in the area and the number and extent of the excavations into consideration, it is unlikely that such a feature would have remained unnoticed if it had existed.

The Later Bronze Age in West-Friesland is contemporary with the urnfields in the northern and eastern part of the Netherlands (Lanting & Mook 1977). Cremation may have been practiced in the area in this period, but no urnfield is known. The absence of urnfields may be a consequence of the scarcity of land and intensive land use during the occupation period (Woltering 1985). However, a much stronger argument against cremation as the method of treating the dead is the scarcity of fuel in this treeless landscape. A considerable amount of fuel is necessary for the cremation of a human body and dung or peat will probably not generate the required temperatures. In cases where the corpses were burned in the grave pit (for example, in Hoogkarspel barrow II, section II.C.2.7) wood was used as fuel. Cremated human bones from Grootebroek and Hoogkarspel still contained considerable amounts of organic matter (chapter VIII).

In a number of barrows, however, primary and secondary graves consisted of cremations. So cremations were carried out in the area, but they date from the earliest phase of occupation. Finds of charcoal indicate that wood was used in burning the bodies. Secondary interments in the barrows are inhumations, which suggests that cremation had declined in importance.

Lanting & Mook (1977) point to the possibility of flat graves as grave form in this period. However, only one such grave from this period is known. This grave in Het Valkje, which contained two individuals, may be somewhat anomalous: two girls aged 14-20 were interred in a ditch rather than a grave pit (section II.C.2.6). Burial of the dead in or close to the houses, of which this double grave may be an example, may have been practiced in this period (Woltering 1985). If, however, this method of burying was predominant in the later period, a larger number of graves could be expected than the single example known. On the other hand, it might explain the occurrence of the isolated bones in the settlement features.

The excavations have produced a number of isolated human bones, found in various kinds of ditches and pits. These represent only a fraction of the total number of human bones that must have been 'produced' during the period of occupation. The taphonomy of the isolated human bones is not clear. The absence of traces of gnawing suggests that the bones were not present on the soil surface for any length of time. Cutting marks are also absent, so defleshing of bodies and cannibalism appears unlikely.

Only some of the barrows originally present in the area were investigated. Many have disappeared and can only be recognized on aerial photographs. It is likely that a number of secondary interments in the upper parts of barrows will have disappeared together with greater or lesser segments of the barrows themselves. This is also suggested by information from inhabitants of the area, communicated by various authors (for instance, Van der Waals 1961). It is unlikely that the disappearance of barrows is a major cause for the lack of burials from the late period of occupation. The inclusion of two barrows of the early period in a terp of the late period, as in Hoogkarspel (Bakker & Brandt 1966) suggests that in the late period at least some of the barrows had lost their original ritual function. In Het Valkje, a barrow dated 3275 ± 35 BP (GrN-7472) was levelled before the building of a house which was dated to 3035 ± 30 BP (GrN-8560).
Other archeologically untraceable methods of disposing of the dead may have been practiced. To mention some, the placing of the dead on rafts which were allowed to float to the sea, or the transportation of the dead to the dune area where abundant wood was present for cremation.

C.1.4. Subsistence

Abundant material is present for the assesment of human subsistence in West-Friesland in the Bronze Age. Largely due to the high water table and the clayey, calcareous soils, organic material and soil traces are well preserved.

The earliest clues to the agrarian activities of the Bronze Age people were found in the barrow excavations in 1942. Below the barrow, Van Giffen found ard furrows, and in fact a considerable part of his 1944 paper on the Zwaagdijk barrows is dedicated to ards and ard traces. Comparable traces, which are clearly visible due to the contrast between the dark soil of the arable layer and the light subsoil, turn up in almost every excavation in the area.
A second indication for the importance of agriculture are the numerous flint sickles from West-Friesland which are also extensively discussed by Van Giffen (1944). The typical 'sickle gloss' of these flints is explained by the polishing effect of cereal straw on the cutting edges of the harvesting tools. However, other non-agricultural activities, such as the cutting of reeds for thatched roofs, may result in similar microwear traces.

Paleobotanical and zooarcheological studies were carried out in various sites in West-Friesland. Both crop growing and animal husbandry were practiced by the Bronze Age inhabitants. Wild animals and fish were of minor importance as food resources (IJzereef 1981) as was, probably, the gathering of products of the wild though this is less easy to prove. Forests were absent in the area (Van Geel et al. 1983) and the creek ridges were fairly densely occupied with farm houses and fields, thus leaving the low-lying wet areas as the only possible environment for uncultivated plants. Roots and other parts of plants growing in this part of the ecosystem may be rich sources of energy (Lievense, pers.comm.). The degree of exploitation of the low-lying areas is not known.

The geology of the area caused a spatial separation of the two main agricultural activities. The creek ridges were suitable for cereal cultivation. The ditch systems present in the area are confined to the ridges and probably represent the boundaries of arable fields (Bakker et al. 1977). The low-lying, grassy areas presented good possibilities for animal husbandry. However, fallow arable on the ridges may also have been used as grazing area.

Zooarcheological studies indicate that cattle dominated animal husbandry. Smaller animals, pigs, sheep and goats were present in the studied sites, but are of lesser importance as food sources (IJzereef 1981). Small numbers of dogs were present, but probably not eaten. These domestic animal species differ in dental morphology and in morphology and physiology of their intestinal tracts. They are adapted to ingestion and digestion of different foods and differ in feeding strategies. Herbivores can be grazers, browsers or intermediate feeders (section V.A), adapted to feeding on plant material of low or higher quality. Omnivores consume and digest a certain amount of non-vegetable food. The differences in relative numbers between the animal species present in the settlements (table II.4) are probably a reflection of the environments of the sites, such as the area of creek ridge relative to the area of low-lying grazing grounds (compare Prummel 1979). The latter ratio is dependent on the geology, but also on the ground water level, and thus, in this region, comprises aspects of space and time. Andijk differs slightly from the other sites in the low percentages of pigs and the high percentage of cattle. Zwaagdijk resembles Andijk, but here only a small bone sample was present.

Unfortunately, data on other sites are not available yet. In the site Velsen-Hofgeest, game was probably rather more important than in the West-Frisian sites (section II.C.2.10).

The correspondence between high percentages of sheep/goat and of dog suggests that dogs may have had a function in sheep/goat herding.

Table II.4. Relative amounts of bones of domestic animals in some sites. See also section II.C.2.2. Data from Clason (1964), Van Mensch & IJzereef in Bakker et al. (1977), Prummel (1979), Van Mensch & IJzereef (1975), IJzereef (1981) and Therkorn (pers.comm.).

site	no. of bones	percentages: cattle	pig	sheep/goat	dog
Zwaagdijk 1961	276	83.7	4.0	10.1	2.2
Hoogkarspel Watertoren	302	75.5	7.3	8.9	8.3*
Hoogkarspel Tolhek	5448	80.7	8.0	9.7	1.4
Andijk	1144	86.2	3.5	8.9	1.4
Het Valkje					
early period	>5000	78.5	6.7	13.5	1.5
late period	>5000	62.8	9.1	24.3	3.8
Schagen-Muggenburg	1641 #	71.5	3.4	17.6	1.0

* due to the occurrence of some complete dog skeletons, this percentage may be too high
# including 6.1.% bones of horse

Near Grootebroek, some small clay animals were found (Van Regteren Altena et al. 1977). Their function, toy or ritual object, is not clear. Besides cattle, small clay pigs are present, but neither the numerically more important sheep/goat (table II.4) nor the dogs are represented. If only the animals regularly present in the settlement were modelled, this might agree with the idea that cattle and pigs were for various reasons kept in or close to the houses. In such an animal husbandry system, sheep/goat, that are well adapted to herding would be grazed at some distance from the farms. Pigs presumably were kept near the houses because of the absence of woodland. They could feed on domestic refuse and on fallow fields, probably also playing a role in tillage (Ten Cate 1972). Reasons for keeping cattle close to the farms may be less clear. However, cattle, at least the modern breeds, need more attention from the farmer in order to prevent them running wild. A second motive might be the supply of milk. Besides, the size of the houses suggests that cattle were stalled at night or in the winter, possibly also for their manure production.

The analysis of seeds, fruits and other plant remains from the sites in the area yielded information on the cereal species and the other plants that were cultivated. Weeds present in the samples are indicators for the methods employed in cereal cultivation.

The main cereal species were hulled barley (Hordeum vulgare) and emmer (Triticum dicoccum). In the later occupation phase, hulled barley became the predominant grain species (Buurman 1979). Occasionally, grains of naked six-row barley (Hordeum vulgare var. nudum) and einkorn (Triticum monococcum) are found (Buurman 1979).

The cereals were probably grown in mixed cultivation. Weeds in the samples from Hoogkarspel show that cereals were grown on sandy soils, eg. the creek ridges, probably as summer crops (Bakker et al. 1977). The small ring ditches and figure-of-eight ditches, which are restricted to the sandy to sandy loamy area enclosed by ditches, probably had a function as grain ricks (Bakker & Metz 1967, Buurman 1979). Such ditches are absent in an unparcelled part of a ridge west of Hoogkarspel-Watertoren (excavation 1978, Bakker 1979) and in the clayey basins.

Flax (*Linum usitatissimum*) was found at two sites in the area (Bakker et al. 1977) and this plant was probably also cultivated locally (Buurman & Pals 1974).
In addition to the cultivated cereals, seeds of certain weeds may have been gathered and consumed, as is suggested by relatively large quantities of seeds of fat hen (*Chenopodium album*), fig-leaved goosefoot (*Chenopodium ficifolium*) and cock spur grass (*Echinochloa crus-galli*) found in pits of pit circles (Buurman 1979).
A further discussion on available vegetable food items is presented in section IX.E.

A model of the subsistence of the West-Frisian Bronze Age farmers has been described by Brandt and IJzereef (Brandt & IJzereef 1980, IJzereef 1981). The model shows that agriculture, i.e. cultivation of cereals and animal husbandry, is capable of supplying food in sufficient quantity to support the relatively dense occupation of the area. The plant food production, (i.e. the area of the grain fields) per farm is probably limited only by the available amount of human labour.

An important aspect in the models is the production of milk. IJzereef (1981) calculated the relative amounts of vegetable and animal food in terms of energy which would be available for the human population under various agricultural regimes for farms in the area around Het Valkje. Milk production in connection with the cultivation of cereals may be the most productive agricultural system considering the limitations of human labour and the area of land available for stock breeding and crop growing.
Important variables in the models are the cereal grain yields and the milk production per cow per annum. Yield ratios (seed/yield) of 1:3 or 1:4, as calculated for medieval situations by Slicher van Bath (1960), seem much too low for the fertile soils in this area. IJzereef (1981) estimates that a 1:30 yield ratio would seem to be more acceptable within the other variables in the model. The fields were probably manured.

For the milk production, IJzereef (1981) estimates that per cow per annum, i.e. per lactation period of c. 200 days, a surplus of some 100 litres may have been available for human consumption.
For our study, the model of IJzereef supplies important reference material for the dietary and agricultural extrapolations on the basis of the bone trace element concentrations (chapter XI).

C.2. Sites from which bones were analysed

In the following section, the sites from which human and/or animal bones were taken are described briefly. Three sites, Schagen-Muggenburg, Velsen and Valkenburg (prov. of South-Holland) fell outside the limits of time and/or as defined in section C.1.

The **bold** printed catalogue numbers refer to the catalogue of the human skeletal material in Appendix 1, on which also the estimations of age and sex are based.

C.2.1. Zwaagdijk: barrows and flat graves

Zwaagdijk: barrows

The tumuli near Zwaagdijk were the first Bronze Age barrows to be excavated in West-Friesland (Van Giffen 1944). Van Giffen excavated three barrows (nrs. I, III and IV) of a complex originally consisting of at least 12 barrows. A number of these mounds had been levelled in preceding years. In fact, when Van Giffen got to hear of it, it was the find of a bronze sword decorated with gold wire in one of these barrows was the direct cause for his interest in the area. The sword is now lost, as is the gold decoration wire (Van Giffen 1944: fig. 16).

The barrows I and IV were almost completely excavated while two trial trenches were dug into barrow III. This barrow had two building phases, both with a circular (?) ring ditch. No human remains were found.

The two-period barrow I was almost completely excavated. The first phase was surrounded by a more or less circular ditch with a diameter of circa 10 m. The grave of this phase, orientated circa NNW-SSE, consisted of cremated human bones (**1**). The dead person was probably burned on the soil surface, and subsequently covered by a barrow. In the second period, the barrow was surrounded by a ditch layed out in the form of a trapezium with axes measuring about 20 m. The primary grave of the second phase consisted of a cremation (**2**). In the upper part of the centre of this barrow, two later interments in extended E-W position were present (**3, 4**). Both were probably female.

In barrow IV only one building phase was recognized, but the double peripheral structure, a ring of post holes and a circular ring ditch, might indicate that the barrow was built in two phases (fig. II.3a). With barrow XIII at Zwaagdijk (Van der Waals 1961), and a barrow at Hoogkarspel (section II.C.2.7) these are the only excavated barrows with a post circle in West-Friesland.

No primary graves were present. Six inhumations were found in the top of the barrow. Van Giffen's initial assumption that the uppermost individuals (**5, 6, 8**), interred in the centre of the barrow in an extended E-W position, were medieval warriors of count William II, as the local legend would have it, appears unlikely in the light of the later research. The state of conservation of the bones of these individuals is no different from that of the other individuals. Furthermore, at least two of the individuals (**5, 6**) were probably females, whose E-W orientation is consistent with that of other inhumed females (section II.C.1.3.). A further three individuals were present a little deeper in the centre of the barrow. These skeletons were orientated approximately N-S or S-N. One of these individuals (**10**) was a child of less than 10 years old. The two other individuals , **7** and **9**, were probably males. The position of the bodies is not clearly indicated by Van Giffen (1944).

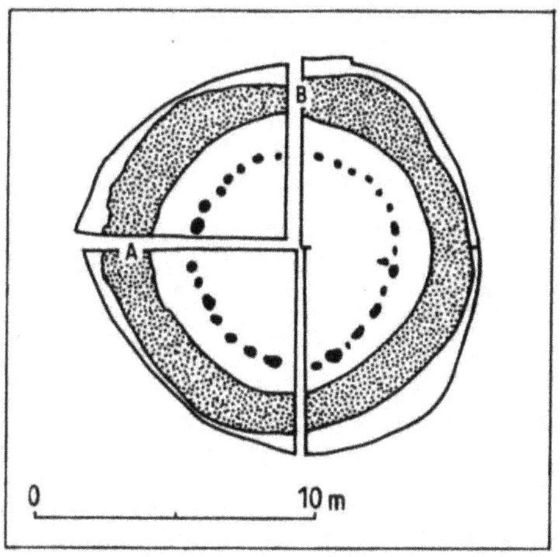

figure II.3a Excavation plan of barrow Zwaagdijk IV (Van Giffen 1944).

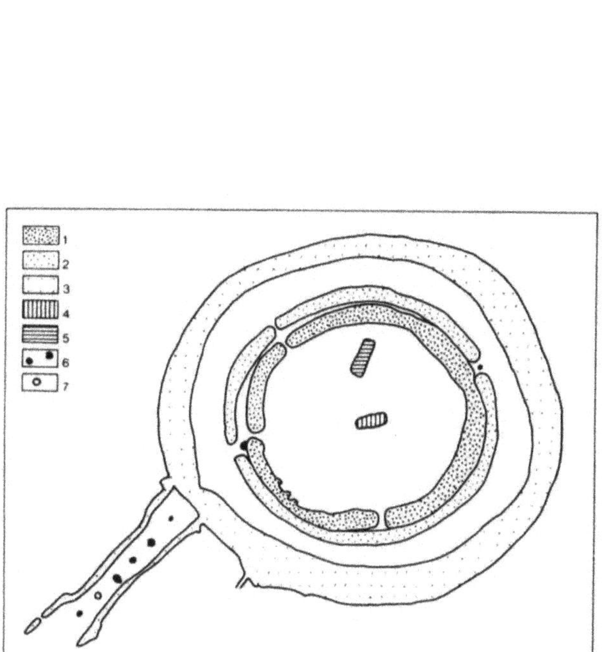

figure II.3b Excavation plan of barrow Grootebroek III. Legend: 1 ring ditch first period; 2 ring ditch second period; 3 ring ditch third period; 4 grave first period; 5 grave second period; 6 post holes; 7 post hole (presumed) (Van Giffen 1953, drawing and legend from Woltering 1985).

Zwaagdijk: flat graves

In 1961 some burials were uncovered about 500 m west of the group of barrows near Zwaagdijk (Van Giffen 1944) during ground levelling activities. Five graves were found in the resulting rescue excavation carried out by the ROB (Modderman 1964). Only some bones could be saved from one of the graves; the position of the skeleton was not recorded (**41**). Three other individuals, two adults (**43, 44**) and a child (**45**), were found close together. The adults were interred in extended positions, the child lay on its back with legs folded above the chest. Skeleton 3 (**43**) is one of the richest graves known from West-Friesland: apart from the bronze rapier (Butler 1964), amber beads (Runia 1986), two pieces of stone (sandstone and worked flint) and a small animal bone, probably a diaphysis fragment of the tibia of a mammal the size of dog or sheep, were found in the grave. The animal bone has a somewhat polished surface. A further skeleton (**42**), also layed out on its back, was found some 30 m NW of this small group of three individuals. This individual is characterized by a number of pathological features. A preliminary description of the skeletons has been published by Huizinga (1964).

In the same plot of ground in which the skeletons were found, a small excavation yielded some settlement traces: ditches, post holes and a figure-of-eight ditch, obviously dating from the Bronze Age. Charcoal from one of the ditches yielded a 14C date of 3200 ± 60 BP (GrN 4243). Animal bones from this small excavation were used as reference material for the human bones from the Zwaagdijk flat graves and barrows. These animal bones have been described by Clason (1964, compare table II.4).

C.2.2. Grootebroek: barrows

Three barrows south of Grootebroek were excavated in 1949 (Van Giffen 1953). Only the eastern half of barrow II was preserved and excavated but no human bones or cremations were found.

Three construction phases can be recognized in barrow I. The earliest barrow, with a diameter of c. 16.5 m, was the smallest and contained a shallow central grave pit in which the corpse had been cremated (**11**). This grave was dated at 3000 ± 140 BP (GrN 160, Lanting & Mook 1977). The second phase, encircled by a narrow, slightly rectangular ditch, contained an excentrically situated grave with cremated bones (**12**). In the third phase, an excentrically situated grave with a cremated woman (?, **13**) and an inhumed small child (**14**) was present. This grave contained a bronze ring.

Furthermore, two inhumation graves were present in barrow II: an extended S-N orientated skeleton (**15**) and a second skeleton, interred on the right side with contracted legs, and facing S-W (**16**). According to Van Giffen, these were medieval interments. However, the state of conservation of the bones and the position of the bodies suggest a Bronze Age date.

Barrow III is characterized by intrigueing ditches and post holes (fig. II.3b). The two earliest phases are enclosed by almost perfectly concentric, circular, interrupted ditches. The third and latest phase has a broad, uninterrupted ring ditch with a conspicuous avenue of two ditches and a central row of post holes (fig II.3). It is tempting to work out an astronomical function for this barrow (compare Woltering 1985). The oldest phase contained a 'Leichenbrandgrab' (**17**), the second phase an inhumation (**18**) in an extended, almost N-S or S-N position. The third and latest phase of the barrow contained a cremation grave (**19**). A second inhumation,

NNE-SSW extended, was present in the centre of the barrow (**20**). According to Van Giffen, this was a late secondary interment.

C.2.3. Oostwoud: barrows

The barrows in Oostwoud have been explored and discussed by archeologists repeatedly since the first excavation campaign by Van Giffen in 1956. Two barrows were present: tumulus I encircled by a ring of pits has a diameter of c. 18 m; and tumulus II with a diameter of c. 20 m and a more complex structure and history.

The barrows yielded the largest complex of Neolithic/Bronze Age human skeletal material in the western Netherlands (table II.5). Uptil now, no physical-anthropological study on the Oostwoud skeletons has been published; the material merits more thorough study than my, rather superficial, inventarization in Appendix 1.

Table II.5. Synopsis of inhumations in the Oostwoud barrows. Catalogue numbers refer to Appendix 1, excavation numbers to Van Giffen (1962) and De Weerd (1966). Abbreviation 'C' in column position of the body stands for a crouched burial.

cat. no.	exc. no.	sex	age	position of body	position in barrow	grave gift
25	230	male	25-35	extended E-W	central	-
26	231	female	25-35	extended E-W	excentric	-
27	127	?	15-20	C. L side E-W	excentric	-
28	228	male	20	C. L side E-W	excentric	-
29	229	male	25-30	?	excentric	-
30	232	female	25-35	C. R side N-S	central ?	-
31	233	female	33-45	?	?	-
32	235	male	adult	?	?	-
33	236	male	>40	C. L side E-W	central	marten bones
34	239	male	20-25	C. L side E-W	excentric	-
35	242	male	17-25	C. L side E-W	excentric	-
36(1)	243	female	35-50	C. R side E-W	excentric	-
36(2)	247	female	25-35	C. R side NNW-SSE	excentric	-
37	516	male	25-35	C. L side E-W	excentric	-
38	533 *					
39	#					

* this number and no.35 represent parts of one and the same individual
# this skeleton could not be traced back

In tumulus I, two inhumations lying on their backs in extended, E-W positions were found, one (**25**) almost in the centre of the barrow, the other (**26**) some 5 m to the south. According to Van Giffen, these are secondary graves, but no other, primary grave was found. A complete skeleton of a pig was found in the S-E quarter of the barrow. This pig was not mentioned and described by Clason (1967), probably because it was of recent date (Van Wijngaarden-Bakker, pers.comm).

Skeletal material of at least 12 individuals was found in tumulus II (fig. II.4). The skeletons were excavated by members of the Laboratorium voor Anthropobiologie in Amsterdam. The position of almost all skeletons was recorded; males were interred on left side in a crouched position, females in

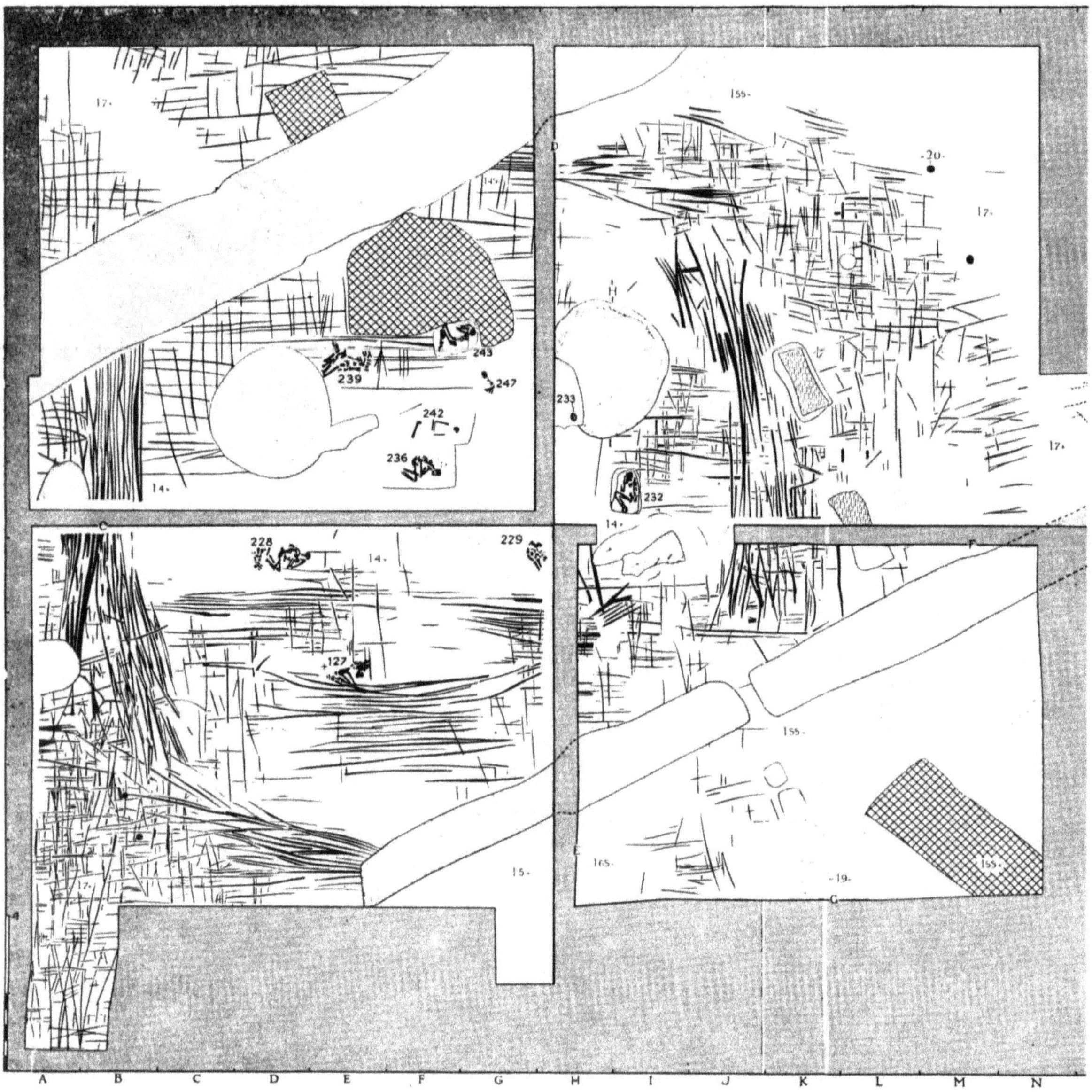

figure II.4 Excavation plan of Oostwoud barrow II, excavation 1955-1956 (Van Giffen (1962). Top of figure is N. Numbers of skeletons correspond with excavation numbers in table II.5.

the same position, but on the right side. Similar graves were found in connection with Late Neolithic occupation traces on river dunes (Louwe Kooymans 1974).

A synopsis of the features of these barrows uncovered after 1957 is given by Lanting (1979). Lanting's view that 236 (**33**) rather than 232 (**30**) is the primary grave of barrow II is interesting in the light of the results of our examination of the skeletal material. Skeleton **33** was a relatively old male, with a number of obvious pathologies, whereas **30** was a 25-35 year old female.

Some radiocarbon dates for the barrows and the levee on which the barrows are situated are available (table II.6).

Table II.6. Radiocarbon datings of the Oostwoud barrows

no.	material	barrow	skeleton	cat.no	date BP
GrN-797	charcoal	I			3025 ± 80
GrN-8801	collagen	II	232	30	3530 ± 25
GrN-6650C	collagen	II	516	37	3945 ± 55
GrN-8721	shells from gully next to levee				4085 ± 40
GrN-8722	peat below clay next to levee				4210 ± 30

The chronology of some of the inhumations in the NW quarter of tumulus II is somewhat obscure. According to Lanting (1979), the grave found in 1963 (De Weerd 1966, **37**) is a Late Neolithic flat grave connected with a c. 8 m wide ring of post holes. However, the bones found scattered above the western part of this grave (533, **38**) are complementary to the bones of skeleton 242 (**35**, Van Giffen 1962, fig. II.4). The two catalogue numbers **35** and **38** represent a single individual, as can be conclusively proved by chemical analysis (table II.7). The excavation plan of Van Giffen suggests that **35** was found in situ, with contracted legs and lying on the L side, facing S. If De Weerd's 1963 skeleton (**37**) is earlier than **35/38**, how did the bones of **38** came to be scattered? A possible explanation, namely careless excavation by Van Giffens workmen, leaving the part (i.e. **38**) of **35/38** disturbed in the soil, is out of the question because **38** was excavated from soil that had not been disturbed recently. Burial **37** is therefore probably antedated by burial **35/38**.

Table II.7. Comparison of skeleton 242 (**35**) and skeleton 533 (**38**). Chemical data are in mg /kg bone ash.

cat. no.	no.	sex	stature	chemical analysis: skeletal part	Sr	Ba	Zn
35	242	male	181	femur	862	131	261
38	533	male	181	tibia	871	123	235

No grave gifts were found except some bones of a marten (Martes sp.) near skeleton **33**. The marten bones, including part of the skull and some of the long bones, were present in the storage case containing skeleton **33**. Consequently, they were not examined and described by Clason (1967). The skull of the marten is visible behind the head of **33** on fig. 5 of Van Giffen (1962). The bones of a hare or rabbit mentioned by Van Giffen in relation to skeleton **30** are lost (Clason 1967:16), and were not present in the storage box of skeleton **30** either. Van Giffen's (1962) fig. 9 of skeleton **30** does not show any hare or rabbit bones. Though this does not prove anything, and though it appears unlikely that Van Giffen mistook a marten skull for a hare skull, I am inclined to doubt whether a hare or rabbit was found near **30** at all.

Two bones of a fox (Vulpes vulpes) were found together with the disturbed bones of **38**; whether these were interred in relation to this skeleton is uncertain.

C.2.4. Enkhuizen, De Tent: barrow

A Bronze Age tumulus near 'De Tent', municipality of Enkhuizen, was partly excavated in 1960 (Lehmann 1963). The barrow was encircled by two, probably concentric, ditches. The oldest, broader ditch was connected to another ditch that may be part of a larger complex of ditches, as is the case in the Hoogkarspel barrows (Bakker et al. 1977). The later ditch was rather narrow and probably more or less rectangular. The diameter of the barrow in both periods was about 20 m. Few finds were made. The dating of the barrow in the Bronze Age is based on geological considerations: the peat on the flank of the barrow and the 'kiek' clay over the barrow (compare section II.B). The centre of the barrow was not excavated, and no primary grave or secondary interments were present in the excavated part of the barrow. Some small human bones and bone fragments were found (**40**).

The residual part of this and a nearby barrow were left intact during the execution of the land reallotment program in this area (Jaarverslag ROB 1974).

C.2.5. Andijk: settlement traces and barrows

Traces of Bronze Age occupation were excavated near Andijk in 1973 (Van Haaff 1973). Besides some 25 house plans situated on or near a sandy creek ridge, the remains of two barrows were found. A house plan measuring c. 18 x 6 m is shown in Van Haaff (1973). No excavation report on this site has yet been published yet. Van Mensch & IJzereef (1975) studied human and animal bones from the site (table II.4). Human bones (**54**) were present in the ring ditch of one of the barrows as well as in other ditches.

C.2.6. Bovenkarspel-Het Valkje: settlement traces, barrow and inhumations

Following the trial excavations in Andijk in 1973, subsequent large scale excavations were carried out north of Bovenkarspel near Het Valkje. No definitive report on this excavation has yet been published, but IJzereef (1981) in his study of the animal bones from the site gives some information on the settlement traces that were found.

The excavated area at Het Valkje is situated on a broad, N-S running sandy and loamy creek ridge (fig. II.5). Numerous house plans were excavated on the flanks of the ridge.

IJzereef (1981) uses the preliminary periodization of the settlement at Het Valkje. For our study, we use the simplified periodization with a division in an Early (phase 1-4, C14 dated 3275-2845 BP) and a Late (phase 5-7, C14 dated 2760-2620 BP) Period of occupation. In the Late Period, houses were situated on small terps surrounded by ditches.

The agricultural potential of the area gradually deteriorated throughout the period of occupation as a consequence of the rising water table. In the Late Period, the area suitable for house building, crop growing and grazing was considerably smaller than in the Early Period. The shift in agricultural strategy forced upon the farmers by the rising water table is reflected in the animal bones recovered (IJzereef 1981, 1983). In the Late Period, relatively more sheep/goat and dog were present in comparison to cattle than in the Early Period (table II.8). The ratio cows/(bulls + steers) in the Late Period is higher than in the Early Period. This suggests a shift towards dairying (IJzereef 1981).

Table II.8. Percentages of numbers of bones from domestic animals in Het Valkje (IJzereef 1981). Cattle female/male ratio calculated from IJzereef 1981:53. From each period, over 5000 animal bones were studied.

period	cattle	female/male ratio	pig	sheep	goat	dog	horse
Early	78.5	1.29	6.7	12.7	0.8	1.5	0.1
Late	62.8	2.24	9.1	22.7	1.6	3.8	-

Paleobotanical analysis of grain samples shows that in the two periods different grain species were dominant. In the Early Period barley (Hordeum vulgare) and emmer (Triticum dicoccum) were equally important. In the later period Hordeum vulgare was the predominant grain species (Buurman 1979).

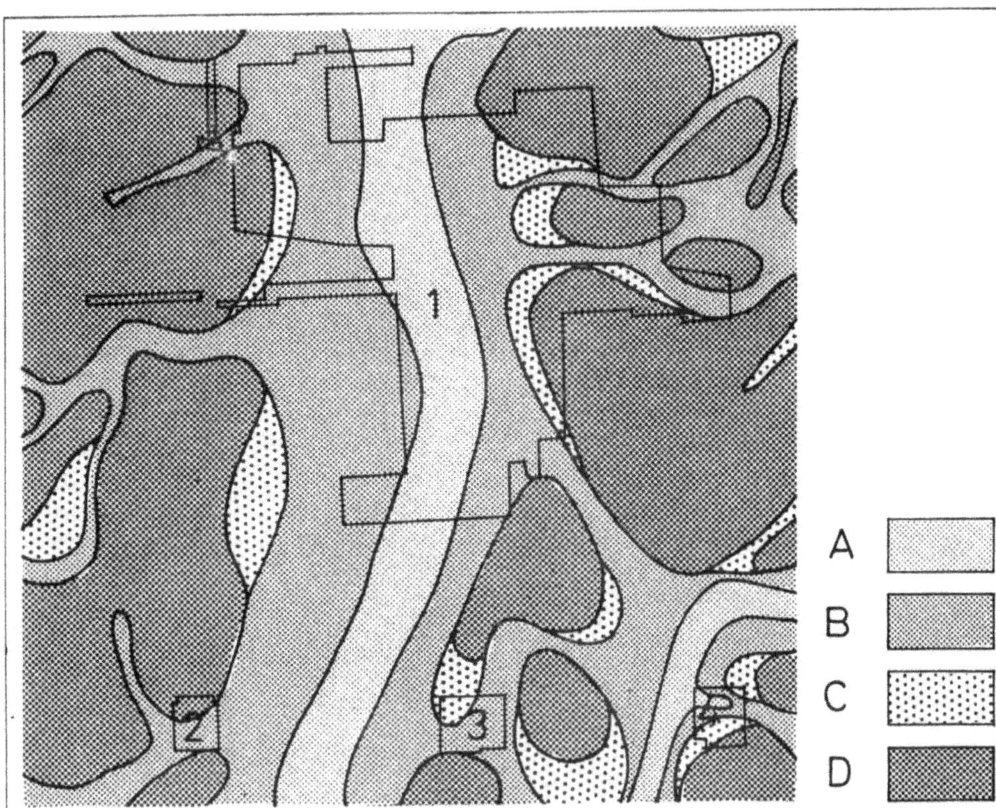

figure II.5 Soil map (1 km^2) of Het Valkje and surrounding area. (1) excavation Bovenkarspel-Het Valkje, (2-4) excavation Bovenkarspel-Monument. Soil units: A sand (ridge); B sandy loam; C loam on clay; D clay (basin). Adapted from IJzereef (1981).

The site has yielded a number of isolated human bones. These bones, mainly long bones, were found in ditches and pits. They have been catalogued by IJzereef (1981: Appendix) and were reexamined for the present study (App.1). Though the remains of a barrow were found, no inhumations or cremations remained from the Early Period. Charcoal from the ring ditch was dated to 3275 ± 35 BP (GrN 7472). This date may be somewhat too early (Lanting & Mook 1977). From the Late Period, skeletons of two individuals were found together in a ditch (55 1-2-45, C14 dated 2710

$\pm$ 35 BP, GrN 7509). Together with a child's skeleton from a disturbed grave, these represent the only inhumations from Het Valkje.
In 'terrein Visser', a small excavation south of Het Valkje, an almost complete skeleton (**57**, 'the witch of Bovenkarspel') was found in a ditch (Maat, in press). For our study, samples from this skeleton were placed in the group of samples from Het Valkje.

A preliminary report on the analysis of human and animal bones from this was been published elsewhere (Runia 1987a).

C.2.7. Hoogkarspel: barrows and settlement traces

Traces of prehistoric settlements were excavated both to the north and to the south of the village of Hoogkarspel. South of Hoogkarspel a number of excavations were carried out by the IPP in the years 1965-1969 (Hoogkarspel-Tolhek: Bakker & Brandt 1966, Bakker & Metz 1967, Bakker et al. 1968, Bakker et al. 1977) while to the north (Hoogkarspel-Watertoren) some barrows and settlement traces were investigated by the IPP and IPL (Bakker 1959, 1966, Modderman 1974, Bakker et al. 1977, fig. II.6).
The earliest excavation to be carried out near Hoogkarspel concerned a barrow (Hoogkarspel I, Bakker 1959, Bakker et al. 1977). A cremation was found in this barrow as well as a few human skull fragments from the ditch. These could not be examined.

The western half of a second barrow situated north of the village (Hoogkarspel Ia) was excavated in 1972 by the IPL (Modderman 1974, Bakker et al. 1977). A trial trench had already been dug through part of the barrow by Bakker during his excavation of barrow I (Bakker 1959). Barrow Ia has three almost concentric ring ditches. The two earliest phases of the barrow were related to cremation burials. In the storage bag containing one of the cremations were a few small uncremated bones, probably of an infant. The almost complete skeleton (**51**), interred on its back in an extended E-W position probably represents the last phase of the barrow, which was dated 3035 $\pm$ 55 BP (GrN 6837). In the storage box containing this skeleton was the proximal part of a tibia of a kitten (<u>Felis silvestris</u>). This might represent a grave gift.
In 1973, the remaining part of the barrow was investigated (Bakker et al. 1977). A fragment of a human skull was found (**53**, Bakker 1974, Bakker et al. 1977) in the third ring ditch but could no longer be traced in the storage depots and was therefore not available for analysis.

The later excavation campaigns in Hoogkarspel-Watertoren were primarily intended to map the settlement features such as the ditches and house plans (Bakker et al. 1977). The working strategy and the machinery allowed little time for the collection of artifacts. This may be one of the reasons why only one human bone was found in this part of the settlement (**53**).
Brandt (in Bakker et al. 1977) recognises certain individual agricultural holdings which consisted of a house site and plots of land surrounded by a ditches. Small ring ditches were present on some of the plots. The ditches of the barrows situated here (Hoogkarspel I, Ia) form part of the extensive system of ditches connected to these agricultural holdings which are clearly confined to the lighter soils of the creek ridge (Bakker in Bakker et al. 1977, fig.II.6)

In 1978 the area west of the 1973 excavation was investigated (Vons-Comis 1978, Bakker in Woltering 1979). Here, the remains of a number of barrows were found. In a barrow with a ring ditch an almost complete human skeleton (**56**) lay in a small (c. 1.3 x 0.4 m), secondary, grave pit. The body was placed on its back, with the legs crossed and contracted above the body, head S, feet N. The head was placed somewhat upright, the face turned a little to the west.

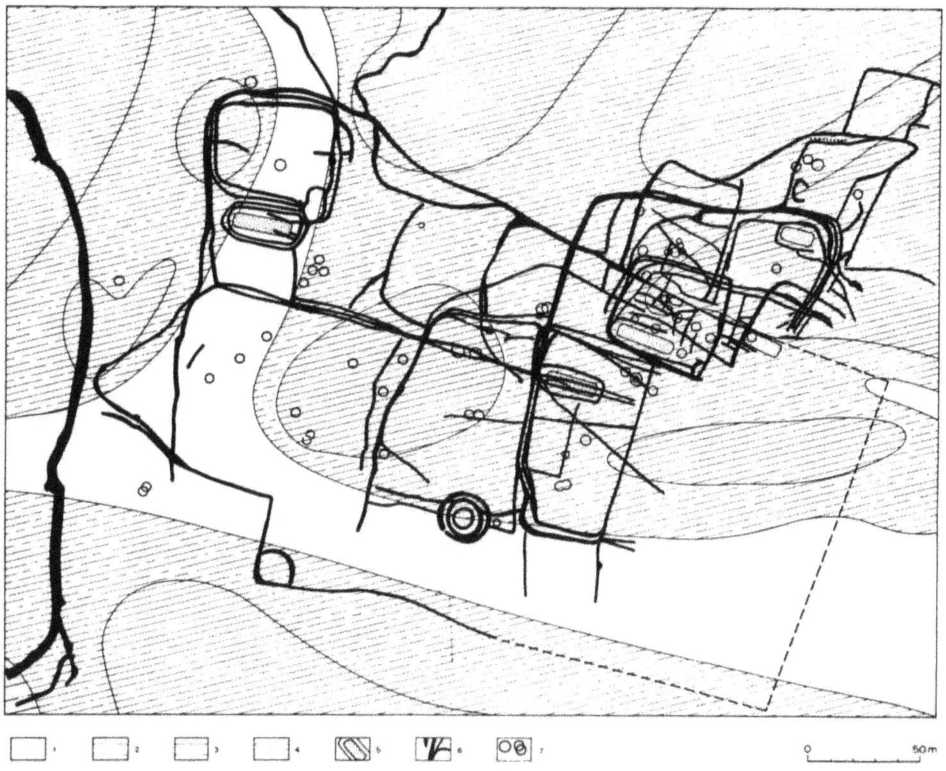

figure II.6 Settlement traces of the site Hoogkarspel-Watertoren, N of the village of Hoogkarspel. 1 sand; 2 sandy loam; 3 sandy loam on clay; 5 house site; 6 ditch; 7 small ring ditches (Bakker et al. 1977, drawing from Woltering 1985).

The excavations carried out by the IPP to the south of Hoogkarspel yielded settlement traces and barrows (Hoogkarspel-Tolhek). The settlement traces consist of numerous ditches of various kinds, some house plans and some house terps. In this site, the conspicuous small ring ditches, figure-of-eight ditches and rings of pits were extensively studied for the first time (Bakker & Metz 1967). These features probably had an agricultural function (Buurman 1979, compare section II.C.1.4.).

Two barrows were found, barrow II with a circular and barrow III with a more or less rectangular ditch (Bakker & Brandt 1966). A secondary grave pit in barrow II contained the remains of a woman (?, **46**) which had been cremated, and also the remains of an inhumed infant (**47**). This grave was dated to 3020 $\pm$ 40 BP (GrN 5050). In the late settlement period, a house terp was raised over the two barrows. The 'terp phase' was dated around 2650 BP (GrN-5048, GrN-5051).

No other graves were found besides the barrow, though a number of isolated human bones were present in the ditches (**48**).

Animal bones from the settlement traces near Hoogkarspel were studied by Van Mensch & IJzereef (1977) and Smits (cited in Prummel 1979, table II.4).

C.2.8. Westwoud: settlement traces

In the summer of 1984, some traces of Bronze Age occupation in the path of a road under construction were investigated by W. de Vries-Metz. In a Bronze Age ditch, a number of animal bones were found in addition to pottery sherds. Some of these bones were analysed, because here it was certain that the bones came from one and the same ditch. Some soil samples were also taken but have not yet been analysed.

C.2.9. Schagen-Muggenburg: settlement traces and flat graves

Part of a native settlement of the Roman period (c. 2nd-3rd century AD) was excavated in 1983-1984 (Therkorn 1984). The excavation yielded only one house plan besides numerous pits and hearths. The pits contained, among other things, charred grain. Besides native pottery, some sherds of imported Roman pottery were found.

In the earlier phase of occupation, houses were built on peat. In a later phase, the surface of two probable house sites was raised using peat (turfs). Due to oxydation of the peat, the terps have been reduced to a layer of c. 15 cm thick with a high concentration of pottery. The oxydation of the peat has resulted in the disappearance of almost all the post holes.

Inhumations of four human individuals were found (**59**) besides the completely interred skeletons of some dogs and a horse. A cluster of seven large urns, each containing a cremated human individual was also excavated.

A final report on this excavation and the economic basis of the settlement is in preparation (Therkorn, IPP). The finds of, for example, large quantities of charred grains and ear fragments of <u>Hordeum vulgare</u> and <u>Triticum dicoccum</u> (C.D. Troostheide, pers. comm.) and agricultural implements may be indicative for the agriculturally based economy of the site. It is likely that <u>Hordeum vulgare</u> and <u>Triticum dicoccum</u> were grown on the peat around the settlement or on salt marsh soils in the neighbourhood (Van Haaster 1985). The relatively large number of horse bones (table II.4) and the presence of some exceptionally large cattle specimens may suggest that some of the animal husbandry products were traded. On the other hand, a number of large hearth places and some slags may indicate that the inhabitants of this site were employed in 'industrial' activities of some kind.

C.2.10. Velsen-Hofgeest: settlements traces and barrows

In the Velserbroekpolder (gemeente Velsen), south of the Hofgeesterweg, settlement remains dating to the Bronze Age were excavated (Beemster & Brandt 1986). These traces may be contemporary with the barrows excavated in 1972/1978 (Woltering 1979).

Velsen-Hofgeest is situated on the south-western edge of the inlet of the Oer-IJ estuary, shielded from the sea by the broad sandy coastal barrier (Hallewas 1981). Near the site, low-lying salt marshes and higher, sandy areas covered with woods must have been present (Jelgersma et al. 1970).

No data on the subsistence economy of this site are available yet. The main food resource was to all probability agricultural production, though the location of the site, near the inlet of the Oer-IJ, may suggest that seafish formed part of the diet. The settlement is roughly contemporary with the Bronze Age occupation in West-Friesland with similar house plans and pottery. As was the case in West-Friesland, sandy soils were used for crop growing, as is indicated by the presence of ard scratches and dark layers of 'arable soil'. Velsen-Hofgeest differs from the West-Frisian sites in the presence of forests in the neighbourhood. Besides, compared to West-Friesland, the area of clayey soils appears to be relatively small. The maps of Hallewas (1981) show extensive areas of peat east of Velsen-Hofgeest.

No exact zooarcheological data on the site are available. However, in an excavation carried out in 1986 close to the 1984 site, approximately 80% of the bones were cattle bones, whereas sheep/goat represented only some 10%. In addition, a small amount of game (deer and others) was present (L.L. Therkorn, pers. comm.).

A number of animal bones from Velsen-Hofgeest were randomly chosen for analysis from the excavated bone material.

The only human bone present in this site, a skull fragment (R half os frontale of adult person with sutura metopica) was also analysed and a series of samples was taken from the six inhumations present in one of the nearby barrows (barrow A, Woltering 1979 and pers. comm.).

These bones have been studied by dr. W.R.K. Perizonius (Utrecht) and are not described in Appendix 1. It is probable that the primary grave of the first period of the barrow which was encircled by closely spaced posts, was a cremation. The second period of the barrow was enclosed by a narrow, circular ditch. Four inhumation graves were present in this phase. A crouched inhumation of a female interred on the R side and looking N, probably represents the primary grave of this phase. Three more inhumations, extended on their backs were present in the barrow: a male (SE-NW) and two females (NE-SW and SE-NW, respectively). A further skeleton, a female, extended NE-SW, was present in a pit that cut the circular ditch. The sixth skeleton, a male, extended SW-NE, was found just east of the barrow.

In the orientation of the bodies, this barrow appears to be different from the barrows in West-Friesland, where all extended female burials are orientated E-W (table II.3).

D. THE BONES

D.1. The human bones

D.1.1. Strategy

The number of bones present per individual is variable. Some skeletons are almost complete, others are represented by only a single fragment of bone. For studies such as the present one, the number of individuals to be analysed should be as large as possible. It was therefore decided to sample not only the more or less complete skeletons, but also isolated bones. A second reason to do this is the difference between the contexts in which the isolated bones and the skeletons were found.

In the group of the isolated bones, each individual is represented by only one sample. The majority of the isolated bones are long bones (femur, tibia, humerus) often incomplete. These long bones were invariably sampled except when the fragment was too small. Other isolated skeletal elements, e.g. fragments of skull or small long bones (ulna, radius, fibula) were sampled only if this was justified by the fragment size and anthropological value.

For reasons of comparison and diagenesis, it is obvious that we must strive to sample and to analyse the same skeletal element in each individual. Long bones are the most suitable for sampling and analysis for both practical and chemical reasons. The thick cortical bone of long bones is less affected by soil conditions, and on account of their robustness one or more long bones are usually present for most of the individuals.

Comparison between trace element levels within individuals is possible through the analysis of samples of various skeletal elements from each individual. Furthermore, this method permits comparison with isolated non-long bone samples. Another reason for analysing more bones per individual is that as a consequence of faster bone replacement in certain skeletal elements, this might yield clues on dietary changes shortly before death.

D.1.2. The samples

As far as possible, a sample from one of the long bones, femur, tibia or humerus, was taken from each individual. Additional samples were taken from the skeletons from one or more other bones (skull, vertebrae, ribs). An overview of the human bone samples analysed is given in table II.9.

D.1.3. Age, sex and status groups

One of the aims of the present study is the assessment of differences between groups of individuals. Besides an obvious separation into groups on the basis of settlement periods, groupings based on sex, age and status are possible.

A division into two status groups is obvious, the one group consisting of the inhumations, the other of the individuals represented by isolated bones. However, besides status differences, these groups also represent different phases of occupation. The inhumations stem from the earlier occupation period while the isolated bones occur in features from the later period (section II.C.2). Within the high status group, i.e. the inhumations, a further division is possible on the basis of location of the grave and the grave gifts. However, due to the limited number of inhumations this would result in groups consisting of no more than a few individuals. Due to individual variations in trace element levels, such a division will not produce meaningful results and has therefore been avoided. Possible status differences should however be kept in mind.

Table II.9. Synopsis of samples of human bones from the sites in West-Friesland. The sex separation includes individuals termed 'probably male' and 'probably female' and is based on Appendix 1.

site	no. of samples		no. of	male	female	unknown
	long bones	other	individuals			sex
Zwaagdijk						
barrows	7	5	8	3	4	1
flat graves	5	4	5	2	2	1
Grootebroek	3	2	5	2	2	1
Hoogkarspel						
settlement	11	3	14	2		12
inhumations	3	3	5	1	2	2
Oostwoud	12	23	13	8	4	1
Enkhuizen						
De Tent		2	2?			2?
Bovenkarspel						
inhumations	3	4	3		3	
Het Valkje	11	11	20	8	3	9
Andijk	11	8	max. 19	5	4	max. 10
Schagen						
Muggenburg	4	9	5	3	1	1
Velsen						
barrow	6	4	6	1	1	4
settlement		1	1		1	
Valkenburg	4		4			4
totals	80	79	max. 110	35	27	48

The status groups may be divided into age and sex classes, a procedure rarely possible in the group of isolated bones since neither age nor sex of the majority of individuals can be established.

In the group of the inhumations in flat graves and barrows, 29 individuals were grouped according to sex and age on the basis of information in Appendix 1. (table II.10).

The age class division (<10, 15-25, 25-35 and >35) was chosen for various reasons. The limited number of individuals does not allow narrower age groups. The limits of the age groups correspond to age group boundaries in the tooth wear age estimation scheme of Brothwell (1981). Individuals estimated as 'adult' were placed in the group 15-25.

The grouping results in a fairly equal distribution of the individuals over the groups. However, the distribution of samples from the same barrow over the groups is not equal. For instance, in the age group of 15-25 almost all females, but none of the males come from the Zwaagdijk barrows. This uneven distribution might cause bias due to geographical differences in trace element concentrations and therefore has to be taken into account in the assessment of the trace element levels in the various age and sex groups.

Table II.10. Division into age and sex groups of the individuals from flat graves and barrows. Based on Appendix 1.

age group	barrow	cat.no
0-10	Zwaagdijk IV-15	10
	Grootebroek I-2(2)	14
	Zwaagdijk 5	45
	HK 2	47

age group	female barrow	female cat.no	male barrow	male cat.no
10-15	-		-	
15-25	Zwaagdijk IV-11	6	Grootebroek I-7	15
	Zwaagdijk I-16	3	Oostwoud II-228	28
	Zwaagdijk I-17	4	Oostwoud II-235	32
	Grootebroek I-4	16	Oostwoud II-239	34
	Zwaagdijk 1	41	Oostwoud II-242	35
			Zwaagdijk 3	43
25-35	Zwaagdijk IV-10	5	Zwaagdijk IV-12	7
	Oostwoud I-231	26	Zwaagdijk IV-14	9
	Oostwoud II-232	30	Oostwoud II-229	29
	Oostwoud II-247	36(2)	Oostwoud I-230	25
>35	Oostwoud II-243	36(1)	Oostwoud II-236	33
	Hw 71	56	Zwaagdijk 2	42
	HB	57	Hoogkarspel Ia 228	51

D.2. The animal bones

D.2.1. Strategy

For reasons explained in section I.B.1, the analysis of animal bones in addition to human bones is essential in trace element studies. A number of animal bones were therefore sampled from each of the sites. In most sites in the area, bones of herbivorous animals, cattle and to a lesser extent sheep/goat, are present in sufficient quantities. Bones of omnivorous animals, pigs and dogs, are in many cases also present, though in smaller numbers. No strictly carnivorous animals are present in the bone material from the excavations.

From the larger sites, cattle metapodia were selected for analysis. It is possible to sex these bones using the criteria described by IJzereef (1981). Thus, for these sites the comparison between trace element levels in cows and bulls/steers is possible.

Because of the relatively and numerically small number of bones from pigs and dogs, it was not possible to maintain the restriction to long bones only and other skeletal elements such as mandibles and ribs were also sampled.

D.2.2. Samples

An overview of the samples of prehistoric animal bones is given in table II.11. In addition to these bones, some fresh cattle bones were sampled and analysed. A series of fresh cattle bones was obtained through the aid of drs. P.L. Bergström (IVO Zeist). A second series of fresh cattle bones was obtained from the Amsterdam Abattoir.

Table II.11. Numbers of chemically analysed animal bones from the West-Frisian sites

site	cattle male	female	total	pig	dog	sheep/ goat	horse	fish
Zwaagdijk			6	3	2	3		
Grootebroek			6					
Oostwoud			7	1				
Enkhuizen De Tent			5	1				
Bovenkarspel Het Valkje	15	17	32	15	14	15		6
Andijk	10	10	20	7	2	10		
Hoogkarspel			19					
Schagen Muggenburg	12	14	32	9	7	11	1	
Velsen			10	2	2	5		2
Westwoud			8	1	1			
totals	37	41	145	38	29	44	1	8

D.3. State of conservation

The state of conservation of the bones can be assessed using macroscopic, microscopic, mineralogical and chemical characteristics.

Macroscopic appearance

Most of the bones appear to be unaffected or only slightly so by the period of burial. A minor part of the material concerned is weathered, but most of the bones have a rather smooth, undamaged cortex. The colour of the bones has changed from the original yellow-white hues to brown, grey-brown or yellow-brown colours at present. Many bones display dark brown mottling (plate 1).

When samples were sawn out of the bones with an electric bandsaw (section III.A), most gave off a nasty smell resembling the smell of heated fresh bones. This, and the weight loss when ashed indicate that at least some of the organic fraction is still present in the bones.

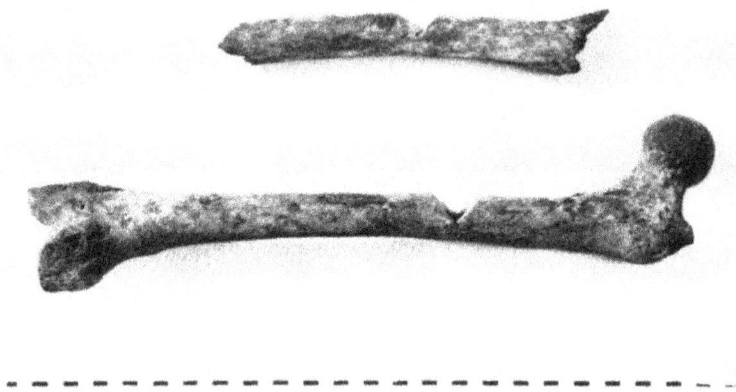

plate 1 Examples of human bones used in this study: a complete femur and a femur diaphysis from Het Valkje. Triangular samples have been taken from each.

Microscopic appearance

Two thin-sections of randomly chosen bones used in this study were made by the Anatomisch-Embryologisch Laboratorium of the Rijksuniversiteit Leiden (dr G.J.R. Maat). No etching or colouring was used. The thin-sections were studied with a microscope using normal and polarized light. Some pictures were taken to show the histological structure still present in the bones (plate 2). The major part of the interior of the bones consists of birefringent bone tissue ordered in haversian systems. Some opaque (iron or other) compounds have been deposited along the cortex of the bone and in the Haversian channels, but the interior of the bones appears practically unaltered. Opaque, more or less dendritic patterns are visible in the bone (plate 3) which probably result from biogenous decomposition by fungi or bacteria (compare Piepenbrink 1986) and mainly affect the organic bone fraction.

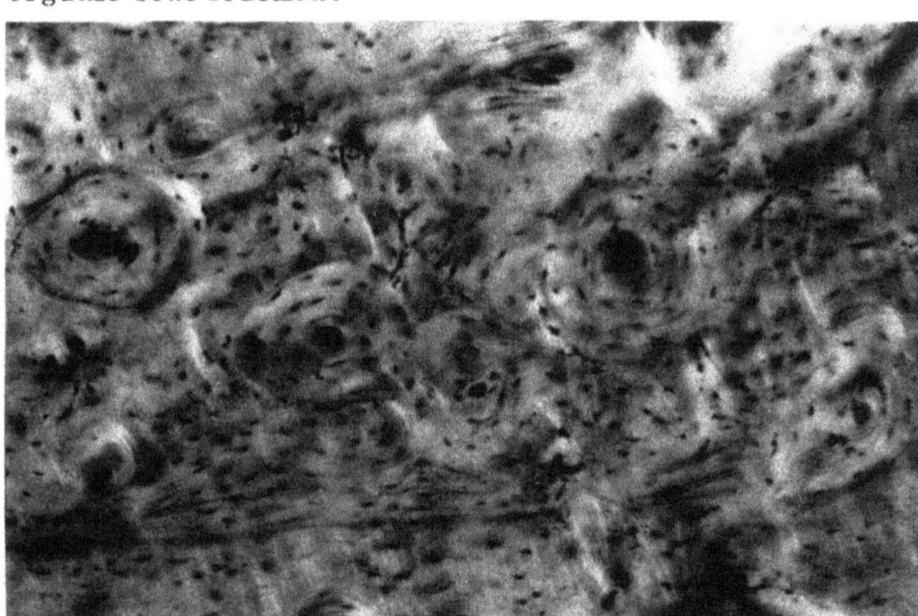

plate 2 Thin section of one of the bones used in this study, showing haversian canals and circularly arranged bone tissue (half polarized light).

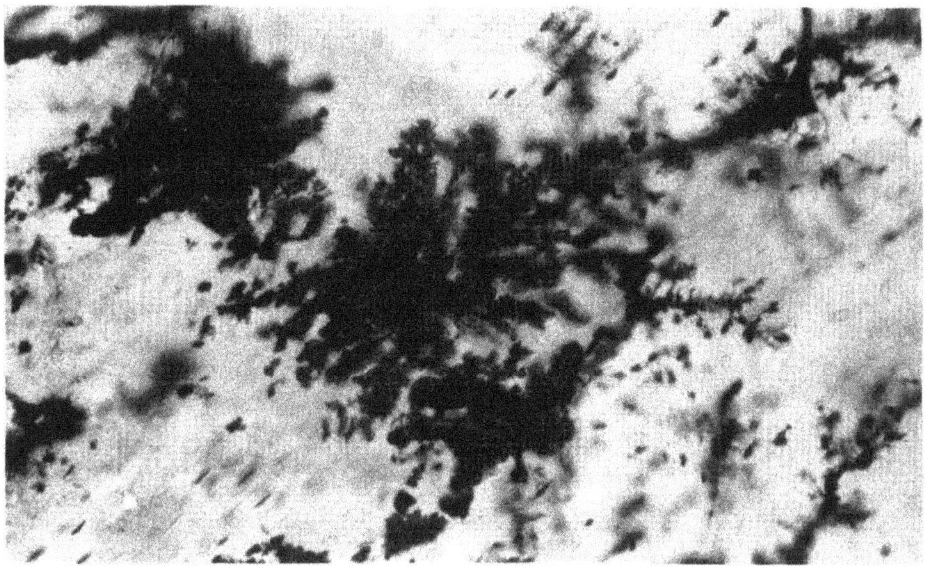

plate 3 Thin section of one of the bones used in this study, showing opaque dendritic structure near the outer cortex (half polarized light).

Mineralogy

As can be inferred from the microscopic appearance of the bones, the mineralogical components of the bones, i.e. the hydroxyapatite crystals, are hardly affected by the soil solution. To check this assumption, some X-ray diffractograms of powdered excavated bone were made by B. de Leeuw (Universiteit van Amsterdam). The diffractograms showed the pattern of broad lines typical for bone hydroxyapatite. No other minerals were detected.

Chemistry

The chemistry of the bones, and especially the amount of Fe and the relation between amounts of Ca and P, is an indication for the state of conservation. These aspects will be discussed in chapter IV.

D.4. Cremations

D.4.1. Strategy

The interred remains of cremated humans have been found in addition to the inhumations at a number of sites in West-Friesland. No information on trace elements in cremated bone is available (section I.B.1.6), and it was therefore decided to explore the potential of cremated bone for paleodietary studies by analysing a limited number of calcinated remains from those sites from which samples of non-burnt bone were taken. The sites are described in more detail in section II.C.2.

D.4.2. The samples

Samples of cremation remains from four sites were taken (table II.12):

Grootebroek

Two samples were taken from each of four cremations. The cremation from the third phase of barrow III is not mentioned by Assies (in Van Giffen 1953: 21) and was not present in the box with the other cremations. The four analysed cremations are **11**, **12** and **13** from the three phases of barrow I, and **17** from the first phase of barrow III. The woman (?) from the third phase of barrow I was incompletely burnt. In this case, burnt and partly burnt or charred bone can be compared (Van Giffen 1953)

Hoogkarspel

From barrow Hoogkarspel Ia two cremations were available for analysis besides an almost complete skeleton. One of the cremation samples was taken from an incompletely burnt (charred) long bone fragment. In this case, the effect of burning on bone trace element concentrations could be monitored.

Schagen-Muggenburg

In the 1984 campaign, a cluster of seven urns, each containing human cremation remains, was excavated (Therkorn 1984). A sample of cremated bone was taken from each urn.

Valkenburg

The large-scale excavations of a cemetery and settlement traces of the Roman Period near Valkenburg (prov. South-Holland) yielded numerous finds of cremations (Bult & Hallewas 1986, Hallewas 1986). Inhumations were also found in the same site. In view of the potential of this large site for comparisons between cremation and inhumation analysis, a pilot study was carried out and a small number of samples was analysed.

Table II.12. Numbers of samples of cremated bone material from various sites

site	samples	individuals
Grootebroek	8	4
Schagen-Muggenburg	7	7
Valkenburg (S-H)	4	4
Hoogkarspel	2	2
total	21	17

III
ANALYTICAL PROCEDURES IN BONE ANALYSIS

A. ANALYTICAL PROCEDURE

Analysis of bones and other materials was carried out at the Netherlands Energy Research Foundation (ECN) at Petten. The general procedure of the analysis of bone samples is described in this chapter with details on the analysis of specific elements presented in the subsequent chapters. The procedures in the analysis of cremations and soil and plant material will be described in chapter VIII and IX.

Bones were superficially cleaned at the excavation. In the laboratory, samples were sawn out of the selected bones using an electric band saw or a simple carpenter's saw. Bone samples were cleaned in an ultrasonic bath with warm demineralized water. After drying, samples were ground in a disc mill (Siebtechnik), with tungsten-carbide vessel and discs. The disc mill proved to be highly satisfactory for grinding the tough and compact bone. The excessive heating of the samples due to long milling times, as encountered in ball mills, was no problem in this type of mill: some 15 seconds of grinding were enough to reduce tough bone to a fine powder. However, cleaning the grinding vessel itself is rather time consuming.
Sieving was not necessary. Bone powder was stored in polyethylene sample tubes.
A second method for grinding bone was employed: the bone sample was mechanically broken in small pieces. These bone pieces were ashed and subsequently ground in an agate mortar.
Fresh cattle bones were boiled and manually cleaned prior to sampling and ashing. After ashing, the ash was ground in the disc mill.
Bone powder (c.q. pieces) was ashed in 2-4 gram portions in quartz dishes in an electric furnace (6 hours, 750°C).

Bone ash was digested using PTFE pressure vessels with stainless steel containers. Approximately 0.25 g of bone ash was weighed accurately into the vessels and heated with a mixture of concentrated HNO_3 and HCl for 6 hours at 175°C.

The hydrochloric acid attacks the stainless steel pressure containers. To avoid this, digestion with a $HNO_3/HClO_4$ mixture was tried. For fresh bone samples, this gave analytical results comparable to the mixture with HCl, but in case of prehistoric bone material, concentrations of Sr and other elements were slightly lower when the $HClO_4$ mixture was used. Strontium concentrations in the nitric-hydrochloric acid digestion were closer to the concentrations determined by isotope dilution (IDMS, see below) than the concentrations in HNO_3-$HClO_4$ digestions. It was, therefore, decided to continue using the HNO_3-HCL mixture despite the extra work involved in cleaning the pressure containers. Apart from the samples from Andijk, all bone samples were digested with the HNO_3/HCl mixture.

The sample solutions were transferred to polyethylene flasks and gravimetrically diluted with demineralised water. After dilution, concentrations of P, Fe, Ba and Sr were measured using Inductively Coupled Plasma Atomic Emission Spectrometry (ICP-AES, Jobin-Yvon type JY38 PI-VHR). Calcium and Zn were determined using Atomic Absorption

Spectrometry (Perkin-Elmer 3030 and Jarrell-Ash 811). In the Sr, Ba and Fe determination, Merck Titrisol was used as a standard.

Isotope Dilution Mass Spectrometry (IDMS) was performed on a number of bone samples by the ECN Mass Spectrometry department. Bone ash was digested in a mixture of nitric and hydrochloric acid in PTFE pressure vessels (180 ^{o}C, 16 hr) together with 44Ca and 86Sr spikes. After evaporation and cation exchange, mass spectrometry (triple filament, thermic ionisation) was carried out. Results have coefficients of variation of 1 %.

B. ACCURACY AND REPRODUCIBILITY

No duplicate samples were analysed, but a number of samples were digested and analysed twice or more to obtain an insight into the reproducibility and accuracy of the analyses. The results of these tests for the various elements are discussed in the chapters IV-VII, respectively. Twenty-five samples were analysed by isotope dilution (IDMS) for Ca and Sr content. Results of IDMS measurements are discussed in chapter IV and V.

IV
ANALYSIS OF BONE:
THE MACRO ELEMENTS CALCIUM, PHOSPHORUS AND IRON

A. INTRODUCTION

In this chapter the analysis of the macro elements Ca, P and Fe is discussed. The concentrations of these elements are of interest in relation to possible diagenetic alterations of bone mineral and bone trace element concentrations. The concentrations of the major element in bone mineral, Ca, form the background against which the concentrations of other elements are reviewed.

B. CALCIUM AND PHOSPHORUS: THE APATITE BUILDING STONES

B.1. General

Calcium and phosphorus in combination with oxygen make up hydroxyapatite (here abbreviated HAP) which constitutes the mineral phase of bone. Theoretically, Ca and P are present in an atomic ratio of 10 to 6. In vivo bone Ca/P ratios often are below the theoretical value of 1.67, probably as a result of the presence of other ions on Ca sites in the apatite or of the presence of defects in the crystal lattice (Jowsey 1977).
Hydroxyapatite is a member of the large group of apatites and has the ideal formula $Ca_{10}(PO_4)_6(OH)_2$ (Posner 1969). In apatites part of the Ca and P can be substituted by other ions, such Sr, Pb, Ba, Zn for Ca and As and V for P. Part of the hydroxy groups can be replaced by CO_3, F or other ions.
HAP is stable at pH values higher than approximately 7 and specific concentrations of HPO4 and Ca. At other HPO_4 and Ca concentrations other phosphate minerals such as octocalcium phosphate ($Ca_4H(PO_4)_3$*3H2O) and brushite ($CaHPO_4$*2H2O) are stable. At pH values below 7, a number of Fe, Al or other phosphate minerals such as variscite ($Al(OH)_2PO_4$) and strengite ($Fe(OH)_2H_2PO_4$) are stable (Lindsay & Vlek 1977)

Throughout this paper atomic Ca/P ratios are used. Published Ca/P mass ratios have been converted to atomic ratios by multiplying by 0.774.

B.2. Experimental

Phosphorus concentrations were measured in the bone ash solutions using ICP-AES at 213.6 and 214.9 nm. For the Ca concentrations measurements 1:200 dilutions of the original bone ash solutions were prepared gravimetrically. The Ca concentrations in these solutions were measured using AAS at 422.7 nm.
Coefficients of variation in multiple independent analyses of reference samples were approximately 1 % for the P analyses and 1.8 % for the Ca determinations.
The concentrations of Ca were determined in 25 reference samples using Isotope Dilution Mass Spectrometry as described in section III.A. The correlation between IDMS and AAS Ca determinations is 0.98 (n=25).

B.3. Results and discussion

In total, 32 samples of fresh cattle bones were analysed. Mean Ca concentration in the ash of fresh bones samples was 38.68 ± 1.14 % (CV=2.9 %, n=32) and the mean P concentration 18.05 ± 0.44 % (CV=2.4 %, n=32). The mean atomic Ca/P ratio in these samples is 1.66 ± 0.07 (CV=4.1%, n=32). This corresponds exactly with the theoretical value for HAP.

The concentrations of Ca and P in the excavated bones are slightly lower than in fresh bones: 35.96 ± 3.61 % Ca and 16.03 ± 1.52 % P in bone ash (table IV 1,2). The difference with fresh bones is probably a result of deposition of iron and other elements in the bones: the mean Fe content in ash of the excavated bones is 2.37 ± 1.63 % (table IV.3).

The differences in mean Ca and P concentrations in animal species are small but, probably as a consequence of small standard deviations, in some cases significant at the 95% level (Student's t test). The Ca/P ratios, however, do not show differences between animal species. This agrees with findings of Grupe (1986) for age groups in humans: both Ca and P levels show variations, but Ca/P ratios are within a narrow range.

Table IV.1. Concentrations (mass % in bone ash) of Ca in bones from West-Frisian sites. Groups with the same letters in the column 'significance' do not differ at the 5 % level (Student's t test)

species	n	mean	SD	CV(%)	significance				
human long bones	80	37.27	2.08	5.6	A	B			
human other bones	79	32.20	5.10	15.8					E
cattle	144	37.49	1.64	4.4	A				
pig	36	36.70	2.32	6.3		B	C		
dog	36	35.20	3.61	10.3				D	
sheep/goat	44	36.01	2.41	6.7			C	D	

The mean atomic Ca/P ratio in the prehistoric bones is 1.74 which corresponds to 10.44 atoms of Ca per 6 atoms of P. Some Ca must therefore have been deposited in the bones or else P has been leached out of the bones slightly more than Ca. The results for the fresh bone samples do not suggest that systematical analytical errors are involved.

Table IV.2. Concentrations (mass % in bone ash) of P in bones from West-Frisian sites. Identical letters in column 'sign.' indicate that groups do not differ at the 5 % level (Student's t test). In the last column, the mean atomic Ca/P ratio (= 0.774 * mass ratio Ca/P) is given

species	n	mean	SD	CV(%)	sign.				atomic ratio Ca/P
human *	80	16.52	.69	4.2	A	B			1.75
human §	79	14.39	2.20	15.3				D	1.73
cattle	145	16.59	.54	3.2	A				1.75
pig	37	16.19	.86	5.3		B			1.75
dog	36	15.54	1.62	10.4			C		1.75
sheep/goat	44	16.41	1.03	6.3	A	B			1.70

* long bones
§ other bones

The chemical and microbiological deterioration of buried bone is apparently a complex process, the outcome of which depends on a number of factors. As stated by Nelson & Sauer (1984), every burial context is unique. This is illustrated by the Ca/P ratios of excavated bones from various sites (table IV.3), which indicates that either Ca or P is present in too high relative quantities. This indicates that Ca was either leached out of, or deposited into, the bone. Phosphorus, in one or another compound, appears to be rather immobile due to the low solubility of many P compounds (Bolt & Bruggenwert 1976).

Table IV.3. Synopsis of published Ca/P ratios in excavated and fresh bones

author	no. of samples	- Ca/P ratio - mass	atomic	no. of Ca ions per 6 P ions
Grupe (1986)	106	1.96	1.52	9.1
White & Hannus (1983)	24	2.37	1.83	11.0
	16	1.77	1.35	8.1
Kyle (1986)	37	2.81	2.17	13.1
this paper	459	2.24	1.74	10.4
fresh cattle bones	32	2.14	1.66	10.0

A model for the decomposition of bone in soil was formulated by White & Hannus (1983). This model comprises the microbiological decomposition of collagen which results in the release of H+ ions that thereupon replace Ca in HAP. Calcium ions may then either be leached out of the bone or remain present in the bone in another mineral form. This process possibly also comprises the formation of brushite. Brushite has a Ca/P ratio of 1 and has been identified in excavated bones (Piepenbrink 1986). This process may be operative even in calcareous soils, because the acids are formed inside the bone. However, oxygen and water have to be present. That this process is unlikely to have been of significance in the bones studied here may be concluded from the high Ca/P ratios.

Kyle (1986) found a strong negative correlation between Si and Ca concentrations in bones. Superfluous Ca appears to be present in the bone in combination with Si and other elements. Kyle used regression lines for trace element and Si concentrations in estimating concentrations not due to contamination. Strontium concentrations appeared to be correlated with Si and Ca concentrations. Regression analysis resulted in an adjusted mean concentration of 1320 ppm Sr in bone ash compared with a measured, 'contaminated' value of 1790 ppm.

The deviation from theoretical Ca/P ratios is very high in the samples of Kyle (1986). Some alterations in Ca concentrations may have occurred in the bones from West-Frisian excavations though these are relatively small (table IV.3). We did not analyse for Si concentrations but Fe concentrations may be used similarly for extrapolations to 'original' trace element levels (section IV.C). It may be expected, however, that in the specific case of the West-Frisian bones, diagenetic changes will have been minor.

C. IRON

C.1. General

Only traces of iron are present in fresh bones, whereas soils contain relatively high amounts of Fe. Iron in excavated bones must therefore result from contamination, and Fe concentrations may thus be used in the assessment of diagenetic changes of bones. Concentrations of trace elements that are correlated with Fe concentrations are suspect. It is for this reason that Fe concentrations in the bones from West-Friesland were measured.

C.2. Experimental

Iron concentrations in the bone ash solutions were measured using ICP-AES at 259.9 nm. Multiple analysis of reference samples yielded coefficients of variation of approximately 0.5-2 %.

C.3. Results and discussion

The Fe content in the fresh bones is very low, all Fe concentrations being lower than 0.02% (n=32). Analytical errors may be relatively large due to these low concentrations,

Considerable amounts of Fe are present in the excavated bones (table IV.4). The lowest Fe concentrations are found in the cattle bones and the human long bones. The bones of the smaller animals in general contain higher amounts of Fe. This agrees with micro- and macroscopic observations on the bones. The dark stains and the opaque intrusions are concentrated near the surface of the bones (section II.D.3). Small bones, obviously, have a relatively large surface area.

Table IV.4. Iron concentrations (mass % in boneash) in bones from West-Frisian sites. Identical letters in column 'sign.' indicate that levels do not differ at the 95% level (Student's t test)

species	n	mean	SD	CV(%)	sign.
human long bones	80	2.01	1.63	68.9	C D E
human other bones *	103	2.73	2.52	92.1	A B
cattle	145	1.94	.72	36.9	E
pig	37	2.40	.87	36.9	B C
dog	36	3.19	1.75	54.9	A
sheep/goat	44	2.32	1.31	56.5	B C D

* including cremations

The data suggest that 'other human bones', the category comprising ribs, vertebrae and other non long bones may be less suitable for chemical analysis.

The concentrations of Ca and Fe appear to be correlated negatively. This probably is a result of the decreasing Ca content which in its turn is the consequence of increasing bone weight due to deposition of Fe.

Correlations of concentrations of Fe with other elements are discussed in chapter V-VII.

V
ANALYSIS OF BONE:
STRONTIUM.

A. STRONTIUM/CALCIUM DISCRIMINATION IN MAN AND ANIMALS

A.1. Introduction: calcium and strontium in the food chain

In paleodietary research we are dealing with Ca and Sr concentrations in human and animal bones. The concentrations of Ca in bone in general show little variation. *In vivo* Sr concentrations in bones are the result of a series of processes that begin with the interactions between Ca, Sr and other elements in the soil, are followed by discrimination processes in the food chain and end with the Sr/Ca discrimination in the human body during the formation of bone mineral. The physiological and/or physico-chemical discrimination processes in the food chain determine the Sr/Ca ratios in the components of human diets.

For the interpretation of Sr levels in prehistoric human bones these processes, or rather their effects, must be understood. Furthermore, knowledge of the range of available and utilized food items is essential.

The impact of a particular food item on the overall Sr/Ca ratio of a human diet is a function of three factors: (1) the relative quantity in which it is consumed, (2) its Ca content and (3) its Sr/Ca ratio relative to the Sr/Ca ratios of the other food items. In this chapter, data on the Sr/Ca ratios in groups of non-vegetable food items are presented. These ratios should be reviewed in relation to the accessory Ca concentrations per unit of energy (table V.1). Strontium/calcium relationships in plants and in vegetable food items are dealt with in a similar way in chapter IX.

The Sr/Ca discrimination in mammals, including man, is of interest, on the one hand because it includes the terminal step in the Sr/Ca discrimination in the food chain to human bone, on the other hand because mammals and their products form a considerable portion of the human diet.

A.2. Mammals and man

A.2.1. The Observed Ratio

The relationship between Sr and Ca in mammalian bodies has been studied by a number of researchers. The terminology introduced by Comar et al. (1957) is commonly used to express the discrimination against Sr on various trophic levels. The overall discrimination is expressed as the Observed Ratio, which is equal to

$$OR = (Sr/Ca\ sample) / (Sr/Ca\ precursor)$$

The OR is the result of the discrimation processes in various organs of the body, which are expressed as Discrimination Factors (DF):

$$OR = (DF1) x (DF2) x ... x (DFn).$$

Table V.1. Energy values and Ca contents for some groups of food items. Calculated from data on modern foods (a: Paul & Southgate 1978, b: NVT 1983). Values (means ± standard deviation) per 100 g edible product.

group	n	energy value kJ per 100 g	Ca content mg per 100g	Ca content mg per 100kJ	ref.
mushrooms	1*	53	3	6	a
edible fungi	2	69	18	24	b
leafy vegetables	13	75 ± 31	116 ± 159	142 ± 133	a
leafy vegetables	11	83 ± 45	79 ± 54	123 ± 103	b
roots	7	131 ± 67	54 ± 29	45 ± 18	a
roots	7	135 ± 70	53 ± 22	46 ± 22	b
wholemeal flour	1*	1351	35	3	a
cereal grains	4	1402 ± 94	51 ± 15	4 ± 1	b
fruits	11	144 ± 56	21 ± 16	20 ± 17	a
fruits	8	151 ± 31	23 ± 15	15 ± 10	b
pulses $	4	1140 ± 9	80	7	b
nuts	5	1886 ± 679	114 ± 82	6 ± 3	a
nuts	3	2061 ± 966	110 ± 67	6 ± 2	b
honey	1*	1369	5	0.4	b
dressed carcasses	4	1349 ± 108	7 ± 0.4	0.5	a
meat	1*	825	10	1.2	b
cows' milk	1*	272	120	44	a
cows' milk	1*	284	125	44	b
chickens' eggs	1*	612	52	8.5	a
chickens' eggs	1*	639	60	9.4	b
fish	9	567 ± 255	24 ± 11	4.9 ± 3.1	a
fish	1§	479	20	4.2	b
marine shellfish	8	390 ± 127	136 ± 84	41 ± 27	a
marine shellfish#	4	295 ± 72	108 ± 55	36 ± 13	b
seaweeds		?	?		
snails		?	?		
insects		?	?		

$ per 100 g dry product
* mean value based on many analyses
§ mean value for fresh water and sea fish, 5 g fat/100g
\# crab, lobster, mussel, shrimp

Although the Observed Ratio is now commonly used, the term 'bone retention factor' was introduced earlier by Alexander et al. (1956). The bone retention factor, Fb, is defined as the Sr/Ca ratio in bone divided by the Sr/Ca ratio in diet. It is therefore mathematically equal to the OR.

For our purposes the overall Sr/Ca discrimination between food and the body tissues is of prime interest. Within the body there appears to be no difference in Sr/Ca ratios in the plasma, the soft tissues and in the bone (Comar 1963, fig. V.1).

Observed Ratios have been established for man and a number of mammal species (table V.2). Various techniques may be used in the assesment of OR's. For instance, the total Sr and Ca intake in food and excretion in urine and faeces can be measured. Other techniques use one or two radioactive tracers. Some researchers have established O R's by comparing human bone Sr levels with average Sr/Ca ratios of foods within a limited area (Knizhnikov & Marei 1967, Tanaka et al. 1981). A comparable method was used for fresh white tailed deer (Price et al. 1985a).

Table V.2. Adult Sr/Ca Observed Ratios for a number of mammal species. Techniques are (a) comparison of generalized dietary Sr/Ca ratios with bone Sr/Ca; (b) Sr and Ca isotope study ; (c) comparison of Sr and Ca in diet and excreta; (d) comparison of Sr/Ca ratios in diets and bone

species	OR	technique	reference
man	0.12	a	Tanaka et al. 1981
man	0.20	a	Knizhnikov & Marei 1967
man	0.25	a	Rivera 1964 §
man	0.25	a	Bryant et al. 1958
rat	0.27	d	Alexander et al. 1956
mouse	0.35	d	ibid.
guinea pigs	0.22	d	ibid.
desert rats	0.16-0.22	a	ibid.
rat non-milk diet	0.23	b	Wasserman et al. 1957
milk diet	0.61	b	ibid.
goat	0.28	b	Comar et al. 1961
cow	circa 0.25	b	ibid.
white tailed deer	0.204	a	Price et al. 1985a
rabbit	0.25	b	Rosenthal & Harbor 1965§
rabbit	0.21	c	Rosenthal et al. 1972

§ cited in Rosenthal et al. 1972

A mean value of 0.20-0.25 for the O R bone-diet in adult mammals and man is commonly accepted (Comar 1963, 1967, Price et al. 1985b, Van Wijngaarden-Bakker 1986).

A.2.2. Age effects

Discrimination against Sr in the intestinal tract is small in very young mammals. At low ages the values of O R's are significantly higher than in older animals. In humans, adult discrimination rates are present within a few years after birth (Bryant et al. 1958, Lengemann 1963, Tanaka et al. 1981). In any case, skeletal material of children of less than a few years old is scarce in archeological contexts.

At higher ages the adult O R values appear to remain at a constant level. Data by Tanaka et al. (1981) show a slight increase in bone Sr concentrations with age (compare also Bryant & Loutit 1964). No such effect is, however, apparent in the data of Bryant et al. (1958).

For practical paleodietary studies the assumption that no physiological age effect exists in the Sr/Ca discrimination in mammals and man would appear to be acceptable.

A.2.3. Effects of pregnancy and lactation

In prehistoric societies many of the females of reproductive age were probably either pregnant or lactating (Hassan, 1981). Physiological effects of pregnancy and lactation on female Sr/Ca discrimination have therefore to be understood in order to compare Sr levels in bones of males and females of reproductive age. Besides this, the relation between Sr/Ca ratios in the diet and in the milk in mammals is of interest.

The Sr/Ca relationships in milk producing animals such as cows and nanny-goats have been studied because milk is an important factor in the transfer of radioactive Sr fallout to man.

Values of the OR milk-diet are close to 0.1 for a number of species (Comar et al. 1961, Comar 1963, Kahn et al. 1965). With OR body-diet values of 0.20-0.25 this implies OR milk-body values of 0.5-0.4. Foetal Sr/Ca ratios are close to a tenth of Sr/Ca ratios in maternal diet (Knizhnikov & Marei 1967) thus corroborating to the value of 0.4-0.6 for the OR foetus-mother reported by Comar (1963). Other published OR foetus-mother values are within the latter range (Bryant & Loutit 1964, Tanaka et al. 1981).

Pregnant and lactating mammals excrete relatively more Ca than Sr to the foetus and in the milk. In consequence one might expect relatively high Sr levels in tissues of pregnant and lactating females. This is, however, not corroborated by experimental data. Female white tailed deer have lower bone Sr concentrations than male deer (Price et al. 1985a). This might be the result of alterations in the discrimination in the intestinal tract of females. In pregnant and lactating females the discrimination against Sr is possibly decreased in comparison to normal situations as a result of the increased demand for Ca and the resulting increased efficiency of Ca uptake (Sillen & Kavanagh 1982, Price et al. 1985a).

A.2.4. Effect of high Ca levels and lactose

Milk is characterized by a high Ca content (table V.1) and a low Sr/Ca ratio, which is 1/10 of the Sr/Ca ratio in the diet of the milk producing animal. No effect of high dietary Ca levels on the OR body-diet has been found in laboratory studies with Ca supplemented food (Wasserman et al. 1957, Comar et al. 1961).

Lactose, on the contrary, has a well established positive effect on the uptake of Ca and other ions from the intestinal tract (Dupuis & Fournier 1963, Allen 1982). Apparently, the discrimination against Sr is decreased by lactose (Lengemann, 1963). This is substantiated by the difference in the values of OR body-diet in rats and man on milk and non-milk diets (Wasserman et al. 1957, Comar & Wasserman 1958, table V.2). However, the quantitative effect of lactose on the OR body-diet of the consumer remains obscure in cases where milk is a minor dietary component.

A.2.5. Grazers and browsers

Ruminants can be separated in groups according to their feeding habits: grazers, browsers and intermediate feeders (Van de Veen 1979, Van de Veen & Van Wieren 1980, compare Groenman-van Waateringe 1986). Grazers or bulk-and-roughage feeders ingest large quantities of vegetable matter, mainly grasses. Browsers or concentrate selectors feed more selectively and concentrate on foods of higher quality such as herbs and fruits. Intermediate feeders behave as grazers or browsers depending on the

availability of food. Examples of grazers are cattle (*Bos taurus*), sheep (*Ovis aries*) and plains bison (*Bison bison*), examples of browsers are elk (*Alces alces*), white tailed deer (*Odocoileus virginianus*) and goat (*Capra hircus*). Reindeer (*Rangifer tarandus*), european bison (*Bison bonasus*) and red deer (*Cervus elephus*) are examples of intermediate feeders.
The feeding behaviour of the animals in the groups is reflected in the anatomy and functioning of their digestive tracts. Grazers are adapted to digest large quantities of food which pass relatively slowly through the intestinal tract. This results in digestion and uptake of a relatively large part of the cell wall material that is present in the food. Browsers, on the contrary, have intestinal tracts that are adapted to a relatively fast passage of high-quality food. Of the ingested material, it is mainly the cell contents which are digested, whereas most of the cell wall material passes the intestinal tract undigested and is excreted.

For trace element studies these differences should be understood because they influence many Observed Ratio measurements. This difference between grazers and browsers will probably not be detected in studies where Sr and Ca tracers are added to food in the form of soluble salts. Few data on Distribution Ratios (section IX.C) on the plant cell level are available. In the light of the data assembled in chapter IX, it appears however likely that differences between Sr/Ca ratios in cell contents and in cell walls do exist. As a consequence, overall Sr/Ca ratios in fodder often will not represent the Sr/Ca ratio in the fraction that can be digested by the animals. In studies in which bone and fodder Sr/Ca ratios are compared (for instance, Price et al. 1985a), this effect might bias the calculation of the Observed Ratio. In fact, the OR

(Sr/Ca ratio in bone)/(overall Sr/Ca ratio in fodder) (1)

is determined in this kind of field studies. The OR

(Sr/Ca ratio in bone)/(Sr/Ca ratio in digestable fraction) (2)

is probably in better accordance with laboratory studies. The white tailed deer, the species studied by Price et al. (1985b), is classified as a concentrate feeder by Van de Veen (1979). In cases like this, analysis of excreta would be a useful addition to the analysis of food and bones. If differences between the overall Sr/Ca ratio in plant material and the Sr/Ca ratio in the digestable fraction exist, these may bias the extrapolation from Sr/Ca ratios in baseline species to regional vegetational Sr/Ca ratios. When a herbivorous baseline species is used, the relation between OR's (1) and (2) should be known. It is to be expected that the difference between these OR's for grazers will be small.

The grazer-browser effect may result in differences in Sr/Ca ratios in the bones of animals that feed on plants with equal overall Sr/Ca ratios, even if these animals exhibit equal Observed Ratios as determined by double tracer studies. Besides food selection, the differential digestion of food may be one of the causes for differences in Sr/Ca ratios in herbivorous single animals in a region. It is not clear to what extent this process is operative, for instance in the case of anomalous Sr concentrations in sheep/goat bones when compared to cattle (compare Runia 1987a). Both sheep and cattle are grazers, but goats are not. Unfortunately, sheep and goat bones are almost indistinguishable from each other in archeological bone assemblages.

A.3. Birds

Both the flesh of birds and their eggs can be consumed by humans. In certain cultures these foodstuffs constitute a considerable part of the human diet. Ostrich eggs, for instance, are eaten by modern hunter/gatherers (Mann 1981). Pre-contact New World cultures had the turkey as the only domesticated animal species besides the dog (Zeuner 1963). In wet environments in temperate regions such as the western part of the Netherlands during the Neolithic and Bronze Age, waterfowl and their eggs are abundantly available and may seasonally be of major importance as food for hunter/gatherers and, probably to a lesser extent, farmers. Some waterfowl bones were found in the Bronze Age sites in West-Friesland (IJzereef 1981). The relative importance of waterfowl and other eggs in the human diet remains, however, obscure. For Dutch prehistory this point is of major interest, because estuarine landscapes were the very environments in which prehistoric cultures in the Holocene part of the country thrived.

Data on Sr/Ca relationships in birds are not available. Some work has been done on the effect of radioactive and stable Sr in chickens' diets on the production and firmness of eggs (Mraz et al. 1967), but we do not have data on the discrimination against Sr in the egg production. Eggs may be of some importance in the Ca supply of humans, because Ca levels per unit of energy are relatively high (table V.1).

A.4. Marine and fresh water fish

Few data on Sr/Ca discrimination in marine and freshwater fish are available. Fish are able to take up Sr and Ca directly from the water via gills and skin, and from food in the intestines, though the latter mode of mineral uptake is considered to be of minor importance (Kornberg & Davis 1966, Chipman 1966).
Fresh water differs distinctly from sea-water in trace element concentrations. Rosenthal et al. (1970) calculated average Sr/Ca ratios of 8 mg/g for fresh water and 20 mg/g for sea-water. Sea-water has a relatively constant Ca concentration of 400 mg/l whereas fresh water has low and variable mineral contents.

Observed Ratios tissue-water for various fresh water and marine animals as calculated by Ophel & Judd (1967) and Rosenthal et al. (1970) ranged from 0.19 to 0.82. OR's appeared to be similar in animals occupying comparable ecological niches (Rosenthal et al, 1970). In my view, this points to a fish bone Sr/Ca ratio dependent on food Sr/Ca ratios rather than on water Sr/Ca ratios. Ophel & Judd (1967) tested a similar hypothesis by analysing bones and stomach contents of carnivorous perch and herbivorous carp from Lake Huron. Though the analysed stomach contents and bones are not from the same fish specimen, these data were used in calculating OR body-diet values (table V.3). Unlike the OR body-water, these OR's appear to be similar: 0.47 and 0.49 for perch and carp, respectively. This suggests that dietary Sr/Ca ratios determine bone Sr/Ca ratios in fish, which is in contradiction with current views on the uptake of Ca and Sr by fish where the uptake of minerals by the intestinal tract is considered to be of minor importance (Chipman 1966, Kornberg & Davis 1966). Further research is needed in order to establish more unequivocal relationships between Sr/Ca ratios in fish, food and water.

Table V.3. Relationships between Sr and Ca (atoms of Sr per 1000 atoms of Ca) in Lake Huron perch and carp. Data from Ophel & Judd (1967), tables IV, V and VI.

species	n	Sr/Ca ratio stomach	bone	Observed Ratio bone-water	bone-diet
perch	3	0.77 ± 0.07			
perch	10		0.36 ± 0.07	0.19	0.47
carp	3	2.57 ± 0.18			
carp	3		1.25 ± 0.6	0.66	0.49

Marine foods have high Sr/Ca ratios compared with terrestrial foods. A (paleo)diet with seafood will have a relatively high Sr/Ca ratio. This should be taken into account when analyzing bones from contexts in which fish was potentially part of the diet (compare Kyle 1986). Even small amounts of foods with deviant Sr/Ca ratios may considerably affect the Sr/Ca ratio of the total diet (Runia, 1987a,b).

No bones of marine fish were found in Bronze Age sites in West-Friesland. The amount of marine foods in the diet of Bronze Age farmers is discussed in chapter IX. Some remains of fresh water fish were described by IJzereef (1981). These bones are to some extent the result of natural thanatocoenose. Fresh water Sr/Ca ratios will probably be relatively close to Sr/Ca ratios in terrestrial animals in the same region.

A.5. Marine and fresh water molluscs and crustacea

Marine molluscs such as mussels (Mytilus edulis), oysters (Ostrea edulis) and cockles (Cerastoderma edule edule) may be important as food resources for coast-dwelling humans.

Marine mollusc shells have been studied for their Sr contents and Sr/Ca relationships. Considerable variations of Sr concentrations occur in mollusc shells. There may be a relationship between water temperature and Sr concentrations (Hallam & Price 1968).

An OR shell-water of approximately 0.2 for some marine molluscs was established by Rosenthal et al. (1970). However, no data on the Sr/Ca relationship in the edible part of the molluscs are presented. Hallam & Price (1968) conclude that some biochemical control system regulates the concentrations of Ca and trace element in the molluscs. It remains, however, unclear at which place in the molluscan body discrimination against Sr occurs. It therefore remains possible that Sr/Ca ratios in the mollusc flesh are higher than in the water as a consequence of preferential secretion of Ca in shell aragonite formation. In short, no quantitative information on Sr/Ca ratios in mollusc meat is available. Despite this, it is evident that marine molluscs have high Ca contents and compared to terrestrial foods, high Sr/Ca ratios.

Freshwater molluscs appear to have OR shell-water values similar to marine molluscs despite the differences in osmotic gradients (Rosenthal et al. 1970). Some freshwater species are edible. As with marine molluscs, no data on flesh Sr/Ca ratios are available.

No marine molluscs were available in Bronze Age West-Friesland, and there are no indications for the consumption of freshwater molluscs (W.J. Kuyper, pers. comm.).

Strontium concentrations in marine and freshwater Crustacean exoskeletons were studied by Rosenthal et al. (1970). Values for OR exoskeleton-water in three species ranged from 0.52-0.82. Again, no data on Sr/Ca ratios in the edible soft tissues are available.

A.6. Reptiles

Reptiles such as turtles and crocodiles may constitute part of human diets (Hayden 1981). Besides their flesh, their eggs may also be eaten. For instance, eggs of large sea turtles deposited in warm beach sands may provide food for coast dwelling humans.
No information on the Sr/Ca discrimination in reptiles is available. In temperate regions this will not cause problems in paleodietary studies because reptiles and reptile eggs are of no importance as foodstuffs.

A.7. Terrestrial invertebrates

Terrestrial invertebrates such as insects and snails may be of some importance as foodstuffs. Present day hunter/gatherers may for instance consume the protein-rich winged male and female termites that once a year leave the termite mounds in great numbers (Hayden 1981). Locusts are eaten in many cultures in tropical and subtropical regions (Brothwell & Brothwell 1969). The insects of the colder regions are of little importance as human food, probably because these insects generally have smaller bodies than their tropical and sub-tropical relatives, and other foods can probably be collected much more efficiently. However, lice in the excreta of Inuit mummies corroborate stories by polar explorers that the Inuit consumed their lice with delight (Hart Hansen 1985). Most likely, this food does not contribute much to the Ca supply of the consumers.
Calcium and strontium relationships in insects have, to my knowledge, not been investigated.

Honey gathered by bees has always been of some significance as food for man and animals (Brothwell & Brothwell 1969). Though Hayden (1981) counts honey as an insect product, it is in fact a plant product that is not processed by the bees. Honey contains some 5 mg Ca per 100 g (table V.1) and its role in human Ca and Sr supply is negligible.

Even now, snails occupy a position of honour in the mediterranean cuisine and in North-Western European diets. Snails like other molluscs probably have some physiologic controlling system for the turnover of Ca because this element is needed for the formation of the shell. We have no data on this system but it is likely that some discrimination occurs. No data on Ca contents of snails are present in NVT (1983) and Paul & Southgate (1978).
In the Bronze Age of West-Friesland snails were of little importance as food item (W.J Kuyper, pers.comm.).

B. EXPERIMENTAL

The strontium concentrations were measured using ICP-AES at 407.7 and 421.5 nm (section III.A).

To gain an insight into the reliability and reproducability of the Sr determination, a number of bone ash solutions were prepared in duplicate or triplicate though for the bulk of the samples this was not done. Two reference samples (St I and St II, cattle bones from Westwoud) were run 6 and 9 times respectively, resulting in coefficients of variation of 0.9 %. Mean coefficient of variation for the ICP Sr determination in independently prepared solutions of bone ash for a given sample was < 1.5 %.

Generally, the correlation between ICP-AES and IDMS Sr measurements is fairly good with a correlation coefficient of 0.996 (n=24). In a single sample, however, the difference between ICP and IDMS determination was 12 %. Probably, this is a result of an interchange of samples.

For the standard samples, ICP and IDMS determined Sr concentrations were 1111 and 1115 (St I) and 1120 and 1125 (St II) mg Sr/kg bone ash, respectively.

A second check on the accuracy of the analysis was the analyses of the IAEA H-5 animal bone reference material. Our result is 180 ± 7.4 (CV=4.1%, n=4) mg Sr/kg bone ash. This corresponds to 102 mg Sr/kg dry bone, the ash content of H-5 being 56.44 %. This is close to the preliminary mean values given by the IAEA (104.85 ± 17.61), but higher than the mean (91.1 ± 1) found by Mahanti & Barnes (1983) who used ICP-AES. The H-5 animal bone sample has a low Sr concentration compared to our Bronze Age samples. The CV found for H-5 (4.1%) is high compared with coefficients of variation found for the other reference samples (less than 1.5 %).

Thus, both the reproducability (indicated by the low coefficients of variation for samples analysed at various moments) and the accuracy (indicated by the coefficients of variation, the correspondence between ICP and IDMS results, and the result for the IAEA H-5 reference material) are sufficient for our purposes. Compared with the coefficient of variation of about 20 % in a population eating the same diet (Schoeninger 1979), analytical errors are negligible.

C. RESULTS & DISCUSSION

C.1. General

Strontium concentrations in some 450 prehistoric bone samples were measured. The mean Sr concentrations for the humans and the animal species are given in table V.4. The standard deviations appear rather large with the coefficients of variation having values of about 20 %.

Plotting the cumulative frequencies of the Sr concentrations on paper with a normal distribution axis results in more or less straight lines (figure V.1). Only in the high and low concentration ranges does some divergence from the straight lines occur. Student's t-test was therefore considered useful to test the significance of differences between mean Sr concentrations (table V.4). Strontium concentrations in the humans are significantly lower than in all of the animal species. Furthermore, significant differences in mean Sr concentrations between the different animal species are also present.

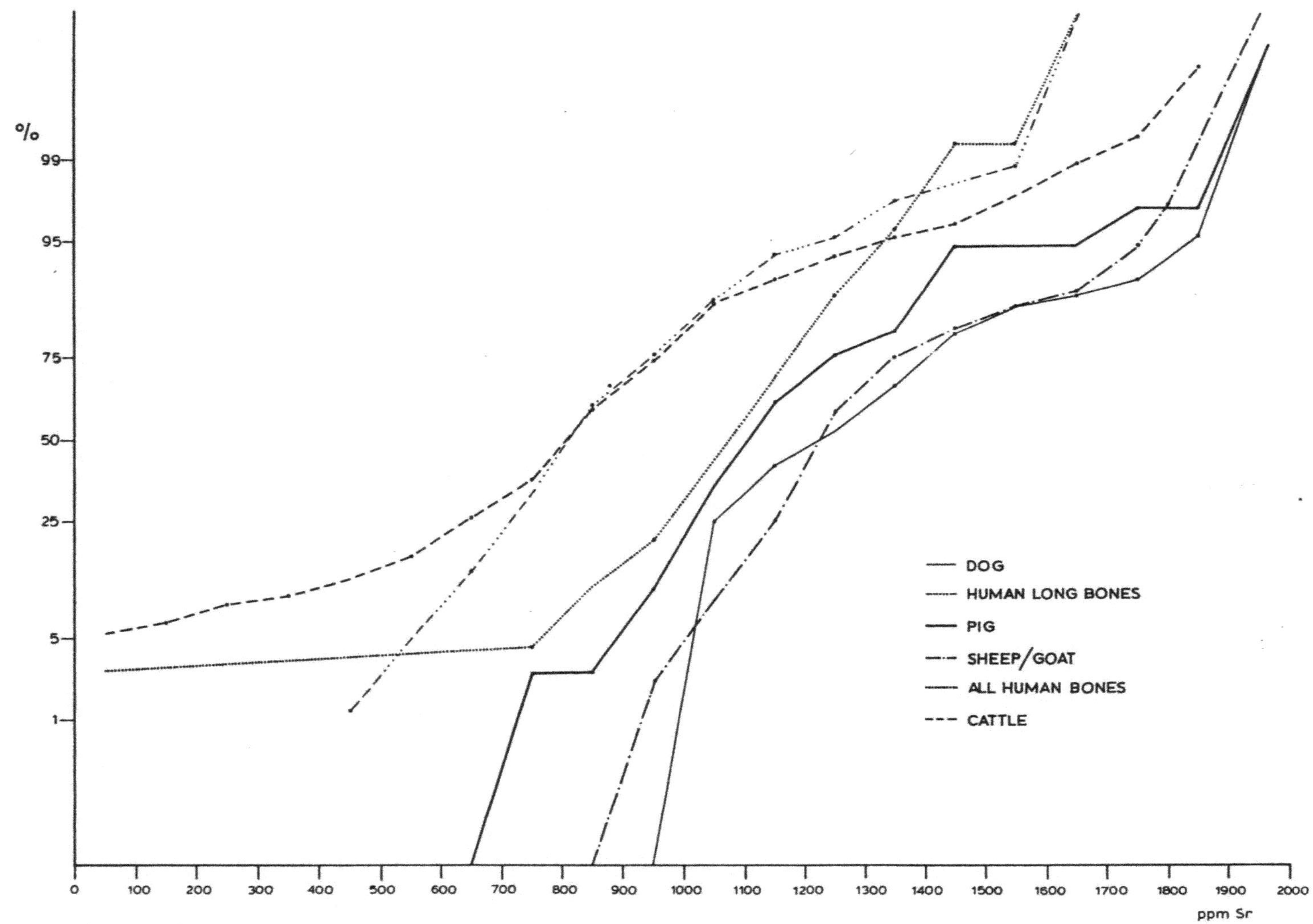

figure V.1 Cumulative frequencies of Sr concentrations in Bronze Age human and animal bones from West-Friesland. Horizontal axis: Sr concentrations (mg Sr/ kg bone ash); vertical axis : cumulative frequency of Sr concentrations, normal distribution.

Table V.4. Strontium concentrations (mg/kg bone ash) in bones from West-Frisian sites: totals for animal species and humans. The last two columns indicate statistical relevance of differences (Student's t test) at 95% and 99% level.

species	n	mean	SD	CV(%)	95%	99%
human *	80	941	208	22	a	A
cattle	145	1145	232	20	b	B
pig	37	1250	221	18	c	B C
dog	36	1373	248	18	d	C
sheep/goat	44	1385	240	17	d	C

* only samples from long bones (femur, humerus etc.)

The Sr/Ca ratios were calculated for the groups of animals. The differences in Sr/Ca ratios between the humans and the animal species show a pattern that does not diverge from that of the Sr concentrations (table V.5)

The data on humans and animals are treated in more detail in the following sections.

Table V.5. As table V.4, for Sr/Ca ratios (mg Sr/g Ca)

species	n	mean	SD	95%	99%
human *	80	2.55	0.67	a	A
cattle	145	3.07	0.66	b	B
pig	36	3.44	0.70	c	C
sheep/goat	44	3.89	0.88	d	C D
dog	36	3.97	0.94	d	D

* only samples from long bones (femur, humerus etc.)

C.2. Diagenesis

Prior to the discussion and interpretation of the Sr concentrations in the bones the extent of diagenetic changes must first be established. Post mortem changes in the concentrations of Sr in bones during prolonged periods of contact between soil and bone have been studied extensively (section I.C). Strontium appears to be one of the very few elements of which the concentration in buried bone is not, or only slightly, changed by diagenetic processes.

In our particular case, there are several indications that diagenetic alterations of Sr concentrations are only a minor factor.

The first indication is formed by the consistency in the distribution of the concentrations (figure V.1), in the coefficients of variation (table V.4), and in the differences between the animal species as described above.

Secondly, the Sr concentrations in the bones are not correlated with the concentrations of Fe (figure V.2) which in prehistoric bones does derive from the soil (chapter IV). In figure V.2, many of the high Fe-high Sr values represent ribs and vertebrae, whereas the low Fe-low Sr points

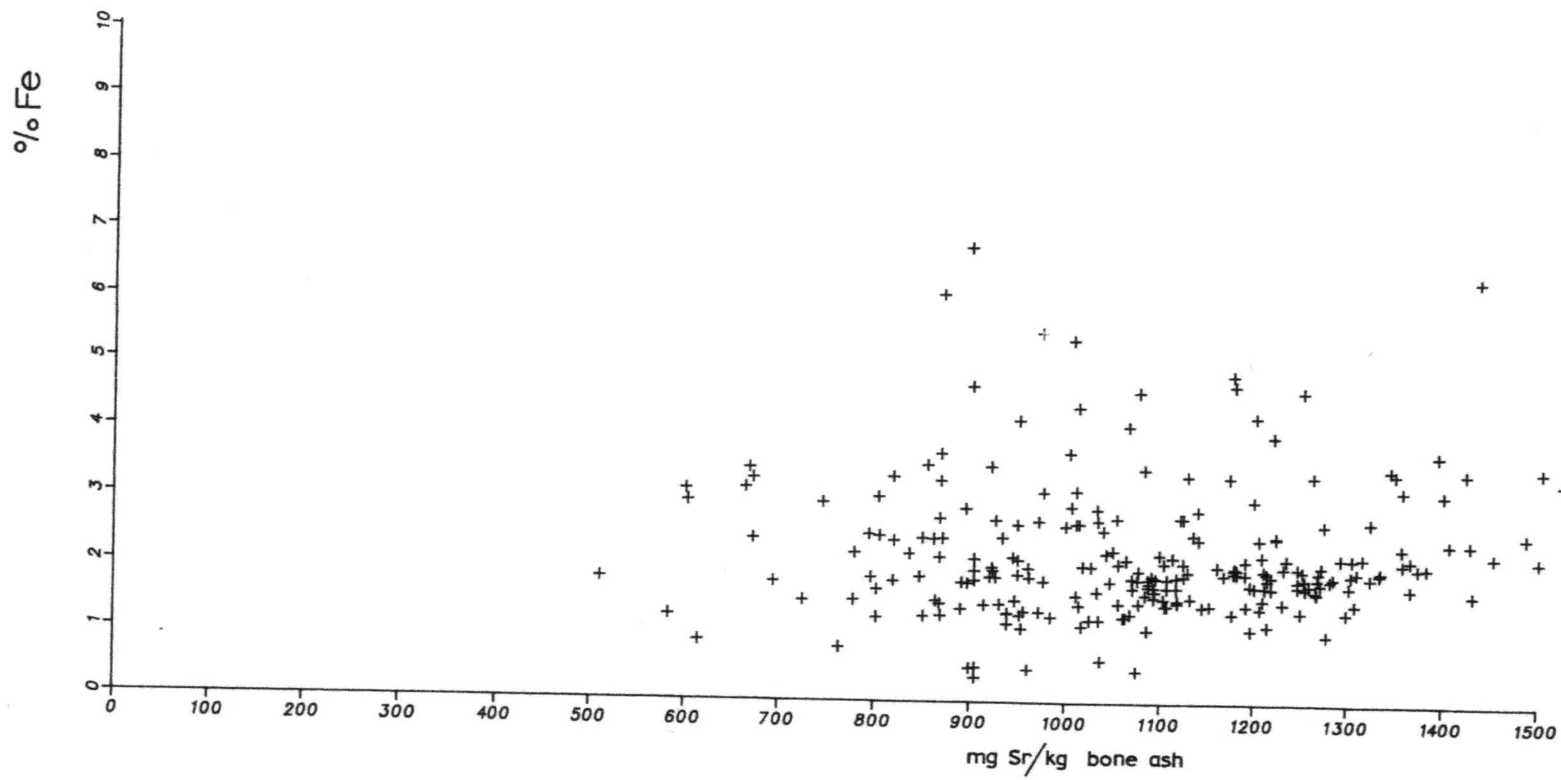

figure V.2 Scattergram of Sr and Fe concentrations of the Bronze Age samples.

represent samples of cremated bones. The remaining cloud of points suggests the independence of Fe and Sr concentrations in the long bones.

Thirdly, analyses of soil samples gave no indications of alterations of bone Sr levels (section IX.B).

However, Sr concentrations in the more or less porous bones such as ribs and vertebrae which have a thin layer of compacta around trabecular bone, may well have changed to some extent. In our study, human ribs and vertebrae were used in exeptional cases when no compact bone from one of the long bones was available, or (for instance, in the Oostwoud-skeletons) as additional samples for the same individuals (section II.D). The results of analyses of these samples are not included in table V.4. Mean Sr concentration in these bones was (n=79) 988 mg/kg bone ash, SD=279. The 28 % coefficient of variation is higher than in the other groups.

Table V.6. Strontium concentrations in animal bones from the larger sites. Concentrations (mean and SD) in mg/kg bone ash. In the last column, Sr concentrations relative to Sr concentrations in cattle bones (as %) are given

site	species	sex	n	mean	SD	CV	rel. to cattle
Valkje Early	cattle	both	18	1112	94	8	100
	cattle	fem.	8	1119	82	7	101
	cattle	male	10	1107	81	7	100
	pig		8	1144	100	9	103
	dog		9	1235	128	10	111
	sheep/goat		10	1315	122	9	118
Valkje Late	cattle	both	14	1101	120	11	100
	cattle	fem.	8	1120	137	12	102
	cattle	male	6	1076	72	7	98
	pig		7	1219	166	14	111
	dog		5	1280	118	9	116
	sheep/goat		5	1439	257	18	131
Andijk	cattle	both	20	1238	87	7	100
	cattle	fem.	10	1260	95	8	102
	cattle	male	10	1216	67	6	98
	pig		7	1275	107	8	103
	dog		2	1180			95
	sheep/goat		10	1255	137	11	101
Schagen	cattle	both	32	1245	174	14	100
	cattle	fem.	14	1306	190	15	105
	cattle	male	12	1232	158	13	99
	pig		9	1550	275	18	124
	dog		7	1633	242	15	131
	sheep/goat		11	1649	253	15	132
	horse		1	1728			139

C.3. Strontium in animal bones

C.3.1. General

The bones of two or more domestic animal species were analysed from seven sites in West-Friesland and one site in the dune area while from the larger sites, bones from four species (cattle, pig, dog and sheep/goat) were studied. In these sites it was possible to distinguish and select bones from cows and bulls/steers (table V.6). In the material from the smaller excavations not all four species were present. As a consequence smaller numbers of bones of fewer species were analysed, and unsexed cattle bones had to be used (table V.7).

A preliminary discussion of part of the data in table V.6 has been published elsewhere (Runia 1987a).

Table V.7. Strontium concentrations (mean and SD) in animal species from West-Frisian sites. In the last column, the relative Sr concentrations, as percentages of the Sr concentration of cattle are given per site.

site	species	n	Sr(mg/kg ash)		Sr/1000 Ca		relative
			mean	SD	mean	SD	Sr conc.
Zwaagdijk	cattle	6	964	69	2.48	0.19	100
	dog	2	1163		3.25	0.03	121
	pig	3	1217	19	3.39		126
	sheep/goat	3	1260	55	3.43	0.18	131
Velsen	pig	2	918		2.49		94
	cattle	10	975	120	2.60	0.31	100
	dog	2	1112		3.05		114
	sheep/goat	5	1226	75	3.29	0.20	126
Grootebroek	cattle	6	1044	151	2.90	0.44	
Oostwoud	pig	1	1011		3.45		87
	cattle	7	1163	73	3.32	0.25	100
Westwoud	pig	1	1124		3.14		94
	dog	1	1196		3.27		100
	cattle	8	1202	96	3.29	0.28	100
De Tent	cattle	5	1253	109	3.54	0.39	100
	dog	1	1429		4.25		114
Hoogkarspel	cattle	19	1267	70	3.39	0.19	

C.3.2. Regional differences

Mean strontium concentrations for cattle in the eight sites range from 964 in Zwaagdijk to 1245 mg/kg bone ash in Schagen. These differences probably reflect differences in original soil and plant Sr contents (or rather, relative abundance of Sr compared to Ca).

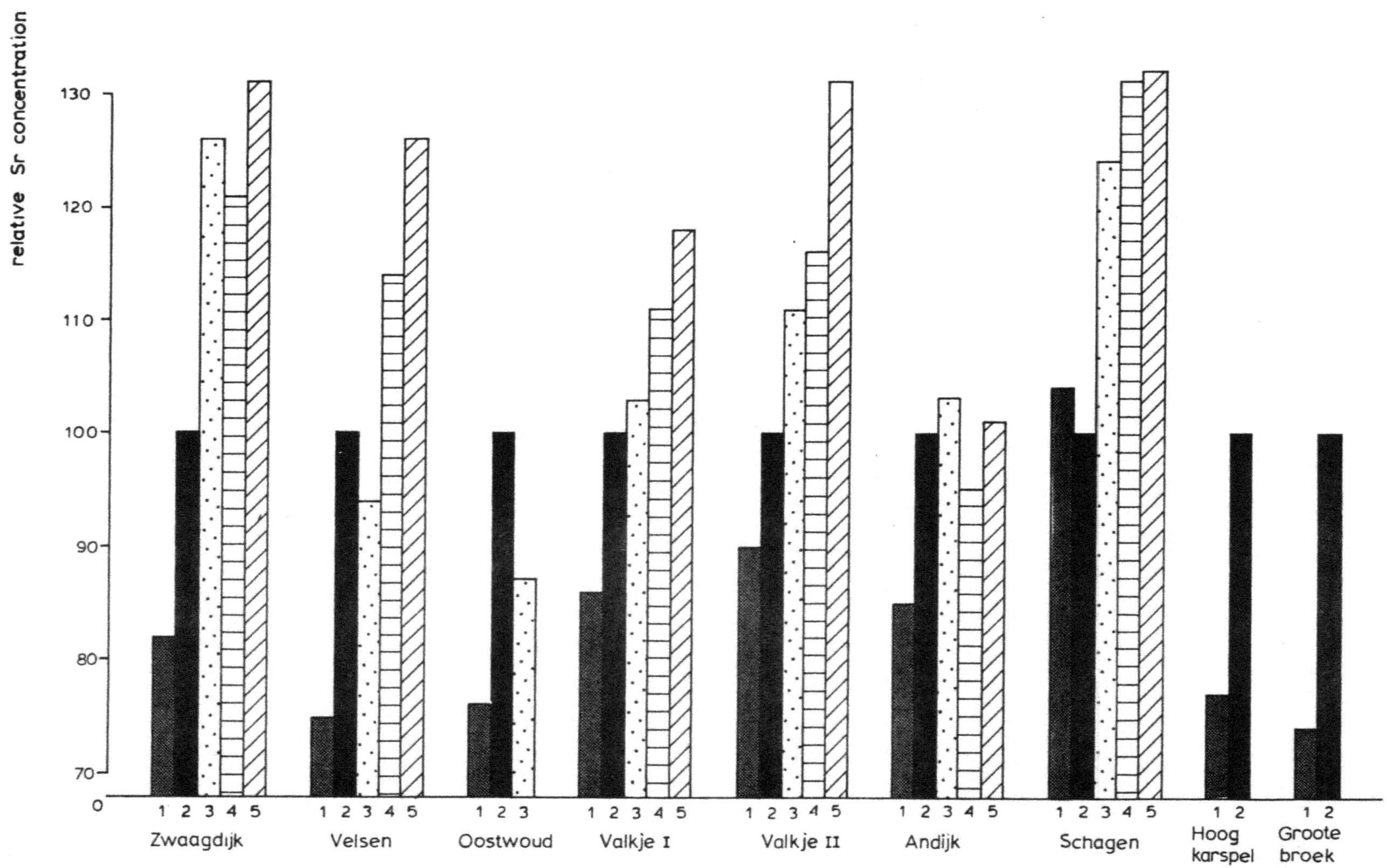

figure V.3 Relative mean Sr concentrations for humans and domestic animals. Vertical axis: Sr concentration as percentage of cattle bone Sr concentration. 1 human; 2 cattle; 3 pig; 4 dog; 5 sheep/goat. Based on table V.6 and V.7.

When the mean Sr levels in cattle bones of the sites are compared with soil maps and paleogeographical maps of the area (Ente 1963, De Mulder & Bosch 1982), a correlation between location of the site and the respective Sr concentrations is not apparent. The only site outside the West-Friesland region, Velsen which lies in the dune area, has somewhat lower Sr levels. The low Sr levels in the Zwaagdijk cattle bones may be a result of other factors. In Zwaagdijk the relative Sr concentrations for pigs, dogs and sheep/goat are rather high compared to the other sites. The same aberrant pattern can be seen in the relative Ba and Zn concentrations (section VI.C.3, VII.A.). This suggests that either the cattle bones from Zwaagdijk do not belong to the same period and/or the cattle may have been raised in a different region (section XI.A). The values of the cattle from Zwaagdijk probably distorts the paleogeographical interpretation of the Sr concentrations.

Soil analysis can be used to establish regional differences in Sr/Ca ratios. As pointed out elsewhere (Runia 1987a), the geological history of the area and the complex interactions of Sr and Ca with adsorbing media in the soil hamper the reconstruction of Bronze Age soil Sr/Ca ratios. Analysis of soil samples from Schagen and Bovenkarspel indicate that relatively large variations in Sr/Ca ratios in the soil do exist in the area (see section X.B.).

C.3.3. Differences between animal species

Strontium concentrations in domestic animal species can be expressed as percentages of cattle bone Sr concentrations because this facilitates comparison between sites (table V.6, 7, figure V.3). Mean values for these relative Sr concentrations were calculated (table V.8).
In some of the sites only a few bones of certain animal species could be analysed (compare table V.7). Despite this limitation a clear pattern appears to be present in the relative Sr concentrations.

Table V.8. Mean relative Sr concentrations: (Sr concentration in species) / (Sr concentration in cattle) x 100% in animal species from various sites. Mean $\pm$ SD based on data in table V.6 and V.7, n refers to the number of sites.

species	n	mean rel. Sr concentration	SD
cattle		100	
pig	8	105	13
dog	8	113	11
sheep/goat	6	123	11

The comparatively high Sr concentrations in omnivorous dogs and herbivorous sheep/goat in Het Valkje were tentatively explained by a model involving the use of different grazing areas for cattle and sheep/goat (Runia 1987a). The cattle and pigs would have been kept in or close to the farm houses on the sandy ridges and grazed on stubble and fallow arable. Sheep and goats guarded by the dogs were presumably kept farther away from the houses in the clayey basins. Analysis of soil samples failed to give conclusive evidence on this model.

Except for Andijk, the pattern of relative Sr concentrations of the animal species is essentially the same for all the sites involved. This need not be surprising, nor be contradictory to the model because all the sites are situated in more or less comparable environments. The site with a 'deviant' pattern, Andijk, is located at the end of the stream ridge system: around the site, the soil map shows narrow ridges and small patches of different soil types (Ente 1963). This aspect is further discussed in section XI.A.

Besides a geographical explanation for the observed pattern a physiological explanation should also be considered. Relatively high Sr concentrations in sheep are not uncommon (Schoeninger 1982, and pers. comm.). There are, however, no indications for different OR body-diet values in cattle, sheep/goat, pig and dog (section V.A). Both sheep and cattle are grazers, whereas goats are browsers. Differential digestion of vegetable material might partly explain the observed difference for the herbivores concerned (section V.A.2.5), but this would not explain the high Sr concentrations in the dog bones.

A further possibility may lie in a different susceptibility of the bones of various species to diagenetic influences on Sr concentrations. The small bones of dog and sheep/goat could be more affected than the cattle bones. This possibility does not explain the relatively low Sr concentrations in the pig bones which are also small in size. Besides this, the consistency of the pattern and the low values of the coefficients of variation fail to support this explanation.

C.3.4. Milk production

In North-Western Europe, cattle, sheep and goats were used for producing milk for human consumption from the Late Neolithic onwards (Sherratt 1981). In West-Friesland we have therefore to reckon with the possibility that in the Bronze Age milk and/or dairy products were part of the human diet. On the basis of zooarchaeological data, IJzereef (1981) postulated an increase of milk production and consumption during the Bronze Age occupation period in West-Friesland.
For bone Sr studies it is essential to know whether milk was part of the diet or not (section I.B.1.3). The production and consumption of milk in prehistoric periods may be inferred from zooarcheological data such as the kill-off pattern of cows and bulls/steers (IJzereef 1981), and archeological data such as the presence of certain types and forms of pottery (Sherratt 1981). It is possible that Sr levels in cattle bones form a new and independent source of information on milk production by domestic animals. It was decided to explore this possibility in cattle bones from West-Friesland.

Cattle bones from four sites were sexed. Results of the analysis of these bones are incorporated in table V.6. Cow bones apear to have slightly higher Sr concentration than bones of bull/steers.

Analyses of recent white tailed deer yielded lower Sr concentrations in the female than in the male deer (Price et al. 1985a). It was tried to establish the influence of prolonged lactation by comparing Sr concentrations in fresh bones of cows and bulls. This attempt was hampered by the Dutch agricultural system. There are abundant milch cows, but hardly any old bulls and non-milked cows. Most of the few remaining bulls are present in the Artificial Insemination stations where they receive high quality food different from the dairy cow fodder.

Results of the analysis of fresh cattle bones are summarized in table V.9. In the comparison of males and females these data are of limited value because the fodder regimes are not known to us. The cows IVO 11-20 and AA 8-9 which are old milch cows exhibit slightly higher Sr concentrations than the younger cows, which have not been milked, and the young bulls. This contradicts the results of Price et al. (1985a). A more detailed study on the effects of milk production on cattle bone Sr concentrations remains to be carried out.

Table V.9. Strontium concentrations in fresh cattle bones. Mean, standard deviation (mg/kg bone ash) and coefficient of variation. IVO samples from an abattoir in the Achterhoek (prov. of Gelderland), AA samples from the Amsterdam Abattoir.

sample	sex	age(years)	n	mean	SD	CV(%)
IVO 1-10	male	ca. 1.5	10	259	50	19
IVO 11-20	female	8-10	10	274	49	18
AA 1-6	female	2-3	6	265	39	15
AA 7	male	1.5	1	322		
AA 8-9	female	5-5.5	2	287		

We may conclude that the mean levels of Sr in cattle bones from West-Friesland do not give any indication either way on milk production. Where only the mean Sr concentrations are used, a certain amount of information is ignored. Assuming that not all cows were milked, it is possible that the relatively large variations in Sr concentrations such as occur in the Late Period of Het Valkje, could be interpreted as the result of milking part of the herd (Runia 1987a). In the Late Period of Het Valkje two cow bones have low Sr concentrations: less than 1000 mg/kg bone ash compared with a mean value of 1101 mg/kg. The resulting coefficient of variation (12 %) is higher than those of cattle in the Early Period (7 % for cows and for bulls/steers) and for Late Period bulls/steers (7 %), but not high when compared to the coefficients of variation for mink raised on identical diets (19 %, Schoeninger 1979) and recent white tailed deer (Price et al. 1985a). In the latter study, no differences in coefficients of variation between males (32.5 %) and females (33.3%) were found. In natural circumstances, stress due to pregnancy and lactation which results in low Sr levels in bone, may be equally present in all adult female animals whereas in a dairying system animals singled out for milk production will be affected relatively strongly. It is, however, unlikely that the few cows with low bone Sr levels at Het Valkje represent the milch cows: one of the bulls from this period also had a low Sr concentration. Moreover, all cows would have been milked.

Besides cattle, sheep and goat may have been kept for their milk. In the Late Period of Het Valkje, sheep/goat have a slightly higher coefficient of variation. This may, however, been caused by mechanisms other than milk production. Sheep/goat bones have not been sexed.

C.3.5. Concluding remarks

Prior to a discussion of the Sr data in connection with other information (chapter XI), some points from the previous discussion should be stressed.

In the first place it should be stressed that it is not possible to draw definite conclusions from the data presented. The lack of a detailed set of reference data from a restricted area hampers the evaluation of the Sr levels in the domestic animal species in Bronze Age West-Friesland. It appears likely that regional differences in soil Sr levels are for a considerable part responsible for the observed pattern in relative Sr levels, but other causes such as differences in physiology must also be considered.

It might be expected that Sr levels in animal bones from a restricted area would reveal a more or less characteristic pattern. However, such patterns remain to be established in present-day reference material by measuring the Sr contents in various animal species living in a restricted area. In pre- and protohistoric contexts it is to be expected that animal bones which do not fit in the pattern are probably allochtonous. The levels of trace elements may be used in the assessment of herding practices and trade contacts.

Questions on prehistoric dairying and its effect on Sr levels in animal bones remain to be answered. The data presented here may be seen as suggestive of milk production but, once again, reference material on the effects of prolonged lactation on cattle bone Sr levels remains to be gathered.

C.4. Strontium in human bones

C.4.1. General

The Sr concentrations in a total of 159 human bone samples were determined: 80 long bone samples and 79 sample of other bones such as ribs, vertebrae and skull. These samples represent 110 individual persons (section II.D). Mean Sr concentrations in the long bones are given in table V.10.

The mean Sr concentration of all long bone samples is 941 $\pm$ 208 mg/kg, for all other human bones 988 $\pm$ 279 mg/kg of bone ash.

Table V.10. Strontium concentrations in human bones. Means and standard deviation in mg/kg bone ash. Only data for long bones and individuals older than 10 years are incorporated in the table. In the last column, concentrations are expressed as % of Sr concentrations in cattle bones from the same site.

site	n	mean	SD	CV	% of cattle
Velsen	6	727	135	19	75
Zwaagdijk barrow	6	750	54	6	78
Grootebroek	3	771	125	16	74
Zwaagdijk flat graves	4	847	127	14	88
Oostwoud	12	889	93	10	76
Valkje Early Period	9	959	94	10	86
Hoogkarspel	11	981	158	16	77
Valkje Late Period	5	987	99	10	90
Andijk	11	1047	147	14	85
Schagen	3	1290	175	14	104

C.4.2. Effect of age and sex

Human skeletal remains from inhumations were grouped according to sex and age (II.D.1.3).

Mean Sr concentrations and Sr/Ca ratios (mg Sr/g Ca) for the age and sex groups were calculated (table V.11) and plotted (figure V.4).

The uneven distribution of individuals in the age and sex groups across the barrows might cause errors due to differences in soil and plant Sr concentrations between various sites. A possible method of avoiding this problem is the normalization of all human Sr/Ca ratios by expressing them as percentages of Sr/Ca ratios of cattle from the same barrow. This normalization leads to mean values and standard deviations, as shown in figure V.5. The main change in the plot following the normalization (compare figures V.4 and V.5) is in the age group 15-25. In the normalized plot, the females of this age group have higher, and the males lower Sr levels as compared to the untreated data. This might be due to the low mean Sr/Ca ratio in the Zwaagdijk cattle, which in turn affects the normalized Sr/Ca ratio of four out of five females in this age group.

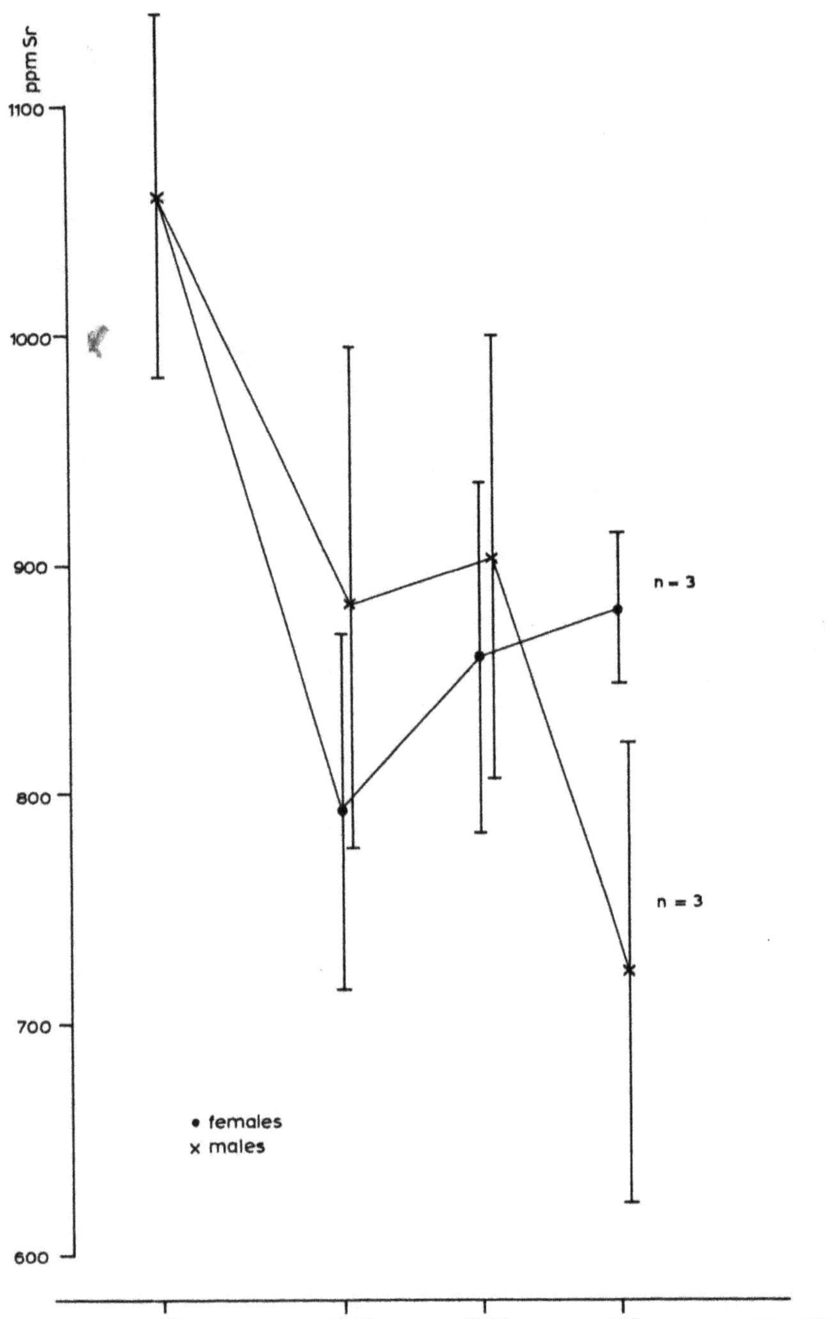

figure V.4 Mean Sr concentrations (mg Sr/kg bone ash) and standard deviations in inhumations (n=29), grouped on the basis of age and sex. Based on table V.11.

Table V.11. Strontium concentrations in mg/kg bone ash and mg Sr/g Ca ratios in groups of inhumations from flat graves and barrows. Sex and age grouping according to section II.D.1.3.

sex	age	n	mg Sr/kg bone ash mean	SD	CV (%)	mg Sr/g Ca mean	SD	CV (%)
??	<10	4	1062	80	8	3.02	0.10	3
female	15-25	5	792	76	10	2.09	0.20	10
	25-35	4	859	76	9	2.39	0.26	11
	>35	3	881	32	4	2.40	0.14	6
male	15-25	6	883	108	12	2.46	0.36	15
	25-35	4	903	97	11	2.72	0.50	18
	>35	3	722	99	14	1.91	0.26	14
total		29	875	126	14	2.44	0.44	18

A further difference between fig. V.4 and V.5 is the value for the males aged 25-35. The somewhat higher value in the normalized plot again results from the low Sr/Ca ratio of the Zwaagdijk cattle affecting the normalized Sr/Ca ratio of two of the four males in this group. As pointed out in section C.3.2., the Sr/Ca ratio of the Zwaagdijk cattle may be too low in comparison to other animal species. By trying to eliminate bias due to geographical factors we apparently introduce new sources of error. This is also illustrated by the sum of coefficients of variation (CV) for the seven groups of table V.11: when working with uncorrected Sr concentrations, the sum of CV values is 66 %, for uncorrected Sr/Ca ratios 76 % while for normalized Sr/Ca ratios the sum is 95 %. This obviously results from the increased number of variables involved in the calculations and it may be regarded as an argument against normalization of human bone Sr concentrations. Normalization of the Sr/Ca ratios apparently does not add to the reliability of the pattern. Geographical differences in Sr levels are, therefore, ignored in the following discussion on Sr levels in the age and sex groups.

The Sr concentrations in individuals of less than 10 years of age are high. Between 15 and 35 years, the mean Sr concentrations in the males are at a constant level of about 880-900 mg/kg bone ash, but at ages over 35 they are distinctly lower. Females have relatively low Sr concentrations in the age range 15-25 years and with increasing age gradually obtain higher Sr levels.

The high Sr concentration in the bones of the young children agrees with empirical data from other sites (Lambert et al. 1979, Sillen & Smith 1984, Grupe 1986a). In two North American Woodland sites, the age group 0-3 years had slightly higher bone Sr concentrations than the other age groups (Lambert et al. 1979). The high Sr concentrations in the young children is probably caused by a combination of physiological and dietary factors as young children are known to exhibit less discrimination against Sr than adults (section V.A.2).

The fall in the curve for males and females after 10 years of age indicates the transition to adult values of Sr/Ca discrimination ratios, which are reached before that age (section V.A.2). Besides this, there may be a

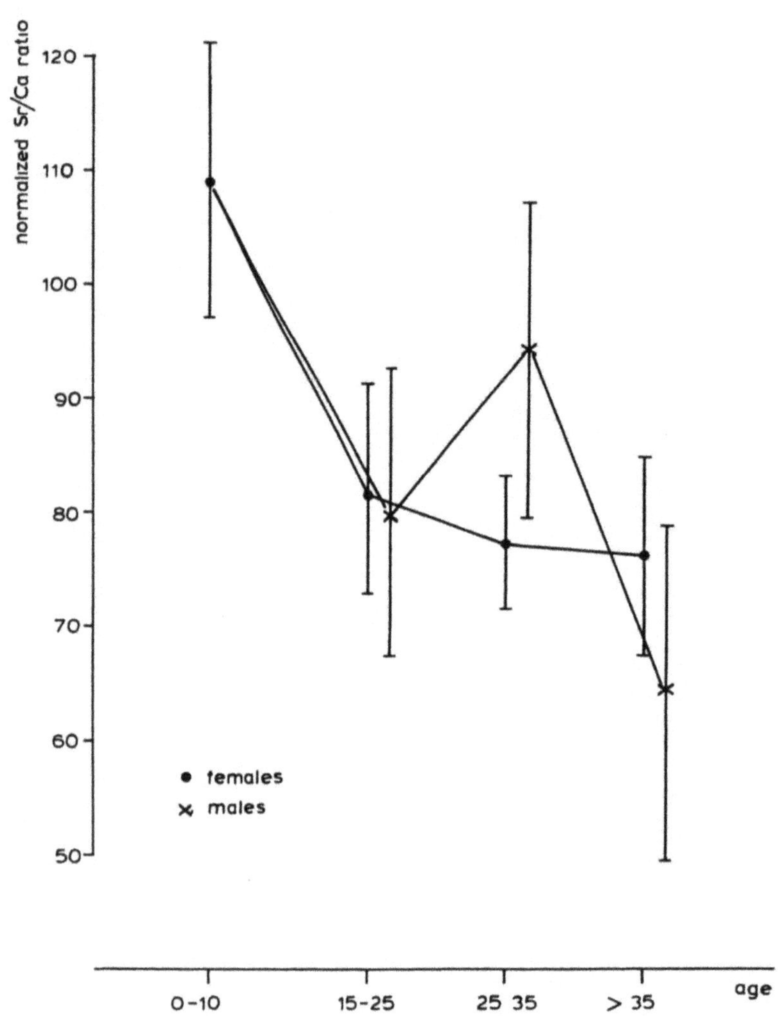

figure V.5 Normalized mean Sr/Ca ratios in inhumations (n=29) grouped on the basis of age and sex. Explanation in the text.

difference in diet between young children and the older children and adults. Unfortunately, no individuals of the age group 10-15 years are present.

Since adult OR values are fairly constant, the diet of the males between the ages of 15 and 35 appears to have been of an almost uniform composition as far as Sr/Ca ratios are concerned.

In comparison to the males, the females show a stronger decrease in bone Sr levels after the age of 10. The lowest Sr concentrations are found in the age 15-25 years, the period of life in which most of the reproduction activities of the females probably occur. Pregnancy and lactation are likely to cause a decrease of Sr concentrations in bone (section V.A.2). The data thus suggest that the difference between male and female Sr concentrations reflect physiological factors related with reproductive activities rather than differences in the diets of males and females.

The low Sr concentration in the small group (n=3) of males over 35 years of age is difficult to explain. They may result from one or more of the following factors: regional variations in Sr levels, physiological causes including the effect of disease, and dietary differences, probably related to status.

The first of these factors assumes that the low mean Sr concentration results from a fortuitous coincidence of age grouping and sites with low Sr levels. In the group of males older than 35 years, the individuals come from three different sites (table II.10). The old male from the Zwaagdijk flat graves (**42**) has a lower Sr concentration than both the male and the female aged 15-25 from this site (**43, 41**). The old male from Oostwoud (**33**) also has a Sr concentration lower than almost all the other individuals from this site. It appears therefore unlikely that the low Sr levels in the old males result from geographical bias.

A change in Sr/Ca uptake and metabolism with advancing age in males is not likely (section V.A.2). At higher ages the difference between male and female Sr/Ca metabolism is probably smaller than at the reproductive age. The females do not show a decrease in Sr concentrations with advancing age. The difference between the older males and females is probably related to differences in diet which may be status determined.

Differences between Sr levels in males and females can also be seen in the stray human bones from three settlements. The value of stray bones is limited as far as estimation of sex and age is concerned, but in a number of cases a tentative diagnosis can be made (Appendix 1). Mean Sr levels for males and females from settlements are assembled in table V.12.

In Andijk the females show somewhat higher Sr concentrations than the males, in Het Valkje mean Sr concentrations for males and females are almost equal. Samples of unknown sex have slightly higher Sr concentrations, which for a part may be the result of the presence of a number of bones from young individuals in this group. The difference in Sr concentrations in males and females in general corroborates the picture of the Sr concentrations in the inhumed males and females.

Table V.12. Mean Sr concentrations in males, females and individuals of unknown sex from two sites. All bone samples (long bones and other bones) are included. Reliability of sexing in certain cases poor. Values in mg Sr/kg bone ash.

site	sex	n	mean	SD
Valkje (total)	(prob.) male	8	949	130
	(prob.) female	5	943	25
	unknown	9	980	132
Andijk	(prob.) male	5	1037	114
	(prob.) female	4	1069	146
	unknown	10	1086	149

C.4.3. Effect of status

General aspects

The material from West-Friesland can be divided in two obvious status groups. A number of inhumations from barrows and flat graves occur in addition to a number of stray finds of human bones from settlement features (section II. D.1.3). Both categories are present at the sites Het Valkje and Hoogkarspel.

Within the category inhumation, a further division in higher and lower status can be based on archeological data, age and sex.

One of the aims of bone Sr analyses is the comparison of groups of individuals of different social standing. In the preceding section we have already touched upon this subject because differences between age and sex groups may also involve a status difference. The sex of the persons has a physiological effect on bone Sr levels quite apart from being a factor in the status-system.

The physiological effects of age and sex probably affects the assessment of status differences between sites because the distribution of males and females of various ages over the barrows is not equal. The mean absolute and relative Sr concentrations have been calculated for each site (table V.10). The Zwaagdijk barrows are of interest in this aspect: the low Sr level in this barrow may be the result of the relatively large number of females.

Inhumations and stray finds of human bones

Mean Sr/Ca ratios for inhumations and stray finds of human bones, respectively, are given in table V.13., with the inclusion of cattle bone Sr/Ca ratios. Sr/Ca ratios in mg Sr/g Ca are abbreviated **Rh** for the human bones and **Rc** for the cattle bones. For each of the sites and groups the normalized Sr/Ca ratio (Rh/Rc * 100 %) is calculated, because this ratio is of interest in dietary extrapolations (chapter XI).

On a total of 31 individuals from graves and 34 individuals from settlement features, both absolute (Rh) and normalized Sr/Ca ratios are lower in the inhumations than in the material from the settlement features. The difference in Rh is significant at the 99 % level (Student's $t = 3.71$, 63 DF).

Within the sites Hoogkarspel and Het Valkje the Sr/Ca ratios of the inhumations are lower than those of the stray finds. These differences are not significant (Student's t test: Hoogkarspel $t=1.84$, 12 DF; Het Valkje Late $t=0.81$, 5 DF). The number of samples in each site is, however, small.

The individuals represented by stray bones from the settlement features are probably mainly in the age group 15-35 years. This assumption would appear to be justified, because bones of young children are more likely to be destroyed in taphonomic processes while people older than 35 years were probably few in number anyway. In order to eliminate this taphonomic bias, the stray bones from the settlements may be compared with the age groups 15-35 years from the inhumations (table V.11, V.14).

Table V.13. Sr/Ca ratios in mg Sr/g Ca for human long bones (Rh) and cattle bones (Rc). Group I consists of more or less complete inhumations, group II consists of stray find human skeletal elements from settlement features.

site	group	Rh n	Rh mean	Rh SD	Rc n	Rc mean	Rc SD	Rh/Rc * 100%
Oostwoud								
barrow II	I	10	2.50	0.42	7	3.32	0.25	75
barrow I	I	2	2.72					82
Zwaagdijk								
flat graves	I	4	2.19	0.15	6	2.48	0.19	88
barrows	I	6	2.00	0.12				81
Grootebroek	I	3	2.06	0.36	6	2.90	0.44	71
Hoogkarspel								
barrows	I	3	2.09	0.41	19	3.39	0.19	62
Het Valkje Late								
flat graves	I	3	2.60	0.10	14	2.83	0.31	92
Hoogkarspel								
settlement	II	11	2.65	0.44	19	3.39	0.19	78
Valkje Early								
settlement	II	8	2.54	0.28	18	2.81	0.21	90
Valkje Late								
settlement	II	4	2.82	0.39	14	2.83	0.31	100
Andijk								
settlement	II	11	2.75	0.40	20	3.35	0.24	82
Velsen								
BA	I	6	1.92	0.32	10	2.55	0.33	75
Schagen-Mug								
inhumations	I	3	3.64	0.69	32	3.37	0.49	108
total *								
inhumations	I	31	2.31	0.39	52	3.07	0.42	75
total								
settlements	II	34	2.68	0.40	71	3.12	0.36	86

* except Velsen and Schagen-Muggenburg

The mean Sr/Ca ratio for the latter group is only slightly higher than the value for all the inhumations, but significantly different from the Sr/Ca ratio of the stray finds from the settlements (Student's t=2.38, 51 DF, 95 % level of sign.). Sr/Ca ratios of inhumed females aged 15-35 years are significantly different (t=3.15, 41 DF, 99 % level of sign.) from the stray find Sr/Ca ratio, while the ratio for inhumed males is not (t=0.80,42 DF).

If we assume that the settlement material consists of both males and females, the males amongst whom have higher Sr levels, this suggests that different mean Sr/Ca ratios are present both for males and females from inhumations and from settlement features.

The obvious explanation for this difference is the composition of the diet, related to the social ranking of the individuals involved. An alternative cause should however also be considered. The inhumations represent individuals from the earliest phase of the Bronze Age occupation of the area (section II.C.1.3) whereas most of the stray finds date from later occupation phases. The different Sr/Ca ratios of the groups may therefore reflect a change in agricultural and dietary potential and practices. This aspect is treated in connection with other data in chapter XI.

Table V.14. Sr/Ca ratios for the inhumations from barrows and flat graves, age group 15-35 years, compared with stray bones from settlement features.

sex/group	n	mg Sr/g Ca	SD	CV(%)
inh. female	9	2.24	0.27	12
inh. male	10	2.56	0.44	17
total inhumations	19	2.40	0.41	17
stray finds	34	2.68	0.40	15

Status and age

After the first few years of human life, there is no age effect on Sr/Ca metabolism (V.A.2.2.). Age effects in bone Sr concentrations in essence are status effects. A special status acquired by age and achievement may result in a different dietary composition.

Within the group of inhumations, the males and females older than 35 years have different mean Sr concentrations. Females and males in this age group had probably acquired a relatively high status as indicated by the fact that they were buried in barrows or flat graves. The Sr levels in their bones suggest, however, that their rank resulted in different dietary regimes for the two sexes. The older males get diets low in Sr, whereas the females remain on a diet with a constant amount of Sr even while growing older.

Still another explanation for the observed difference in the older males and females may be found in the pathological effects on Sr/Ca metabolism. Pathological features are mainly present in the bones of the older individuals (section 4.5).

C.4.4. Strontium in long bones and other bones

In the preceding sections, only long bone Sr levels are discussed. Besides these, Sr concentrations in a series of other bones were measured. As pointed out in I.B.1.3, the comparison between long bone and other bone Sr levels is of interest in relation to dietary questions. Mean Sr concentrations in 'other bones' are assembled in table V.15. The mean 'other bone' Sr level are generally close to the Sr concentration in long bones. A mean value for 'other bone' Sr levels expressed as percentage of long bone Sr concentrations of 105 % can be calculated for 10 sites. Fresh 'other bones' have lower Sr concentrations than long bones (table I.3). The 'other bone' Sr levels are probably to some extent affected by diagenetic processes. This renders the comparison between Sr levels in long bones and the other bones valueless in the discussion of diets. The alternative explanation for the high Sr levels in the other bones would be that all individuals had changed to diets with higher Sr/Ca ratios relatively shortly before their decease, which is very unlikely.

Relatively large differences between long bone and other bone Sr concentrations are found in the Zwaagdijk inhumations and in the individuals from Schagen.

Two inhumations in a single flat grave in a ditch at Het Valkje were of females aged 15-19 years (55 1-2-45). A preliminary discussion on the Sr levels in these individuals was given in Runia (1985). At first, a metatarsal from each was analysed for Sr concentrations. These yielded high concentrations (1263 and 1174 mg/kg), which resulted in the conclusion that these abnormally buried individuals had abnormal Sr levels (Runia 1985). This proved to be incorrect in the light of the subsequent analysis of samples of compact bone from the femurs of these persons. These samples yielded 'normal' values (960 and 926 mg/kg). This illustrates the necessity of using, if at all possible, compact bone for analysis and for caution in explaining aberrant Sr concentrations. The high Sr concentrations in the metatarsals remain, however, to be explained. No other human metatarsals were analyzed. Tanaka et al. (1981, see table I.3) found lower Sr concentrations in bones from the feet than in long bones.

Because Sr levels in the 'other bones' appear to be less reliable than the long bone Sr levels, conclusions on changes in the diet shortly before death remain uncertain.

Table V.15. Mean Sr concentrations in 'other bones', excluding individuals younger than 10 years, in mg Sr/kg bone ash. In the last column, Sr concentrations in other bones are expressed as a percentage of long bone Sr concentrations.

site	n	mean	SD	CV	% of long bones
Velsen	5	729	92	13	100
Zwaagdijk barrow	5	915	135	15	122
Grootebroek	1	694			90
Zwaagdijk flatgr.	3	1003	42	4	118
Oostwoud	23	838	160	19	94
Valkje Early per.	7	936	158	17	98
Hoogkarspel	5	951	42	4	97
Valkje Late period	5	1043	150	14	106
Andijk	8	1100	128	12	105
Schagen	8	1525	240	16	118

C.4.5. Strontium concentrations, pathology and body length

Dental pathology

The relation between bone Sr concentrations and incidence of carious and periapical lesions is of special interest. The composition of the diet, food processing and eating habits influence the incidence of these lesions (Caselitz 1986). Besides this, age, and hence abrasion of the elements, plays a role.

A group of individuals exhibiting clear lesions in dentition and the associated jaw-bone was selected from the material assembled in Appendix 1. In the group of inhumations, 15 individuals have no caries, one individual has carious teeth and eight individuals have caries and associated periapical abcess cavities. In the material from Oostwoud eight individuals are caries free and three individuals have caries and periapical lesions.

In table V.16, Sr levels in the groups of carious individuals are compared with Sr levels in the group without caries. The group with dental pathologies have lower Sr levels than the caries-free individuals. The differences are not significant.

Table V.16. Strontium concentrations (mg/kg ash) in humans with and without caries and periapical abcesses.

group		n	mean	SD
Oostwoud	no caries	8	895	104
	caries & abcesses	3	846	39
total	no caries	15	854	119
	caries & abcesses	7	792	102

Other pathologies

Strontium is not an essential element and though Sr may have some influence on bone growth, no pathological features can be related to high or low dietary Sr levels (Underwood 1977). Still, it may be of interest to compare incidence of certain pathological phenomena and bone Sr levels. In doing this, correlations between age and incidence of pathologies such as arthritis may cloud the picture. For instance, the males older than 35 all have arthritic features, which may have a relation with the low Sr concentrations in this group. Of the old females, **36(1)** has a bowed tibia, **56** a broken and unhealed ulna and **57** a number of pathological features.

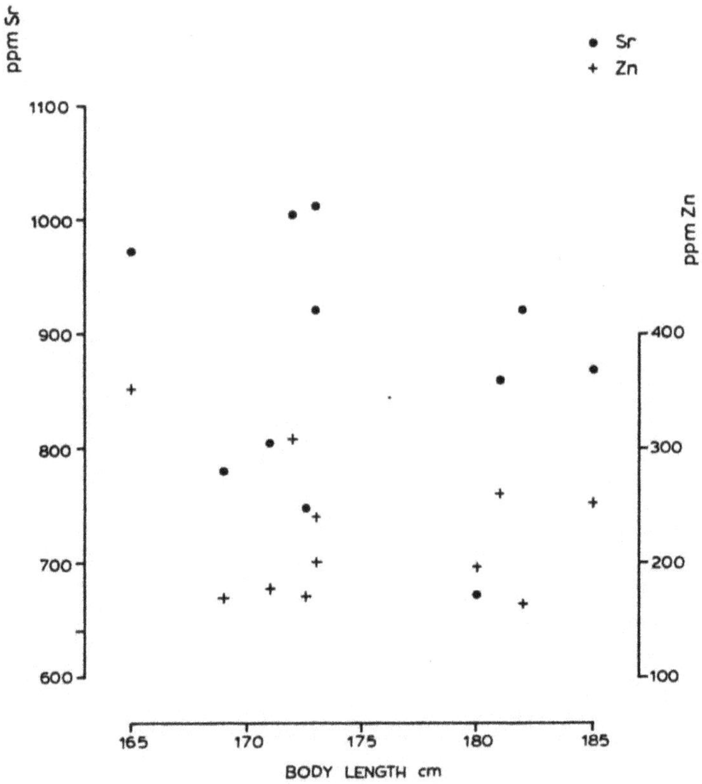

figure V.6 Strontium and zinc concentrations (mg/kg bone ash, vertical axis) in relation to the body lengths (cm, horizontal axis) of inhumed males.

Body length

Human stature to a certain extent reflects general living conditions, which includes health and dietary aspects. Diets containing high amounts of proteins in general will tend to increase body length.

It is, therefore, of interest to compare bone Sr levels with stature. A number of body lengths could be estimated (Appendix 1). Males are between 165 and 185 cm in height, females between c. 155 and 170 cm. Strontium concentrations and body length of the males are plotted in figure V.6. There is no correlation (r=-0.21) between these variables.

C.4.6. Dietary implications

Strontium levels in human bones can be used as indicators of prehistoric diets. Qualititive and quantitative aspects of the diets of the Bronze Age farmers from West-Friesland can, however, not be discussed solely on the basis of human bone Sr levels. Data on the range of potential food items and on their relative Sr/Ca ratios are needed. Besides this, agricultural circumstances and nutritional requirements have to be taken into consideration. Animal food items have already been discussed in section V.A. In section IX.E, Sr/Ca ratios and the archeological aspects of potential vegetable food items will be discussed while the dietary implications of the concentrations of Sr will be treated in a broader context in chapter XI.

VI
ANALYSIS OF BONE: ZINC.

A. ZINC IN FOOD AND METABOLISM

A.1. Zinc in metabolism

The important role of zinc in many physiological processes was recognized only recently (Prasad 1976). Since then the effects of high and low Zn levels on various physiological processes have been studied extensively (Jonxis 1983). Zinc forms part of a number of metalloenzymes that are involved in many metabolic processes both in animals and plants (Riordan & Vallee 1976). Zinc deficiency may manifest itself in a number of symptoms, such as delayed maturation, growth retardation, loss of appetite, poor wound healing and impaired functioning of male and female reproductive organs (Prasad 1976, Underwood 1977). Administration of Zn to patients showing Zn deficiency symptons usually leads to considerable improvement.

Because Zn is an essential element in a number of physiological processes, it is actively handled within the organism. In consequence, there appears to be no direct correlation between dietary Zn concentrations and Zn levels in various tissues (Underwood 1977). When ample Zn is available, it may be incorporated in the bone mineral. In case of insufficient dietary Zn intake, skeletal Zn may be released upon remodelling or breakdown of bone mineral. Under Zn stress and low plasma Zn levels, bone Zn levels may remain high as long as no bone mineral is resorbed. It is likely that there is no age accretion in bone Zn; in this, Zn behaves differently from other, non-essential elements such as lead.

Pregnancy influences plasma Zn levels in the female (Sandstead et al. 1976, Pories et al. 1976), but there appears to be no unanimity in which direction. In a diagram, Sandstead et al. (1976) show plasma Zn levels of patients with various diseases. Zinc levels in pregnant women are significantly lower than normal Zn levels, and appear to decrease post-delivery (Pories et al. 1976). The relatively high concentration of Zn in human milk (Jonxis 1983) may result in decreasing Zn levels in lactating females.
Gilbert (1985) suggests a difference in Zn metabolism in males and females on the basis of differences in correlation between long bone growth, incidence of pathology and bone Zn levels in males and females in some prehistoric Indian populations. In females the Zn resources would be used in the first place for gaining sufficient growth to allow for pregnancy, whereas in males Zn surplus would be used in body maintenance in order to withstand disease. There may be some doubt on this explanation, but it illustrates that bone Zn levels are not a direct derivative of dietary Zn levels. A study of bone Zn levels in a recent population is urgently needed.

The efficiency of the uptake of Zn from food depends on a number of factors. At low plasma Zn levels relatively high amounts of Zn are absorbed from the intestinal tract. Simultaneous presence of Zn and other elements such as Ca, Cu, Fe may adversely affect uptake of Zn (Underwood 1977, Jonxis 1983). The role of phytate and/or fibers, which are mainly present in cereal grains, in inhibiting Zn uptake in the intestinal tract has been frequently discussed (Spencer et al. 1976, Van Barneveld 1983). In cereal grains, Zn, phytate and fibers are mainly present in the bran while the endosperm possesses low Zn levels. A study by Andersson et al. (1983) showed that phytate rather than fibre is responsible for low Zn uptake from wholemeal products.

A.2. Zinc in food

In the fourth edition of McCance & Widdowsons' Tables on the Composition of Foods (Paul & Southgate 1978) the Zn present in various food items are tabulated. Dutch tables on the composition of foods (NVT 1983) do not contain information on Zn levels though some data are provided by Staarink & Hakkenbrak (1984). Mean Zn concentrations combined with energy values and Ca concentrations for certain food items are assembled in table VI.1.

High Zn levels are found in red meat, organs, oysters and other seafoods (Underwood 1977, table VI.1). Vegetable food items generally have lower Zn contents; however, wholemeal products, nuts and leafy vegetables have relatively high Zn contents. Some of the Zn in the vegetable foods may be poorly available due to binding to phytate (Spencer et al. 1976, Underwood 1977). Leafy vegetables appear to have high Zn contents per unit of energy. Animal products are distinct in their very high Zn/Ca ratio, and hence a relatively large part of the Zn in meat may be taken up in the intestinal tract. The concentrations of Fe which may also act as a competative ion in intestinal uptake in general are much lower than Ca concentrations.

In general, carnivores will achieve considerable intake of easily absorbable Zn. This is reflected in their bone Zn concentrations: Rheingold et al. (1983) give values of 90-150 ppm Zn in herbivores and 175-250 ppm in carnivores (table VI.6).
In present-day Dutch diets, some 40 % of Zn intake is present in meat, fish and eggs, some 20 % in milk and dairy products and some 15 % in bread and cereals (Hulshof 1985). Animal products thus supply more than half of the Zn.

Table VI.1. Zinc concentrations in a number of food items. Calculated from Paul & Southgate (1978).

item		---- mg Zn per ----		
	n	100 g	MJ	mg Zn/g Ca
fruits	6	0.1	0.7 ± 0.3	10.3 ± 7.3
fish	7	0.5 ± 0.1	0.9 ± 0.3	21 ± 6
cows' milk	1*	0.35	1.3	2.9
nuts	3	2.8 ± 0.3	1.4 ± 0.1	39 ± 19
meats	4	2.5 ± 0.7	1.9 ± 0.7	342 ± 103
wheat wholemeal	1*	3.0	2.2	86
chickens' eggs	1*	1.5	2.5	29
root crops	5	0.3 ± 0.1	2.6 ± 1.3	7.7 ± 5.3
leafy veg's	12	0.4 ± 0.2	5.1 ± 0.3	6.1 ± 4.0
wheat bran	1*	16.2	19	147
marine shellfish	7	8.9 ± 14.9	35 ± 7	73 ± 90

* mean value for many analyses

As stated before, concentrations of Zn and other elements in food items should be seen in relation to the energy values (concentrations per unit of energy) because these to a certain extent determine the amount (in kg) which will be consumed (Runia 1987b). The data in table VI.1 show, for instance, that the Zn/MJ ratios in nuts are lower than in cereal grains. Nut diets will therefore have lower Zn contents than cereal diets.

A.3. Zinc in bones and soil

Zinc can be present on Ca sites in the mineral matrix of apatite (McConnell 1973, Lindsay & Vlek 1977). It therefore resembles Sr in the relative unsusceptibility to diagenetic influences (compare table I.1). On the basis of comparisons between Zn levels in excavated ribs, soil (Lambert et al. 1979) and femurs (Lambert et al. 1982) from North American Woodland sites, it was concluded that Zn is little affected by diagenetic processes. Earlier, Gilbert (1975, cited in Gilbert 1985) had reached the conclusion that Zn was useful as a dietary discriminator.

In the soil, the divalent Zn cation is predominant but Zn can be present both in positively and in negatively charged compounds (de Haan & Zwerman 1976). Like other ions Zn^{2+} is adsorbed to charged soil particles (clay, organic matter), though it is possibly somewhat less strongly adsorbed than Ca (section IX.A).

B. EXPERIMENTAL

Zinc concentrations in the bone ash solutions were measured using AAS. Measurements were done with correction for background absorption at 213.9 nm in an air-acetylene flame.

Reference samples on which two or more independent Zn determinations were carried out yielded a mean coefficient of variation of about 2 %. Two standards St I and St II yielded 334 ± 6.5 mg Zn/ kg bone ash (CV=1.95%, n=6) and 258 ± 3.7 mg Zn/ kg bone ash (CV=1.43 %, n=9) respectively.
Reproducibility of the analysis thus appears to be fairly good. Analyses of IAEA H-5 animal bone reference material yielded a mean of 171 ± 1.87 (CV=1.1 %, n=4) mg Zn/kg bone ash. This corresponds to 96.5 mg Zn/kg dry bone, which is rather high compared with the preliminary IAEA value of 89.91 ± 15.39 mg/kg and the value of Mahanti & Barnes (1983) of 76.6 ± 0.9 mg/kg.
The relatively small coefficients of variation indicate that the accuracy within our analyses is fairly good. Compared with coefficients of variation encountered in the Zn concentrations in groups of individuals the coefficients of variation in analysis are small and bias due to analytical procedures negligible.

C. RESULTS AND DISCUSSION

C.1. General

Mean Zn concentrations in the groups of analysed bones are assembled in table VI.2. A striking feature of the results is the high coefficient of variation: the highest value (86%) is reached by the cattle. Within sites, smaller coefficients of variation are found (table VI.4, VI.5). However, in comparison with analyses of bones from other sites, the CV values do not appear to be excessively high. Lambert et al. (1979) give coefficients of variation of 8-76 % for Woodland sites, while in the same sites Lambert et al. (1982) found coefficients of variation in Zn concentrations up to 101 %. In such cases it is not surprising that no statistically significant differences between males and females are found.

Table VI.2. Zinc concentrations in human and animal bones. Mean and standard deviation in mg Zn/kg bone ash. Identical letters in the column 'significance' indicate that the mean values do not differ significantly at the 99% level (Student's t-test). In the last column, the relative concentration is given as percentage of cattle bone Zn concentrations.

species	n	mean	SD	CV	significance			relative conc.
human *	80	238	130	55	A			93
cattle	145	256	220	86	A	B		100
pig	37	321	162	50		B	C	125
sheep/goat	44	378	182	48			C	148
dog	36	424	253	60			C	166

* only long bones

Unfortunately, few data on the variation in Zn in bones from animals raised on identical diets are available. Tissue and plasma Zn levels in normal healthy persons appear to have a smaller variation (Prasad 1976, Sandstead et al. 1976). Bones from 11 rats fed the same diet yielded mean Zn concentrations of 380 mg/kg and a coefficient of variation of 6 % (Alexander & Nusbaum 1962). Data in the same paper indicate that the coefficients of variations are higher in groups of humans. Bones of 25 humans from the USA yielded a CV of 39 %, a subsample from Los Angeles a CV of 36 %. Becker et al. (1968) found a CV of 13 % for five fresh human bones, but a CV of 37 % for five prehistoric desiccated Peruvian human bones.

Fresh bone samples from Dutch cattle with unknown dietary regime give a mean coefficient of variation of 15 % (n=29, table VI.3). Connor & Slaughter (1984) report on Zn concentrations in polar bear and caribou, both species exhibiting a large difference between the two analysed specimens (polar bear: 1113 and 247 ppm Zn, caribou 351 and 135 ppm Zn). It is, however, not clear whether these were fresh bone samples.

Table VI.3. Zinc concentrations in fresh cattle bones from the Achterhoek (IVO samples) and the Amsterdam Abattoir (AA samples). Mean and standard deviation in mg Zn/kg bone ash.

sample	sex	age(years)	n	mean	SD	CV(%)
IVO 1-10	male	ca. 1.5	10	100	10	10
IVO 11-20	female	8-10	10	108	20	19
AA 1-6	female	2-3	6	114	9	8
AA 7	male	1.5	1	128		
AA 8-9	female	5-5.5	2	134		
total			29	127	17	15

Zinc plays a role in several enzymes and it is therefore actively processed. This may result in a large variation in the Zn concentrations in bone: it is the balance between dietary Zn levels, and of Zn requirements for the body which affects its deposition in, or removal from bones. For animals which are kept under identical circumstances such as laboratory rats these processes may result in low variations in Zn concentrations (compare Alexander & Nusbaum 1962). However, for humans and unconfined animals considerable variations in Zn concentrations may be expected.

The data on fresh material, however, do not show variations in Zn content as high as reported for some complexes of excavated bones, and post-mortem, diagenetic changes in bone Zn levels should be reviewed as a cause for this variation.

C.2. Diagenesis

Lambert et al. (1984) found Zn to be homogenously non-patterned distributed in soil around buried bones, which would indicate that no Zn had entered or left the bone. Low soil Zn levels are, according to Lambert et al. (1979) an argument in favour of Zn levels in bone being not altered. However, in the soil a number of complex interactions can take place, such as between ions in solution, in minerals, adsorbed on charged particles or bound by chelating agents. Consequently, the comparison of absolute concentrations (by weight) of just one element in soil and bone is an over-simplification. Bone mineral interacts with the soil solution, in which the ionic concentrations are determined by a number of factors. The extent of in- or efflux of Zn in bone is probably partly determined by the Zn/Ca ratio (or rather the total ionic composition) of the soil solution. Bone and soil Zn/Ca ratios rather than Zn concentrations should therefore be used in judging the potential effect of burial on bone Zn levels. In the case of Gibson/Ledders (Lamber et al. 1979) the Zn concentration in the soil is much lower than in the bones (mean value of 41 and 300 ppm respectively). However, the Zn/Ca ratio in the soil (approximately 1.5 mg Zn/g Ca) is higher than in the bone (0.9 mg Zn/g Ca).

In Schagen-Muggenburg soil samples were taken at various points around a human and a dog skeleton. Zinc concentrations and Zn/Ca ratios were significantly different in the subsoil and in the settlement layer (section IX.B.). The subsoil has significantly lower Ca concentrations than the settlement layer. Zinc concentrations in the soil are lower, but Zn/Ca ratios higher than in adjacent bone (skull of Mug 81: 414 mg Zn/kg bone ash and 1.25 mg Zn/g Ca, soil from skull 129 mg Zn/kg and 12.9 mg Zn/g Ca; vertebra of dog 396 mg Zn/kg bone ash and 1.26 mg Zn/g Ca, soil below vertebrae 99 mg Zn/kg and 8.8 mg Zn/g Ca). In this case the Zn/Ca ratios in the soil may be high enough to cause contamination of the buried bone.

A scatttergram with on the Fe content on the one, and the Zn content of the prehistoric bone samples on the other axis was made (Figure VI.1). The concentrations of Fe and Zn are weakly correlated ($R = 0.43$, R squared = 0.19). This indicates that, if Zn concentrations in the bones are altered due to soil contamination, the contamination is not correlated with the iron influx.

In a number of studies bone Zn levels were considered to be of use as dietary indicators (section I.B.1.4). In some cases (for instance, Lambert et al. 1979) the validity of the arguments raised against diagenetic alterations may be doubted. An explanation for the coefficients of variation,

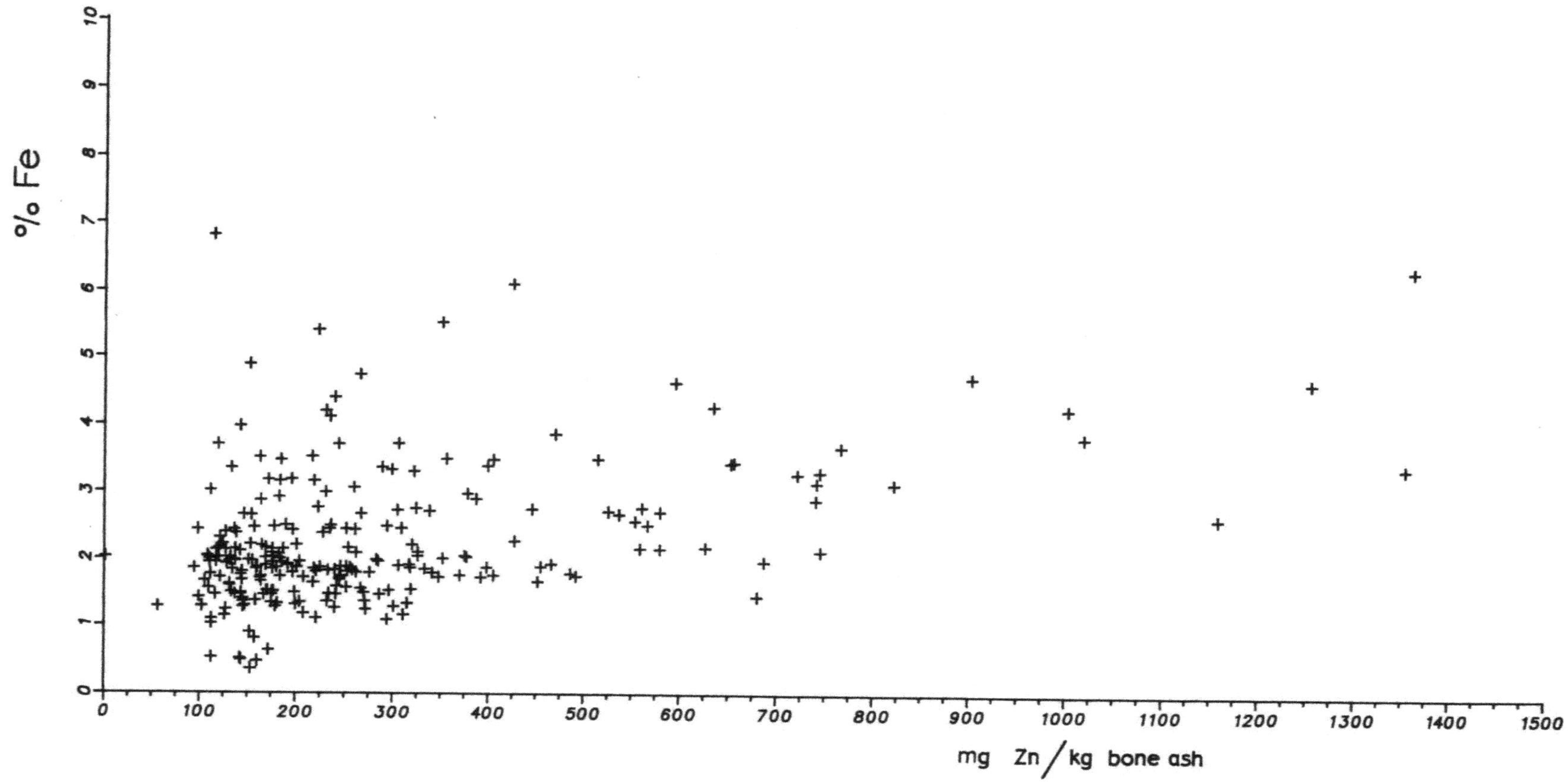

figure VI.1 Scattergram of Zn and Fe concentrations of the Bronze Age samples.

which are large in comparison to those in recent material, is not given. On the other hand, meaningful correlations between bone Zn levels and various parameters (sex, age, species, disease: Gilbert 1985) are strong indications against diagenetic influences on bone Zn levels. Possible correlations between bone Zn concentrations and biological and archeological variables should therefore be investigated cautiously.

C.3. Zinc in animal bones

Mean Zn concentrations for the animal species were calculated for each site (table VI.4, VI.5). There are differences in Zn levels in various sites. The lowest value for cattle is 120 mg Zn/kg bone ash in De Tent, the highest Zn concentrations in cattle are found in Grootebroek (819 mg Zn/kg bone ash).

The homeostatic control of Zn levels in the body starts with regulation of Zn uptake from the intestinal tract (Underwood 1977). Variations in dietary Zn concentrations and Zn intake due to geographical variations in soil Zn contents will partly be counterbalanced by variations in uptake of Zn from the intestinal tract. The differences in Zn levels in cattle bones suggest, however, that regional differences in soil Zn levels are reflected in bone Zn levels.

Differences in bone Zn concentrations between species should more or less reflect the dietary regime of the animals. Rheingold et al. (1983) supply a table with 'typical ranges' of Sr and Zn contents in mammalian bones (table VI.6). These data should be used with caution because details regarding origin and diet of analysed specimen are lacking. In the absence of other studies, this table will, however, be used as reference material for relations between bone Zn levels in various animals species. Our data on fresh cattle bone Zn levels (table VI.3) fall within the range of the herbivores of Rheingold et al. (1983).

Table VI.4. Zinc concentrations in animal bones from various sites. Means and standard deviations in mg/kg bone ash. In the last column the Zn concentrations are expressed as percentages of Zn concentrations in cattle bones from the same site.

site	species	sex	n	mean	SD	CV	relative conc.
Valkje Early	cattle	both	18	144	43	30	100
	cattle	female	8	146	47	32	101
	cattle	male	10	142	40	28	99
	pig		8	249	80	32	173
	dog		9	244	127	52	169
	sheep/goat		10	244	82	34	169
Valkje Late	cattle	both	14	186	69	37	100
	cattle	female	8	191	82	43	103
	cattle	male	6	180	46	26	97
	pig		7	290	141	49	156
	dog		5	360	211	59	194
	sheep/goat		5	559	186	33	301
Andijk	cattle	both	20	212	93	44	100
	cattle	female	10	206	77	37	97
	cattle	male	10	218	105	48	103
	pig		7	433	182	42	204
	dog		2	496			234
	sheep/goat		9	285	99	35	134
Schagen	cattle	both	32	278	199	72	100
	cattle	female	14	216	122	57	78
	cattle	male	12	407	246	60	146
	pig		9	309	136	44	111
	dog		7	478	240	50	172
	sheep/goat		11	454	183	40	163

Table VI.5. Zinc concentrations in animal bones from various sites in mg Zn/kg bone ash. In the last column the Zn concentrations are expressed as percentages of Zn concentrations in cattle bones from the same site.

site	species	n	mean	SD	CV	relative conc.
Zwaagdijk	cattle	6	147	19	13	100
	pig	3	410	242	59	279
	dog	2	598			407
	sheep/goat	3	442	181	42	301
Velsen	cattle	10	189	51	27	100
	pig	2	258			137
	dog	2	290			153
	sheep/goat	5	457	134	29	242
Oostwoud	cattle	7	288	214	74	100
	pig	1	184			64
Westwoud	cattle	8	284	115	40	100
	pig	1	280			99
	dog	1	329			116
De Tent	cattle	5	120	8	7	100
	dog	1	138			115
Hoogkarspel	cattle	19	278	148	53	
Grootebroek	cattle	6	819	513	63	

To facilitate the comparison of mean Zn concentrations between animal species these can be expressed as percentages of cattle bone Zn concentrations (table VI.2, VI.4, VI.5). Some observations should be made regarding the comparison with figures from Rheingold et al. (1983, table VI.6). The mean value for pig, 125 %, agrees very well with the 'omnivore' value of 133 %. The dogs, which probably eat somewhat more animal products than the pigs, have a higher value (148 %) which is also close to the value for the omnivores.

Table VI.6. 'Typical Ranges' of Sr and Zn content in mammalian bones. Adapted from Rheingold et al. (1983). Mean values are approximations. In the last column, Zn concentrations relative to herbivores (as %) are given.

species	ppm Sr range	ppm Zn range	ppm Zn mean	relative Zn concentration
herbivore (cattle, deer, goat, rabbit)	400-500	90-150	120	100
omnivore (rat, beaver, dog, bear)	150-400	120-200	160	133
carnivore (bobcat, wolf, mink, weasel)	100-300	175-250	213	177

The high value for sheep/goat (166 %) is difficult to explain. Unfortunately, reference data on Zn levels in sheep/goat compared to cattle are lacking. The anomalous Zn levels in the sheep/goat bones may be related to the equally high Sr concentrations in these bones (section V.C.3). A diagenetic cause for the high Zn levels is unlikely, because bones from other small animals (dog and pig) appear to be relatively unaffected. This problem will be further discussed in chapter XI.

The relative Zn concentrations in the animal species (table VI.4, VI.5), are graphically presented in fig. VI.2 in combination with the approximate mean Zn levels as derived from Rheingold et al. (1983). A comparable pattern is present within each site. Sheep/goat Zn levels appear to be too high in relation to cattle Zn levels in every site.

The mean Zn levels of pigs, dogs and sheep/goat in Zwaagdijk are very high in comparison to the levels in cattle. As pointed out in section V.C.3.2, this might indicate that the cattle bones from this site do not belong to the same period and/or stem from animals that were raised in another area.

The difference between the Early and Late Period of Het Valkje is intrigueing. When compared to the Early Period, the mean Zn levels of cattle and pigs are slightly higher in the Late Period, whereas those of sheep/goat are more than twice as high. The difference between Zn concentrations in sheep/goat from the two periods is significant on 99% level (t=4.23, 13 DF). This is also clear in figure VI.2. Though dogs in the Late Period have higher Zn levels, the difference with the Early Period is not significant (t=1.19, 12 DF). Relative Zn concentrations in the human bones (table VI.7) score 118 % in the Early and 182 % in the Late Period. A diagenetic cause for this phenomenon is unlikely as all bones come from the same excavation. Possibly, the explanation should be sought in geographical differences in soil Zn levels in relation to herding practices. This option has been discussed in connection with the animal bone Sr levels (Runia 1987a). A further discussion is presented in chapter XI.

No difference in bone Zn levels occurs between cows and bulls/steers in either the excavated bones and in the fresh bones (table VI.4 and VI.3, respectively).

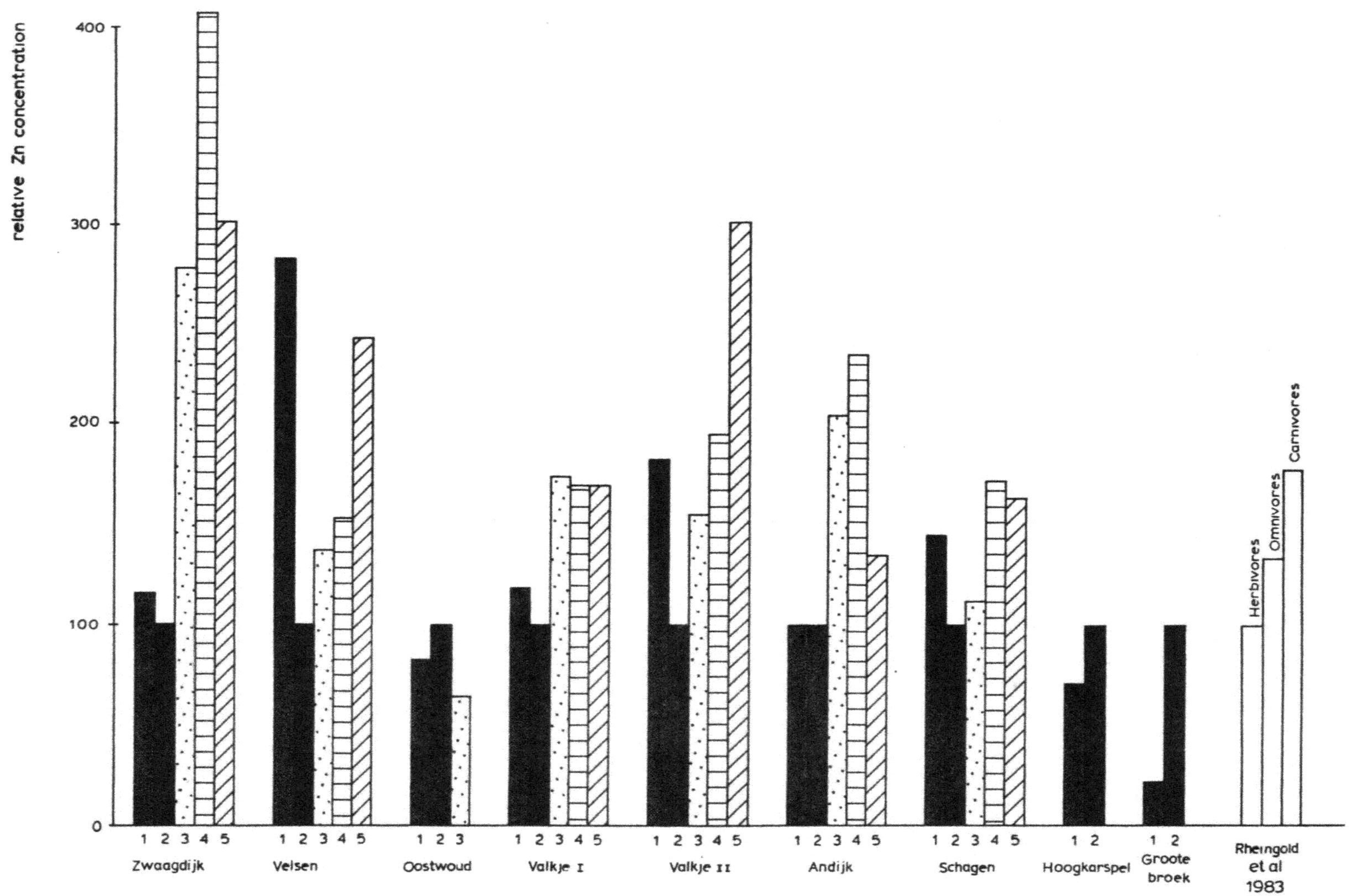

figure VI.2 Relative mean Zn concentrations for humans and domestic animals. Vertical axis: Zn concentration as percentage of cattle bone Zn concentration. 1 human; 2 cattle; 3 pig; 4 dog; 5 sheep/goat. Based on table VI.4, VI.5 and VI.6.

C.4. Zinc in human bones

C.4.1. General

Mean zinc concentrations in the human long bones are given in table VI.7. These values range from 161 mg Zn/kg bone ash in Zwaagdijk to 534 mg Zn/kg bone ash in Velsen. The Zn content of human bone to a great extent depends on environmental Zn levels, as is suggested by the Zn levels relative to cattle bones. Except for the sites Oostwoud, Grootebroek and Hoogkarspel, these values lay in a relatively narrow range close to the value for omnivores (compare figure VI.2). The abnormally high relative value for the samples from Velsen (283 %) may be a reflection of the different environment of this site, which is the only one to be located in the dune area near the sea.

Table VI.7. Mean Zn concentrations in human long bones in mg Zn/kg bone ash. In the last column, the Zn concentration is expressed as percentage of the mean Zn concentration in cattle bone from the same site.

site	n	mean	SD	CV(%)	relative
Zwaagdijk barrows	7	161	29	18	110
Grootebroek	3	169	23	14	21
Valkje Early Period	8	170	36	21	118
Zwaagdijk flat graves	5	180	38	21	122
Hoogkarspel	14	194	59	30	70
Andijk	10	212	74	35	100
Oostwoud	12	234	68	29	81
Valkje Late Period	5	339	101	30	182
Schagen	4	403	108	27	145
Velsen	6	534	150	28	283

Cattle bones were the animal bones to be analysed from the sites Grootebroek and Hoogkarspel. Here, the humans were the only omnivores to be analysed. These cases represent two of the three sites in which human bones have Zn concentrations lower than the cattle bones. In Grootebroek, this is clearly caused by the exceptionally high Zn concentration in cattle bones. The Sr concentrations in these bones are normal (section V.C.3.), and the cause for the high Zn levels remains unclear. Analysis of bones from other species might be useful to solve this problem.

In Oostwoud, the third site in which the mean Zn concentration in human bones is lower than in cattle bones, only one bone from another species (pig) was analysed besides the cattle bones. The Zn concentration in this bone is lower than the mean for cattle. Two of the seven cattle bones from this site appear to have very high Zn concentrations (687 and 554 mg/kg bone ash) compared to a mean of 155 $\pm$ 18 mg Zn/kg bone ash for the remaining five bones. Taking the latter value as reference, the relative Zn content in human bones is 151 %, and in the pig bone 119%. These values agree reasonably well with the other data.

C.4.2. Effect of age and sex

The human bones from graves and barrows were divided in groups according to their age and sex (section II.D.1.3). Mean Zn concentrations and Zn/Ca ratios were calculated for each of the groups (table VI.8) and plotted (figure VI.3).

Table VI.8. Zinc concentrations in groups of inhumations from barrows and flat graves. Age and sex grouping according to table II.10.

sex	age	n	mg Zn/kg bone ash			mg Zn/g Ca		
			mean	SD	CV(%)	mean	SD	CV(%)
??	<10	4	198	39	20	0.58	0.17	29
female	15-25	5	166	32	19	0.44	0.08	19
	25-35	4	200	79	40	0.55	0.20	36
	>35	3	196	32	16	0.53	0.08	15
male	15-25	6	262	55	21	0.73	0.18	24
	25-35	4	177	39	22	0.53	0.16	29
	>35	3	176	4	2	0.47	0.02	3
total		29	201	57	29	0.56	0.18	31

The differences in mean Zn concentrations in the various age groups are relatively small. In the group of 15-25 years, however, the mean Zn concentrations of the males and the females diverge. Lambert et al. (1979) found a relatively large coefficient of variation for approximately the same age group (12-20 years) in a sample of males and females from Gibson, a North American Woodland site (C V values of 76 % for 12-20 years, 54 % for 20-35 years, 36-45 % for the other age groups). This might be the result of different mean Zn levels for males and females in this age group. Physiological reasons for the diverging Zn concentrations may be present in this age. Pregnancy and lactation influence Zn levels (section VI.A.1), and the reproductive activity of the females falls largely in the age 15-25. Besides this, in this period of life sexual maturation takes place, a process in which Zn plays an important role.

Physiological causes for differences between males and females appear to be present. These do not explain, however, the high Zn concentrations in the males aged 15-25. A dietary cause for these high concentrations would appear to be probable.

It is obvious that Zn levels show regional differences (section VI.C.3). These regional differences are unevenly distributed over the age and sex groups and might be considered as a possible cause for the differences in the age groups 15-25. Three of the females in this group come from the Zwaagdijk barrows, four of the males from the Oostwoud barrow II. From the Grootebroek barrow there are a male and a female in this age group, which have 201 and 153 mg Zn/kg bone ash, respectively. Furthermore, a male (254 mg Zn/kg bone ash) and a female (169 mg Zn/kg bone ash) from the Zwaagdijk flat graves is present in this group. It thus appears to be reasonable to accept a difference between males and females aged 15-25 years. This difference may be overemphasized to some extent by regional influences.

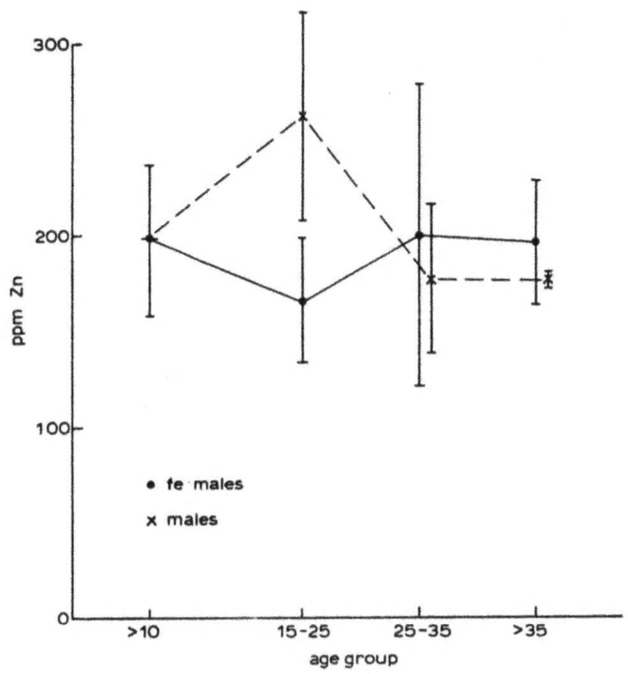

figure VI.3 Mean Zn concentrations (mg Zn/kg bone ash) and standard deviation in inhumations (n=29) grouped on the basis of age and sex. Based on table VI.8.

Mean Zn concentrations were calculated for all inhumations and stray male and female bones from the settlements if they could be sexed (table VI.9). For Het Valkje, the number of bones is very small. In both periods the females have lower Zn contents than the males (n=2). The difference between male and female Zn concentrations is relatively large in Andijk.

Table VI.9. Mean Zn concentrations in males and females from various settlements. Mean and standard deviation in mg Zn/kg bone ash.

site	sex	n	mean	SD	CV
(inhumations)	females	12	185	55	30
	males	13	216	60	28
Het Valkje					
Early Period	females	2	159		
	males	6	183	65	36
	unknown	7	167	36	22
Late Period	females	3	334	60	18
	males	2	398		
	unknown	2	473		
Andijk	females	4	164	37	23
	males	5	319	171	54
	unknown	9	258	98	38

Females with lower Zn concentrations than males were also found by Lambert et al. (1982) in two North American Woodland sites (table VI.10). These authors impute the difference between males and females to dietary factors. The low Zn levels in the females were attributed to a diet low in meat and high in grain. In the case of Gibson, femur and rib Zn levels show a large variation.

Table VI.10. Zinc concentrations in bones from two North American Woodland sites. Data from Lambert et al. (1982).

		femur				rib				rib Zn as
site	sex	n	mean	SD	CV	n	mean	SD	CV	% of femur
Gibson	males	10	242	244	101	23	325	209	64	134
	females	12	361	185	51	33	278	135	49	77
	both	22	307	217	71	86	302	158	52	98
Ledders	males	12	223	83	37	12	375	148	39	168
	females	13	206	109	53	12	225	76	34	109
	both	25	210	98	47	32	308	129	42	147

Apart from the age-dependent effect related sexual maturation and reproductive activities, there appears to be no age-effect in the bone Zn concentrations (figure VI.3 and table VI.8). There are no indications for changes in Zn uptake and metabolism with increasing age. The data therefore indicate that, except for the males in the ages 15-25, there were no major differences in Zn intake between people of various sex and age. Small differences, however, may have been present but will be obscured by the homeostatic control of body Zn levels and other factors.

C.4.3. Effect of status

No differences in Zn levels are present between the two obvious status groups, the inhumations and the stray find bones from settlement traces (section V.C.4.3, table VI.11). This suggests that no large differences between Zn intake between these groups existed. This aspect will be discussed in section XI.C.

C.4.4. Zinc in long bones and other bones

Mean Zn concentrations in 'other bones', which include ribs, vertebrae and skull bones, are presented in table VI.12. Changes in Zn concentrations in bones, whether in vivo or post-mortem in the soil will probably primarily occur in the 'other bones'. In vivo changes in bone Zn levels may be caused by changes in dietary Zn levels or by disease. Zinc stress due to, for instance, pregnancy and lactation may thus show up in a large difference between rib and femur Zn concentrations. A similar effect may result from a major change in Zn intake, for instance, as a consequence of immigration to a new environment. Large differences between Zn concentrations in long bones and other bones may, on the other hand, also result from alterations of Zn concentrations in the soil.

Table VI.11. Zn/Ca ratios for human long bones from various sites. Data for young children are omitted. Grouping refers to status groups I: inhumations; II: stray find bones from settlement traces.

		human			cattle			
site	group	n	mean	SD	n	mean	SD	rel.
Oostwoud								
Neol barrow II	I	10	0.72	0.18	5#	0.44	0.03	164
EBA barrow I	I	2	0.41					93
Zwaagdijk								
EBA flat graves	I	4	0.48	0.11	6	0.38	0.05	126
EBA barrow	I	6	0.43	0.08				113
Grootebroek								
EBA barrow	I	3	0.45	0.06	2#	0.32		141
Hoogkarspel								
BA barrow	I	3	0.54	0.12	19	0.74	0.40	73
Valkje Late period								
BA flat graves	I	3	0.92	0.21	14	0.48	0.18	192
Hoogkarspel								
EBA MBA	II	11	0.52	0.17	19	0.74	0.40	70
Valkje Early period								
EBA MBA	II	8	0.45	0.10	18	0.36	0.11	125
Valkje Late period								
MBA	II	3	0.83	0.33	14	0.48	0.18	173
Andijk								
BA	II	10	0.56	0.20	20	0.58	0.26	97
Velsen								
BA	I	6	1.41	0.38	10	0.50	0.13	282
Schagen-Muggenburg								
Roman Iron Age	I	3	1.00	0.22	32	0.76	0.56	131
total inhumations *	I	31	0.59	0.21	46	0.56	0.32	105
total settlements	II	32	0.54	0.21	71	0.55	0.30	98

* except Velsen and Schagen-Muggenburg
\# exceptionally high values ignored

Comparisons can by made by expressing 'other bone' Zn levels or Zn/Ca ratios as percentages of Zn levels or Zn/Ca ratios of long bones (table VI.12). The percentages range from 73 to 145, with a mean of 117 ± 20 (n=10 sites). This range is smaller than the range in Gibson and Ledders (77 to 168, mean 122 ± 33, n=4, table VI.10), but the means are almost equal. Amongst the inhumations there are a few individuals where other bones were analysed as well as long bones. The number of cases is however too small to judge the effect of sex and age on the difference in long bone and 'other bone' Zn concentrations. Mean ratios (Zn in 'other bones')/(Zn in long bones) are 134 ± 55 % (n=7 individuals) for the females and 128 ± 43 % (n=10 individuals) for the males.

No information on the _in vivo_ relation between Zn concentrations in 'other bones' and long bones is available. The ratios of Zn in 'other bones'/Zn in long bones fall in a relatively narrow range. This can probably be interpreted as an indication that post-mortem changes in (long) bone Zn levels are small. However, the Zn concentrations in various bones from a single individual should be compared with modern reference material.

Table VI.12. Mean Zn concentrations in 'other bones'. Concentrations and standard deviations in mg Zn/kg bone ash. In the last column, 'other bone' Zn concentrations are expressed as percentage of long bone Zn concentration.

site	n	mean	SD	CV	%
Zwaagdijk barrows	5	149	26	18	93
Grootebroek	2	208			123
Valkje Early Period	8	182	64	35	107
Zwaagdijk flat graves	4	247	115	47	137
Hoogkarspel	4	235	114	49	121
Andijk	8	307	157	51	145
Oostwoud	23	303	134	44	129
Valkje Late Period	5	433	163	37	128
Schagen	9	465	175	38	115
Velsen	5	390	234	60	73

C.4.5. Zinc levels, pathology and body height

A number of diseases are accompanied with low plasma Zn levels (Sandstead et al. 1976). Gilbert 1977 (cited by Gilbert 1985) found a negative correlation between bone Zn levels and incidence of pathological features in the skeletal material of prehistoric Amerindian males. Also, body height and Zn levels appeared to be correlated in the males.

Dental pathology

Caries and periapical lesions occur rather frequently in the West-Frisian skeletal material (section V.C.4.5)

Table VI.13. Zinc concentrations (mg/kg ash) in inhumations with and without caries and periapical abcesses.

group		n	mean	SD
Oostwoud	no caries	8	246	53
	caries & abcesses	3	164	37
total	no caries	15	208	58
	caries & abcesses	7	163	26

Mean Zn levels in the groups of carious and caries-free individuals are presented in table VI.13. Caries-free individuals have a relatively high mean Zn concentration. The difference with the other group is, however, not significant (Student's t=1.87, 20 DF). The same is true for the Oostwoud subgroup (t=2.23, 9 DF). Obviously, these differences to some extent reflect the differences between age and sex groups. Most individuals with caries are old, whereas a number of the caries-free individuals are males aged 15-25. The latter group is in any case characterized by high Zn levels.

Other pathologies

Not many individuals with pathological features other than dental lesions are present amongst the skeletal material from West-Friesland. This, and the fact that the pathological features are present in some of the older individuals hampers the assesment of a correlation between pathology and Zn levels.

Stature

The stature of 11 males and three females of the group of inhumations could be estimated. Male statures range from 165 to 185 cm, female statures from c. 155 to c. 170 cm.

For females this group is too small for any assesment of a correlation between Zn levels and stature. For the 11 males, there is no correlation between Zn levels in bone and stature (compare fig.V.6)

C.4.6. Dietary implications

Levels of Zn in bone can be used in dietary extrapolations. However, the active treatment of Zn by the living organism veils any unequivocal relationship between dietary Zn levels and Zn concentrations in the body. High Zn levels in bone are considered to be the result of high dietary Zn levels, and thus of a diet containing foodstuffs with considerable amounts of Zn in easily absorbable form, such as meat and seafood.

Only a small amount of seafood was eaten in Bronze Age West-Friesland (chapter X). The most important sources of Zn in the human diet were, therefore, probably red meat and organs. The role of vegetable foods such as roots and cereal grains as a source of Zn is not very clear, but is probably minor in comparison to meat (section A.2).

The relatively small differences in Zn levels in the age and sex groups suggest that the amounts of meats consumed by members of these groups did not differ much. Only in the age group 15-25 may there have been differences in male and female Zn intake. In this group, female show Zn levels below the mean, a phenomenon which might be attributed to sexual maturation, pregnancy and lactation. Human milk has high Zn levels (Jonxis 1983). The high male Zn levels may, however, be the result of the consumption of foods with high Zn levels.

Further consideration to the dietary implications of the bone Zn levels will be given in chapter XI.

VII
ANALYSIS OF BONE:
MISCELLANEOUS TRACE ELEMENTS

A. INTRODUCTION

Concentrations of barium, lead, arsenic and copper were measured, Ba concentrations in all, and Pb, As and Cu in only some of the bone ash solutions. This took little extra time and was considered to be a useful exercise in order to indicate whether or not these elements, if more extensively studied, might yield evidence of paleoecological value and information on (semi) industrial activities (Van Wijngaarden-Bakker 1986). A disadvantage of the accessory approach to the analyses of the elements Pb, As and Cu is that the analytical circumstances were not optimal. Potential uses of the elements in paleodietary and paleoecological studies, experimental methods and results are described in the following sections.

B. BARIUM

B.1 Introduction

Barium is placed below Sr in the Periodic Table of the elements. Barium therefore resembles Sr and Ca in electronic configuration and will in consequence react similarly to Sr and Ca. In atomic weight and ionic radius Ba is, however, considerably greater than Ca (table I.1). In biological systems, the discrimination against Ba will therefore be stronger than against Sr. The effects of the trophic level, such as are present in the Sr/Ca ratios, might therefore be even more marked in the Ba/Ca ratios. There are, however, no data avialable on trophic level effects on Ba/Ca ratios. It is possible that the relatively large differences between Ba and Ca prohibit clear relationships between Ba/Ca ratios in various trophic levels. The possibility remains that Ba cannot replace Ca in organisms, which Sr, on the contrary, to a certain extent can.

B.2. Experimental

The concentrations of Ba were measured using ICP-AES at 455.3 nm. The reproducibility of the analysis was tested by multiple analysis of a series of reference samples. The average standard deviation in the Ba determinations was less than 2%. The reference samples St I and St II yielded coefficients of variation of 1.8% (n=6) and 1.3% (n=9).

B.3. Results and discussion

B.3.1. General

Mean Ba concentrations in humans and in animal species are presented in table VII.1. Mean values range from 194 mg Ba/kg bone ash in humans to 294 mg/kg in dogs. A conspicious feature of the results are the high coefficients of variation which range from 35 to 52 %. For Ba concentrations, we have little information on variations in living populations. However, samples of fresh cattle bones yielded much lower variation coefficients (tabel VII.2).

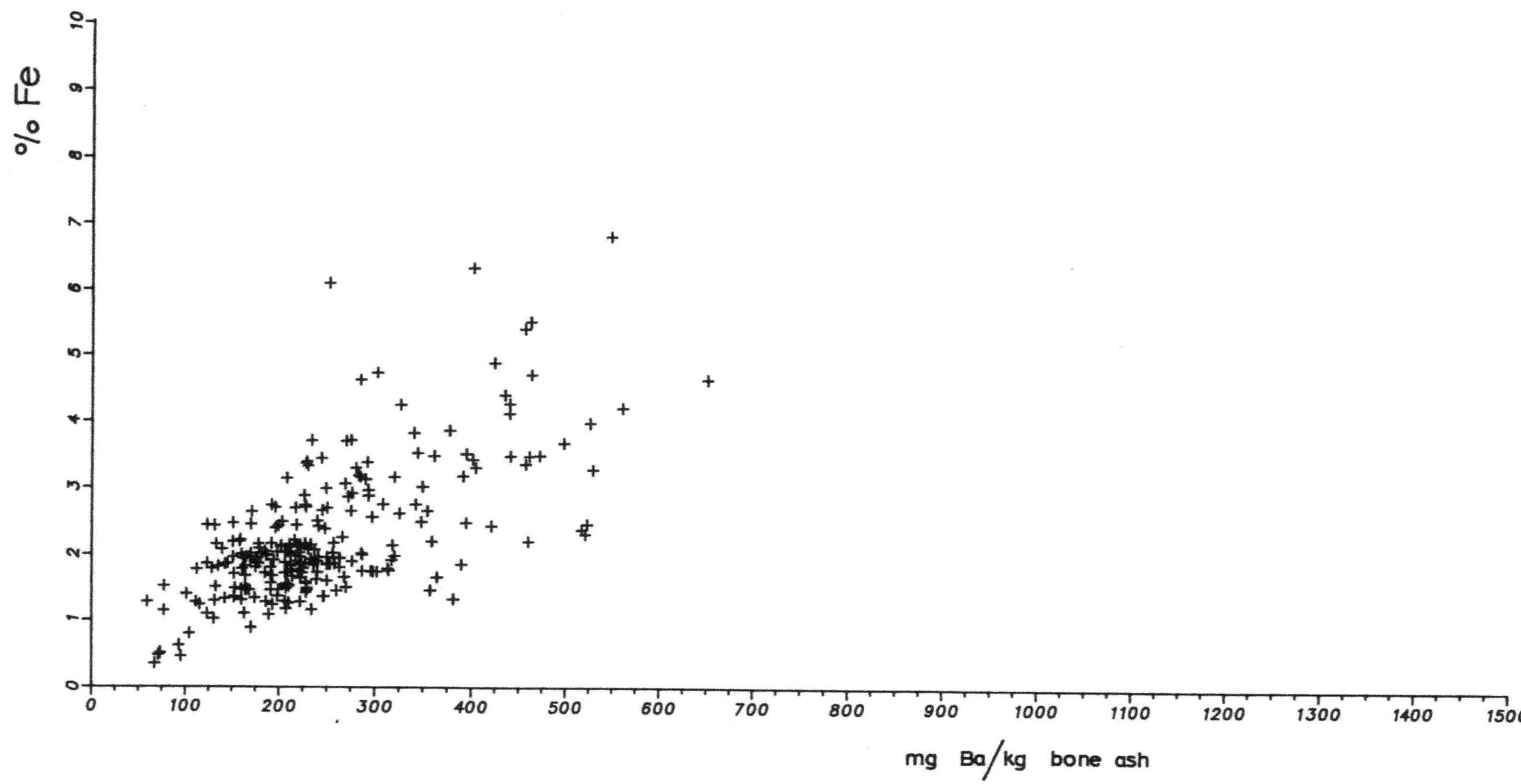

figure VII.1 Scattergram of Ba and Fe concentrations of the Bronze Age samples.

Table VII.1. Barium concentrations in human and animal bones. Mean values and standard deviation in mg/kg bone ash for all sites. Identical letters in the column 'significance' indicate that the values do not differ significantly (Student's t-test, 99% level). In the last column, mean concentrations are expressed as % of mean concentrations in cattle bone.

species	n	mean	SD	CV(%)	significance	rel. to cattle
human *	80	194	101	52	A	89
cattle	145	217	94	43	A B	100
pig	37	251	89	35	B C	116
sheep/goat	44	268	120	45	C	124
dog	36	294	142	48	C	135

* only long bones

Published data suggest that Ba concentrations in bone may become altered diagenetically (Lambert et al. 1984). The Ba and Fe concentrations in bones appear to be correlated in the material from West-Friesland (figure VII.1). This suggests that Ba concentrations have been altered in the soil. Use of Ba concentrations in a paleoecological and paleodietary discussion is, therefore, hazardous. All the same, the Ba concentrations in human and animal bones will be discussed briefly.

Table VII.2. Barium concentrations in fresh cattle bones, mg Ba/kg bone ash.

sample	sex	age (years)	n	mean	SD	CV(%)
IVO 1-10	male	1.5	10	97	26	27
IVO 11-20	female	8-10	10	156	40	26
AA 1-6	female	2-3	6	128	31	24
AA 7	male	1.5	1	185		
AA 8-9	female	5-5.5	2	97		

B.3.2. Barium in animal bones

Mean Ba concentrations in animal bones are presented in table VII.3 and VII.4. Within the sites the coefficients of variation are smaller than in the overall means (table VII.1).

Barium concentrations relative to those in cattle were calculated (table VII.3 and VII.4) and plotted (figure VII.2). Figure VII.2 does not show a particularly clear pattern in relative Ba concentrations, as figures V.3 and VI.2 do for relative Sr and Zn concentrations, respectively. The Ba concentrations in the animal species from each site are fairly close to each other. The different pattern for Zwaagdijk can be interpreted as an indication that Ba levels have been altered diagenetically. Cattle bones from Zwaagdijk combine low Ba contents with low Fe contents. This suggests that the Ba levels in the other bones from Zwaagdijk may have been increased by contamination with Ba from the soil.

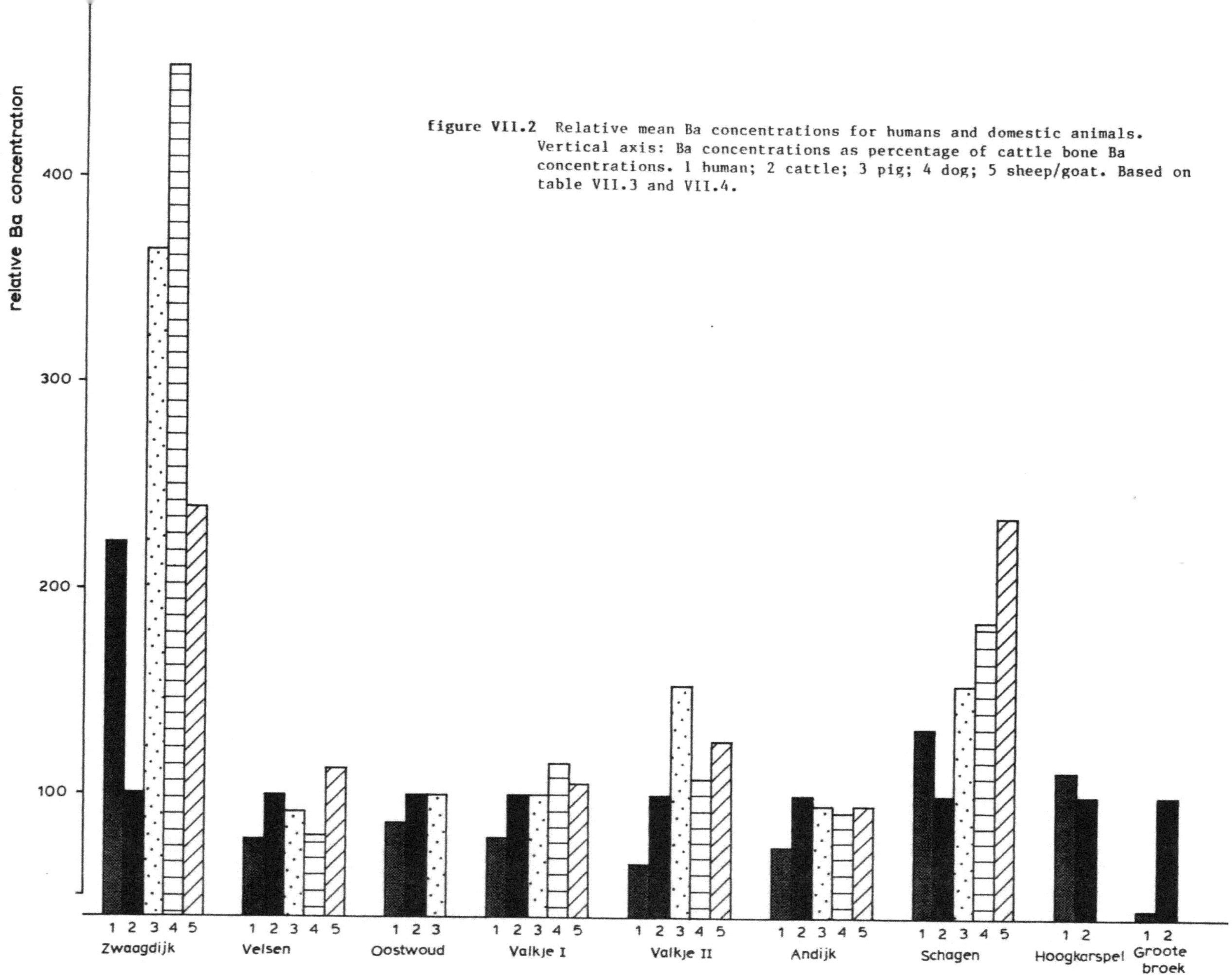

figure VII.2 Relative mean Ba concentrations for humans and domestic animals. Vertical axis: Ba concentrations as percentage of cattle bone Ba concentrations. 1 human; 2 cattle; 3 pig; 4 dog; 5 sheep/goat. Based on table VII.3 and VII.4.

Table VII.3. Barium concentrations in animal bones from the larger sites. Concentrations (mean and SD) in mg/kg bone ash. In the last column, the Ba concentrations are expressed as percentages of those in cattle bones.

site	species	sex	n	mean	SD	CV	relative to cattle
Valkje Early	cattle	both	18	215	42	20	100
	cattle	fem.	8	217	58	27	101
	cattle	male	10	214	21	10	100
	pig		8	214	37	17	100
	dog		9	249	104	42	116
	sheep/goat		10	228	66	29	106
Valkje Late	cattle	both	14	225	66	29	100
	cattle	fem.	8	215	53	25	96
	cattle	male	6	239	78	32	106
	pig		7	346	41	12	154
	dog		5	242	90	37	108
	sheep/goat		5	286	55	19	127
Andijk	cattle	both	20	268	49	18	100
	cattle	fem.	10	263	41	16	98
	cattle	male	10	274	55	20	102
	pig		7	254	22	9	95
	dog		2	247			92
	sheep/goat		10	251	77	31	94
Schagen	cattle	both	32	148	50	34	100
	cattle	fem.	14	139	42	30	94
	cattle	male	12	161	60	38	109
	pig		9	230	126	55	155
	dog		7	276	112	41	186
	sheep/goat		11	349	183	52	236

The strong suspicion of diagenetic influences, of which the relatively large standard deviations and the absence of differences between Ba levels in the domestic animal species are symptoms, renders the Ba concentrations in animal bones unsuitable for paleoecological extrapolation.

Table VII.4. Barium concentrations (mean and SD) in mg/kg bone ash. In the last column the Ba concentrations are expressed as percentages of those in cattle bones.

site	species	n	mean	SD	CV(%)	relative to cattle
Zwaagdijk	cattle	6	79	11	14	100
	pig	3	274	85	31	365
	dog	2	374			473
	sheep/goat	3	189	16	8	239
Velsen	cattle	10	209	55	26	100
	pig	2	190			91
	dog	2	167			80
	sheep/goat	5	236	43	18	113
Oostwoud	cattle	7	319	104	33	100
	pig	1	320			100
Westwoud	cattle	8	178	26	15	100
	pig	1	151			85
	dog	1	150			85
De Tent	cattle	5	315	104	33	100
	dog	1	517			164
Hoogkarspel	cattle	19	218	73	33	
Grootebroek	cattle	6	399	144	36	

B.3.3. Barium in human bones

Barium concentrations in human bones are collected in table VII.5. The 'other bones' which include ribs, vertebrae and skull bones in general have Ba concentrations that are higher than the long bones. No reference data on Ba levels in various skeletal elements are available. The rather large variations in relative Ba levels in 'other bones' suggest, however, that Ba levels were influenced by the soil condition. It is obvious that the Ba concentrations in 'other bones', which are rather porous and have comparatively large surface areas, will be affected more strongly than the long bones.

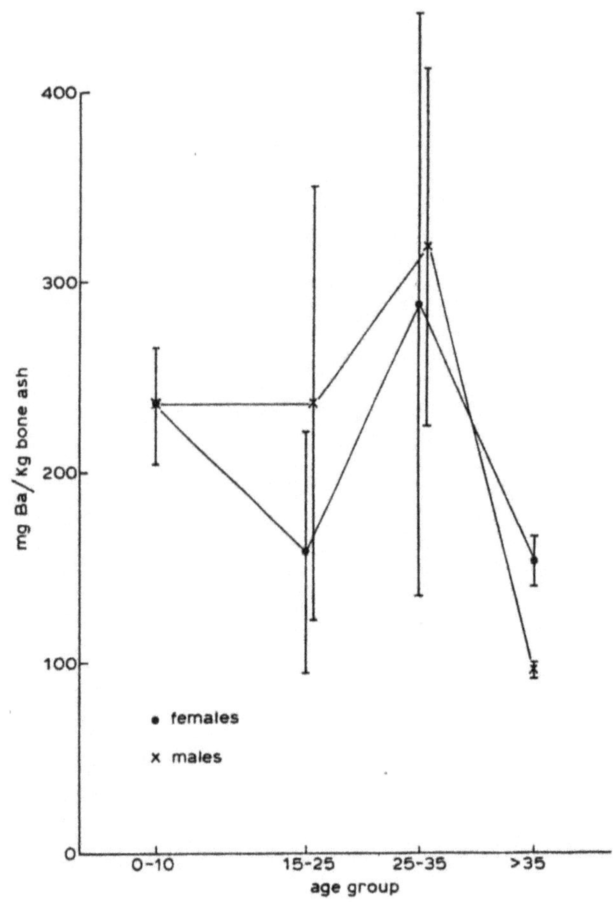

figure VII.3 Mean Ba concentrations (mg Ba/kg bone ash) and standard deviation in inhumations (n=29) grouped on the basis of age and sex. Based on table VII.6.

Table VII.5. Barium concentrations (mg Ba/kg bone ash) in human long bones and other bones from the sites in West-Friesland. In the last column, concentrations in other bones are expressed as percentage of those in long bones.

site	long bones n	mean	SD	CV(%)	other bones n	mean	SD	CV(%)	rel. %
Oostwoud	12	279	139	50	23	305	102	33	109
Zwaagdijk									
barrows	6	178	67	38	5	301	108	36	169
flat graves	4	143	43	30	3	243	19	8	170
Hoogkarspel									
barrow	2	112			1	151			135
settlement	11	241	133	55	3	227	1	0.4	94
Andijk	11	201	27	13	8	197	27	14	98
Het Valkje									
Early Period	9	166	38	23	7	160	57	35	96
Late Period	5	149	21	14	5	217	27	13	146
Grootebroek	3	187	21	11	1	313			167
Schagen-Mug	3	200	115	58	8	463	170	37	232
Velsen	6	164	35	21	5	179	28	16	109

Barium concentrations in age and sex groups of inhumations from West-Friesland (table II.10) were calculated (table VII.6) and plotted (figure VII.3). The variations of Ba levels within the groups are large, which may be the result of differences in soil Ba levels in the various sites from which the skeletons derive.

Males and females older than 35 years appear to have low Ba concentrations. The age groups 25-35 years apear to have relatively high mean Ba concentrations, but this is probably a result of geographical bias.

Table VII.6. Barium concentrations in groups of inhumations from barrows and flat graves. Mean and SD in mg Ba/kg bone ash.

sex	age	n	mean	SD	CV(%)
??	<10	4	235	30	13
female	15-25	5	158	63	40
	25-35	4	288	153	53
	>35	3	153	13	8
male	15-25	6	236	114	48
	25-35	5	318	94	30
	>35	3	96	4	4

B.4. Conclusion

The analysis of Ba concentrations in human and animal bones from Bronze Age West-Friesland apparently yields little information of value to paleoecological and paleodietary problems. The use of Ba in such studies is limited by two major problems. Firstly, Ba concentrations in bones seem to be prone diagenetic influences, which makes the Ba concentrations in excavated bones suspect in many cases.

The second major problem in the use of Ba in paleoecological studies is the lack of knowledge on relationships between concentrations in food and bone, or, more generally, on trophic level effects on Ba concentrations. As a result of diagenetic processes, the analyses of the bones from West-Friesland fail to yield 'patterns' in the Ba concentrations in the various animal species. Such patterns might have suggested possible discrimination processes in the food chain.

C. LEAD

C.1. Introduction

The influence of lead on past and present day societies has engendered considerable interest of late (for example, Bellow 1982, Nriagu 1983a). The adverse effects of Pb from car exhausts and other sources on psychological and intellectual capacities of children and other ecological effects of Pb have been studied (Underwood 1977, Holdgate 1979). Programs to reduce emission of Pb into the ecosphere, such as the introduction of Pb-free car fuels, are in progress. In addition to present day Pb pollution the possibility of Pb pollution and Pb poisoning in Roman times and its relation to the decline of the Roman Empire has attracted attention (Gilfillan 1965, Nriagu 1983a, b). For our study, the discussion on this subject is not very relevant but the information on high Pb concentrations in Roman food items (Nriagu 1983a, b) is of use in the interpretation of Pb concentrations in bones from Roman and native contexts.

Natural Pb levels in soil, water and air are usually very low, and nowadays the major part of Pb in foods probably derives from man-made pollution. This makes recent data on Pb contents of foods less useful for paleodietary purposes. It is to be expected that in prehistoric periods foods were very poor in Pb.

Lead is a typical bone-seeker which means that about 90% of the body burden of Pb is present in the skeleton (Underwood 1977). Relatively high Pb concentrations are found in the liver and other organs whereas muscle tissue has the lowest Pb concentrations (Underwood 1977). Vegetable foods will therefore probably have higher Pb concentrations than muscle meat. Plant roots have relatively high Pb concentrations compared to the shoot as a result of the limited mobility of Pb in plants (De Haan & Zwerman 1976, Underwood 1977).

Lead uptake from the digestive tract is strongly influenced by the concentrations of other elements (Ca, P, Fe, Zn, Cu) and by the Fe status of the individual concerned (J.L. Smith 1976). Lead uptake from food is negatively correlated with Ca/Pb ratios in the intestinal tract. High dietary Pb levels cause a rise in bone Pb levels, even though the levels in muscle tissue remain low (Underwood 1977). Children may take up some 50% and adults about 1-10% of ingested Pb (J.L. Smith 1976, Holdgate 1979). Tissue Pb concentrations increase with age because the uptake of Pb generally exceeds the excretion (Underwood 1977, Drasch 1982). Hodge (1981) mentions a value of 0.6 mg Pb intake per day above which the uptake exceeds excretion. No data on differences in Pb turnover in males and females are available.

In pre-Roman contexts, differences in bone Pb concentrations may be related to dietary habits which involve the consumption of certain food items, such as organ meat and root crops. The interactions with other elements may bias the interpretation of bone Pb concentrations. The natural differences in Pb concentrations will be surpassed by differences due to contamination once Pb compounds or metallic Pb comes into use, for instance in the form of leaden food and wine containers, cooking utensils and water piping. The contamination of drinking water with Pb as a result of leaden water pipes is considered to be slight and dependent on hardness of the water (Hodge 1981), but foods prepared or stored in leaden utensils can contain high amounts of Pb (Gilfillan 1965, Nriagu 1983a).

Uptake of Pb from the lungs may be of importance. Much of the inhaled Pb dust or fumes is deposited in the lungs and becomes incorporated in the body (Holdgate 1979). Industrial activities involving Pb smelting can therefore result in high levels of Pb in bone.

Lead concentrations in prehistoric and historic bones have been analysed in a number of cases (Gilfillan 1965, Mackie et al. 1975, Waldron 1982, Drasch 1982). Diagenetic changes of Pb levels may occur (Drasch 1982, Waldron 1983), though in other cases the Pb concentrations in bone appear to be relatively unaltered (Waldron et al. 1976, Rogers & Waldron 1985).

C.2. Experimental

Lead concentrations in bone ash solutions were measured using AAS with background correction at 283.3 nm in an air-acetylene flame. Lead concentrations in over 100 human and animal bone samples and some 30 soil samples were measured. No duplicates were analysed except for some reference samples. At an earlier stage Pb levels were (inaccurately) measured using AAS without background correction.

C.3. Results and discussion

Lead concentrations in most of the solutions were too low to allow for accurate AAS measurements. The concentration below which readings were unreliable corresponds with a concentration of circa 25 mg Pb/kg bone ash. Lead levels in the majority of the bones are lower than 25 mg/kg bone ash, corresponding to less than 20 mg Pb/kg bone on dry weight basis. No reliable comparisons between Pb levels in humans and various animals can therefore be made. The Pb concentrations in the West-Frisian bones are comparable to concentrations in human bones from a Neolithic barrow (Rogers & Waldron 1985), and slightly lower than levels in recent human ribs (a mean concentration of about 36 ppm was calculated by Waldron (1983) from 12 studies, see table VII.7). Recent bonemeal, probably of animal origin, contained 1.5-8.7 ppm (n=20, Roberts 1983).

Only a few of over 100 bone samples have Pb concentrations higher than 30 mg/kg. The highest levels in Bronze Age bones were found in a bone from Grootebroek (30 mg/kg) and in two human bones from Hoogkarspel (mean 39 mg/kg). Rather higher Pb concentrations were found in some of the bones from Schagen-Muggenburg. A number of animal bones from this site were analysed, but in only five animals (two bulls, two pigs, a horse) were rather higher Pb concentrations found. The humans from Schagen-Muggenburg (n=2, 6 bone samples) show relatively high Pb levels (51 and 96 mg/kg in femurs). The three other humans present also have high Pb concentrations (results of inaccurate AAS measurements). The Pb concentrations are comparable with those in bones from Romano-British cemeteries (table VII.7, Mackie et al. 1975, Waldron et al. 1976), but are lower than the values for skeletons from the Cirencester cemetery (Waldron 1982).

The higher Pb levels in the Schagen bones may either directly or indirectly result from higher soil Pb levels. A study by Waldron (1983) strongly suggests that bones may take up Pb from the soil. Higher natural Pb levels in the Schagen soil, if present, would indirectly result in higher bone Pb levels via the food chain. The latter possibility appears unlikely in the light of the almost identical Pb levels in the subsoil in Schagen (22 mg/kg dry soil, n=4) and Bovenkarspel (24 mg/kg dry soil, n=8), the strong binding of Pb in the soil and low translocation rate of Pb in plants (De Haan & Zwerman 1976). In the settlement layer, Schagen has somewhat higher Pb concentrations than Bovenkarspel (40 $\pm$ 7 mg/kg, n=7 and 29 $\pm$ 9 mg/kg, n=9, respectively).

Table VII.7. Lead concentrations in recent bone samples (mg/kg dry bone) and in excavated bones from various sites.

site	period	part	n	mean Pb conc.	source
Hazelton	Neolithic	rib	11	14.3	Rogers & Waldron 1985
West-Friesl.	Bronze Age	various	46	<25§	this study
Gibson	Woodland	rib	86	34	Lambert et al. 1982
		femur	22	52.4	ibid.
Ledders	Woodland	rib	32	31	ibid.
		femur	2	43.4	ibid.
Cirencester	Roman	rib	109	301.1	Waldron 1982
		ulna	144	189.0	ibid.
York	Roman	rib	77	63.5	Mackie et al. 1975
Poundbury	Roman	rib	161	56	Waldron et al. 1976
Henley	Roman	rib	41	65.7	ibid.
Schagen	native/Roman	femur	2	74	this study
Virginia	AD 1670-1730	various	5	185$	Aufderheide et al. 1981
Virginia	AD 1670-1730	various	11	35#	ibid.
U.K.	recent	rib	31	34.5	Waldron et al. 1976
	recent	rib	??	c.36	Waldron 1983
USA	recent	bonemeal	20*	1.5-8.7	Roberts 1983

§ mg Pb/kg bone ash
$ mg Pb/kg bone ash, planter family
# mg Pb/kg bone ash, slaves
* 20 brands of bonemeal, probably produced from all sorts of animal bones

Contamination by soil Pb may have occurred in some of the bones, but because (1) only a few of the bones in Schagen have high Pb levels; (2) the minor difference between soil Pb levels in Bovenkarspel and Schagen; and (3) the general agreement between Pb concentrations in our samples and Pb concentrations in other recent and older bones (a mean concentration of 34 mg/kg not due to soil contamination was calculated for a mediaeval site, Waldron 1985), we may conclude that the measured Pb concentrations to a large extent represent ante-mortem bone Pb levels. An exception to this are probably the Pb concentrations in the more porous bones (ribs, vertebrae) which are the highest of all (157 and 176 mg/kg in rib compared with 51 and 96 mg/kg in femur in **59** Mug 81 and 82 respectively; 157 mg/kg for a horse vertebra). In living humans, on the contrary, the concentrations of Pb in ribs are probably lower than in femurs (compare Drasch 1982). Interestingly, the bones studied by Waldron (1985) were ribs. In the Cirencester samples rib Pb concentrations were considerably higher than ulna Pb concentrations (Waldron 1982). This may be an indication of diagenetic alterations of bone Pb levels. Analyses of long bones should be preferred to analyses of ribs.

High Pb contents in Roman skeletons have been explained by contamination of their foods and beverages (especially wine) with Pb from containers and pipings (Nriagu 1983a, b). Schagen lies outside the Limes, but most likely had trade links with the Roman Empire (Therkorn, pers comm.).

Trade contacts between Romans and natives are evident from finds of, for example, Roman coins, pottery and statuettes north of the Limes (Van Es 1981, Woltering 1985). Trade in food products is often seen more or less uni-directional: native farmers supply the Roman army with cereals, meat (and hides) and salt in exchange for luxury products. The import of Roman luxury foods may have been underestimated. Wine and processed wine, i.e. defrutum, were probably much valued by the natives. Finds of wine barrels in (native)-Roman contexts are in evidence of wine trade (Van Es 1981, Bloemers 1978). Some of the pottery in native settlements was probably imported not for its own sake but because it happened to contain luxury foods. Wine and 'thick wine' in Roman times often contained considerable amounts of Pb (Nriagu 1983a,b).

A small experiment was carried out to test whether high Pb levels in imported Roman pottery could be measured. A number of sherds from imported and native pottery were placed in weak hydrochloric acid extraction solution in polyethylene bottles. Base and rim sherds were taken from seven pots. The Pb levels in the extraction solutions were determined using AA-BG. Different Pb levels in rim and base sherds would be indicative of contamination due to high Pb levels in the foods that had been stored and/or prepared in the pots.

The result of this experiment was negative. Lead concentrations in the extraction solutions were very low. Base sherds had slightly lower Pb concentrations than rim sherds. There were no differences between native and Roman pottery.

The result of the experiment can not be used as evidence against high Pb levels in the food in Schagen-Muggenburg, because we do not know how the Pb level in sherds is affected by a long period of contact with soil and the soil solution. Lead may have been leached out of the sherds in the soil. Further experiments might be useful.

It can be concluded that it is possible that Pb levels in the human bones from Schagen reflect the Roman influence on the diet, i.e. consumption of imported wine and food, in this settlement.

Fireplaces, (iron) slags, crucibles, coal and some small pieces of metallic Pb were found in the Muggenburg site (Therkorn 1984 and pers. comm.). These finds suggest 'industrial' (s)melting activities (Cordfunke & Diederik 1984). Coal is not suitable for smelting iron ore (Woltering 1985), but it may have been used in melting Pb or in glass production.

Lead was abundantly available in Roman times, being the by-product of silver extraction (Tylecote 1976, Hodge 1981). Considerable amounts of Pb were found in the Roman fortress and harbour at Velsen (Morel, pers. comm.). Natives from Schagen-Muggenburg may have brought Pb from Velsen or other Roman sites to their own settlement for use in some semi-industrial activity. Thus, an alternative explanation for the high Pb levels in bones might be the Pb pollution resulting from these activities.

Still another possible explanation for the high levels of Pb in the human bones from Schagen-Muggenburg might be that the interred individuals were retired auxiliaries who had served in the Roman military force. This alternative is, however, unlikely because one of the individuals with high Pb levels was a man aged 23-25 (**59** Mug 82). The women also had high Pb levels.

Four bones from a true Roman context, the cemetery near the Valkenburg castellum (Bult & Hallewas 1986, Hallewas 1986), were analysed. One femur yielded 28 mg Pb/kg bone ash, three others (inaccurately measured by AAS) have approximately comparable Pb concentrations. This value is closer to the Bronze Age Pb levels than to the values for Schagen. However, as the Romans usually cremated their death in this particular period, the femurs probably did not belong to Roman civilians, which would agree with the careless way in which the bodies were interred (Bult & Hallewas 1986, Hallewas 1986). In the Roman period, Pb poisoning was typically an aristocratic problem. Foods and wines of the lower classes had relatively low Pb concentrations (Nriagu 1983a,b). A correlation between social ranking and Pb intake remained present in historic times (Nriagu 1983b, Aufderheide et al. 1981).

The relatively high Pb levels in some of the pigs of Schagen-Muggenburg may be a consequence of the 'refuse collector' role of pigs. The somewhat higher Pb levels in two of the cattle bones will be discussed elsewhere (Therkorn & Runia, in prep.).

C.4. Conclusion

In pre-Roman contexts, levels of Pb in human bone are of little interest. In West-Friesland, the Bronze Age population had very low bone Pb concentrations.

In the site Schagen-Muggenburg, relatively high Pb levels were found in the human bones and in some animal bones. No unequivocal cause for these high Pb levels can be given, but the alternative causes discussed in section C.3. all suggest contacts with the Roman Empire in one form or another.

In the Roman period, Pb levels in human bones may yield useful indications on the status of individuals, and probably on trade contacts between the Roman Empire and native tribes, within or outside the Limes. Diagenetic influences on bone Pb levels should, however, be tested for.

D. ARSENIC

D.1. Introduction

Arsenic may be the most interesting among the elements that deserve further investigation in relation to their potential usefulness as palaeodietary indicators (Parker & Toots 1980). In the Periodic Table of the elements, As takes the place directly below P, which is comparable to the position of Sr in relation to Ca. In consequence of the resemblance in electronic configuration, P and As atoms will in general show comparable chemical behaviour. Arsenic occurs as a substitute in apatite minerals (McConnell 1973, Lindsay & Vlek 1977) and As/P ratios in bone will probably be affected only slightly during a long period of contact between soil and bone. No data on diagenetic influences on As contents of bones are, however, available.

Most foods contain small amounts of As, usually less than a few mg/kg fresh weight. Certain seafoods (prawns, shrimps) were found to have high As concentrations (up to 100 mg/kg and more), and seafish contains 2-8 mg As/kg (Schroeder & Balassa 1966, Underwood 1977).
The As/P system differs from the Sr/Ca system in that As probably is an essential element (Underwood 1977), which Sr is not, and that As is not a typical 'bone seeker' as is Sr. Observed Ratios for the As/P system are not available. A sex-related difference in As metabolism might be inferred from data in Underwood (1977). Males have significantly higher As concentrations in hair than females (though this may be a result of environmental factors) and in experiments with rats the males were more strongly affected by low As intakes than the females.

Still another aspect of As is its role in early metallurgy. Many Cu ores used in the Copper and Bronze Age contained considerable amounts of As, and As is an important component of early Cu alloys (Tylecote 1976, Butler 1979). Upon heating, Cu ores may lose part of their As because of low boiling points of As oxydes (Schroeder & Balassa 1966, Tylecote 1976). High As levels in human bones may therefore in certain cases be related to Cu mining and manufacturing activities. Bone Cu levels are probably less useful in this respect because of the low uptake of pure Cu and Cu oxydes from the intestinal tract. Scheinberg & Sternlieb (1976) refer to a study of Cu levels in copper miners: despite chronic exposure to environmental Cu concentrations as high as 1 %, the miners had normal Cu levels in liver and serum.

In addition to the methodological limitations, such as the absence of OR values for the As/P system, a practical problem in the use of As is posed by the low concentrations in bone. Furthermore, ashing of the bones may influence As concentrations and As concentrations are difficult to measure using conventional AAS or ICP.

D.2. Experimental

Twenty samples of human and animal bones, ten from each period of Het Valkje were selected for As analyses. Arsenic concentrations in the bone ash solutions were measured using hydride-AAS by the Chemical Department of the ECN at Petten.

D.3. Results

Results of the analyses are given in table VII.8. It is uncertain whether or not any As was lost during the ashing of the bone powder. Together with the limited number of samples, this uncertainty precludes any definite conclusion on the usefulness of As in paleodietary studies here. All the same, the results will be discussed briefly. Further studies on bone As should investigate effect of ashing on As contents of bone and other materials.

Arsenic concentrations in the prehistoric bones are of the same magnitude as in a recent bonemeal (Roberts 1983). The As contents are not related to Fe, Sr or Zn contents of the bones.
Mean As concentrations in the bones are not significantly different in the Early and Late Period. Dogs and sheep/goat appear to have somewhat higher As levels than humans, cattle and pigs. One of the human bones displayed an exceptionally high As content. One can only speculate as to the cause of

this. It is unlikely to be the result of the consumption of seafood, because the Sr content is comparable to the other humans. The Zn concentration in this bone is rather high. A relation with Cu or bronze metallurgy in the West-Frisian context is unlikely. Schroeder & Balassa (1966) recollect having seen mountain people in the Alps eat native As, but this would appear to be unlikely in West-Friesland.

Table VII.8. Arsenic concentrations (mg As/kg in bone ash) in 20 bones samples from two periods of Het Valkje.

species	Early Period	Late Period
cattle	6	9
	25	25
pig	18	18
	10	24
dog	45	33
	11	47
sheep/goat	36	47
	54	72
human	8	29
	15	163

E. COPPER

E.1. Introduction

In plants and animals the essential elemant copper plays a role in a number of enzymes (Marschner 1983, O'Dell 1976, Underwood 1977, Jonxis 1983). Because Cu is used in metabolic processes it is activily treated by organisms (Scheinberg & Sternlieb 1976). This raises problems in establishing straightforward Observed Ratios for the Cu/Ca system. Besides, other divalent ions such as Ca, Zn and Mo compete with Cu in the uptake processes by plants and in the intestinal tracts of vertebrates (De Haan & Zwerman 1976, Underwood 1977). Only a limited part of ingested Cu is taken up by mammals. The uptake is influenced by a number of factors, such as concentrations of other elements, pH, chemical form of the Cu and the presence of chelating compounds such as phytate. Uptake of Cu in its almost pure metallic form and in the form of inorganic Cu compounds (oxydes) is very low (Underwood 1977).

The liver is the main storage organ of Cu and also important in Cu metabolism (Underwood 1977). During intra-uterine life, the foetus builds up a substantial Cu stock (Jonxis 1983). Nowadays, Cu is extensively used as a growth stimulator in stock-breeding as an additive to pig fodder (Scheinberg & Sternlieb 1976, Underwood 1977). Sheep are very sensitive to high Cu levels, which may lead to jaundice (Underwood 1977).

Clay particles and, especially, organic matter, bind Cu in soil, which decreases its mobility. As a result of the low mobility of Cu in plants relatively high Cu concentrations are found in the roots (De Haan & Zwerman 1976).

Almost all foods contain small amounts of Cu. Very low Cu concentrations are found in bread and milk. Rich in Cu are liver, marine crustaceans and shell fish, seafish, and nuts. Intermediate Cu concentrations are found in non-leafy vegetables, fruits and cereals. Upon milling and refining of cereals and flour, much of the Cu is lost.

Few data are available on the diagenetic influences on Cu concentrations in buried bones. Copper ions can probably replace Ca in the apatite crystal lattice (Lindsay & Vlek 1977). Copper was one of the elements analysed by Lambert et al.(1979) in a large number of Woodland bones. A mean concentration of 10.6 ppm in ribs was found. In children aged 0-3, the mean Cu concentration was higher than in older children and adults, of which the age groups have mean concentrations in the range of 7.7-8.9 mg/kg. This seems to reflect the ante-mortem Cu concentrations and may indicate that Cu concentrations were not substantially altered during burial. Lambert et al. (1984), however, concluded that Cu levels in ribs and femurs were not suitable for dietary reconstruction because of contamination with soil Cu.

E.2. Experimental

Copper concentrations in 20 bone ash solutions were measured using AAS. No duplicate samples were measured.

E.3. Results

Copper concentrations in the bones are low (mean 14.8 $\pm$ 9.0 mg/kg, n=18, range 5-31 mg/kg, one sample has 462 mg/kg). Mean value in the human bones (n=4) is 14 $\pm$ 7 mg/kg in bone ash, corresponding to about 11 mg/kg in dry bone. This value agrees fairly well with the concentrations found for Woodland sites by Lambert et al. (1979). The mean value in cattle bones (n=6) is 8 $\pm$ 6 mg/kg, and a dog has 24 mg Cu/kg bone ash. The slightly higher Cu content in human and dog bones in comparison to cattle bones may be caused by consumption of foods containing relatively large amounts of Cu (fish, liver and other organs) by dogs and humans. However, post mortem alterations in the bone Cu may have taken place. The number of analyses is too small to allow for a critical approach of this aspect.

VIII
TRACE ELEMENTS IN CREMATIONS

A. INTRODUCTION

Virtually no data exists on trace element concentrations in cremations (I. B.1.6). It was, therefore, thought useful to analyse a limited number of cremations from sites which also yielded bones for analysis (section II. D.4). In this chapter, the analysis of the cremations is discussed.

B. EXPERIMENTAL

Cremated bone was cleaned ultrasonically and dried as customary for the samples of non-cremated bone. The samples were dried at 105 ^{o}C and ashed at 750 ^{o}C to remove any residual organic matter present in the samples.
The further analytical procedure was identical to the procedure followed for non-cremated bone samples (chapter III).

C. RESULTS

Trace element concentrations were determined in samples from four sites: Grootebroek, Hoogkarspel, Schagen-Muggenburg and Valkenburg (Z-H) (section II. D.4). A synopsis of the results of the analysis is given in table VIII.1.

Table VIII.1. Results of analyses of samples of cremated bones from four sites. Concentrations in mg per kg ash, Ca/P ratio is atom/atom. Means, SD and CV (%) are given

site	n	Sr mean	Sr SD	Sr CV	Ba mean	Ba SD	Ba CV	Zn mean	Zn SD	Zn CV	Ca/P mean	Ca/P SD	Ca/P CV
Grootebroek	8	386	191	50	132	102	77	140	47	33	1.71	.07	4.1
Hoogkarspel	2	244			50			131			1.63		
Schagen-Mug.	7	177	121	69	20	21	109	46	41	90	1.68	.01	0.6
Valkenburg	4	128	23	17	21	27	131	33	28	85	1.69	.00	0.0
total	21	253	179	71	65	85	131	87	67	77	1.69	.05	3.0

The atomic Ca/P ratios of cremated bones are close to 1.67, the theoretical value for hydroxyapatite (section IV. B). Most of the Ca/P ratios lay within a narrow range close to this value. In combination with the mean Ca (37.61 $\pm$ 1.41 %, n=21) and P concentrations (17.31 $\pm$ 0.79 %, n=21), this indicates that practically no Ca or P was leached out, or deposited in the cremated bone. The Fe content is very low (mean 0.39 $\pm$ 0.41 %, n=21), and the white colour of most of the cremations also suggests that no contamination has taken place after burial.

A conspicuous feature of the results are the high coefficients of variation for the trace element concentrations. The variation is clearly higher than in non-cremated bones (chapter V-VIII). This may partly be an artifact of the analysis itself on account of the lower concentrations in cremated bones, but it is clear that much larger variations in trace element levels are found in cremations than in non-cremated bone.

D. DISCUSSION

Comparisons between trace element concentrations in burnt and non-burnt bones can be made in four sites. Incompletely cremated individuals are present in two of these, thus allowing an assessment of the results of burning and burial on trace element levels in bone mineral. The status of the bone samples, i.e. burnt or incompletely burnt, is determined from the external appearance.

The amount of organic matter still present in the samples is a good indication for the status of the samples. This amount is measured by heating the samples to 750 °C and determining the weight loss.

Table VIII.2. Comparison between trace element concentrations in samples of burnt and incompletely burnt bone from one individual, cat. **50**, site Hoogkarspel. Concentrations in mg per kg ash. The weight loss of the samples upon heating to 750 °C is given in the column '% loss'.

sample	status	% loss	Fe %	Sr mg/kg	Ba mg/kg	Zn mg/kg	Ca/P atomic ratio
B207-1	cremated	5.2	0.96	370	88	211	1.63
B207-2	charred	16.1	1.86	796	250	256	1.66

In table VIII.2 and VIII.3, concentrations in bone samples of two individuals each cremated to a different extent are compared. Considerable differences in Sr and Ba concentrations are present within the individuals. The concentrations of Zn appear to be less affected by the burning of the bone. In both individuals, the Sr and Ba levels are correlated with the percentage of weight loss. The burning of bone and the subsequent period in the soil apparently results in lower trace element concentrations.

Table VIII.3. As table VIII.2 for samples from one individual from Grootebroek, cat. **13.**

sample	status	% loss	Fe %	Sr mg/kg	Ba mg/kg	Zn mg/kg	Ca/P atomic ratio
G 2-1	cremated	5.0	0.22	319	87	233	1.70
G 2-2	cremated	11.6	0.96	532	172	149	1.87
G 2-3	charred	11.8	1.79	694	313	197	1.81

In table VIII.4, trace element levels in cremations are compared with levels in non-burnt bone from the same site by expressing the first as a percentage of the second.

The cremated bones have significantly lower concentrations of trace elements than the non-cremated bones from the same site. On the assumption

of approximately equal ante-mortem concentrations in the specimens involved, some explanation for this difference must sought. The difference might be the result of one or more of the following processes:
(1) the trace element levels of the non-cremated bone have increased since the burial of the bone;
(2) the trace element levels of the cremated bones have decreased since the burial of the cremated bones;
(3) during recrystallization of the hydroxyapatite upon cremation of the dead body, the trace element contaminations present in the original, small crystals were excluded from the new, large crystals.

Table VIII.4. Trace element levels in cremated human bone expressed as percentage of trace element levels in non-cremated human bone from the same sites. Based on data in table VIII.1 and sections V.C.4, VI.C.4 and VII.B.

site	n crem.	n bone	---conc. as % of conc. in bones--- Sr	Ba	Zn
Grootebroek	8	3	50	71	83
Hoogkarspel	2	11	25	21	68
Schagen-Mug	7	3	14	10	11
Valkenburg	4	4	16	38	21

The extent of the effect of the first of these processes may be assessed on the basis of the data on trace element concentrations presented in chapter V, VI and VII.B. Though some alterations of the concentrations, especially of Ba, in the bones may have occurred, the conclusion was that the levels of Sr and Zn in excavated bone are more or less representative of the ante-mortem trace element concentrations in the bone mineral.

The large hydroxyapatite crystals that are characteristic for cremated bone (section I.B.1.6) are more resistant against chemical attack in the ground than uncremated bone, leaving the second process unlikely to be the sole process responsible for the observed effects.

The marked variation in the concentrations of cremations when compared to the bones that which were buried under comparable circumstances and for a comparable period, are evidence in support of the third process. The burning of bone probably resulted in a range of trace element concentrations in the newly formed crystals. The concentrations in the new crystals probably depend on various parameters during the cremation such as temperature and amount of oxygen available. Interestingly, the highest variation in concentrations is found in Ba, which, of the three elements concerned, is the one which differs most from Ca in weight and size.

Still another indication for the feasibility of process (3) is the rather strong correlation between weight loss on heating to 750 °C (i.e. the amount of organic matter that was still present in the incompletely burnt bone), and the concentrations of Sr and Zn. For the eight samples from Grootebroek, which came from the femurs and skulls of four individuals, Sr, Ba and Zn concentrations were plotted against weight loss (figure VIII.1). For low concentrations of Sr and Ba, points are almost on a straight line. Coefficients of correlation are 0.96 for Sr and 0.82 for Ba (n=8). There is no correlation between concentrations and weight loss for Zn (coeff. of corr.

0.05), neither is there any correlation between skeletal element (femur or skull) on the one hand and trace element concentration and weight loss on the other.

We may assume that the weight loss reflects the circumstances under which the cremation took place. The weight loss can therefore be used as a measure for the alteration of the bone mineral. The correlation between weight loss and trace element levels suggests that the cremation of bone causes alterations which make it possible for trace impurities to be leached out of the bone. Besides being an indication for the circumstances of cremation, the remnants of the collagen which remain behind possibly act as a binding medium that protects the trace elements against leaching out. It is possible that the trace elements are adsorbed to the collagen remnants.

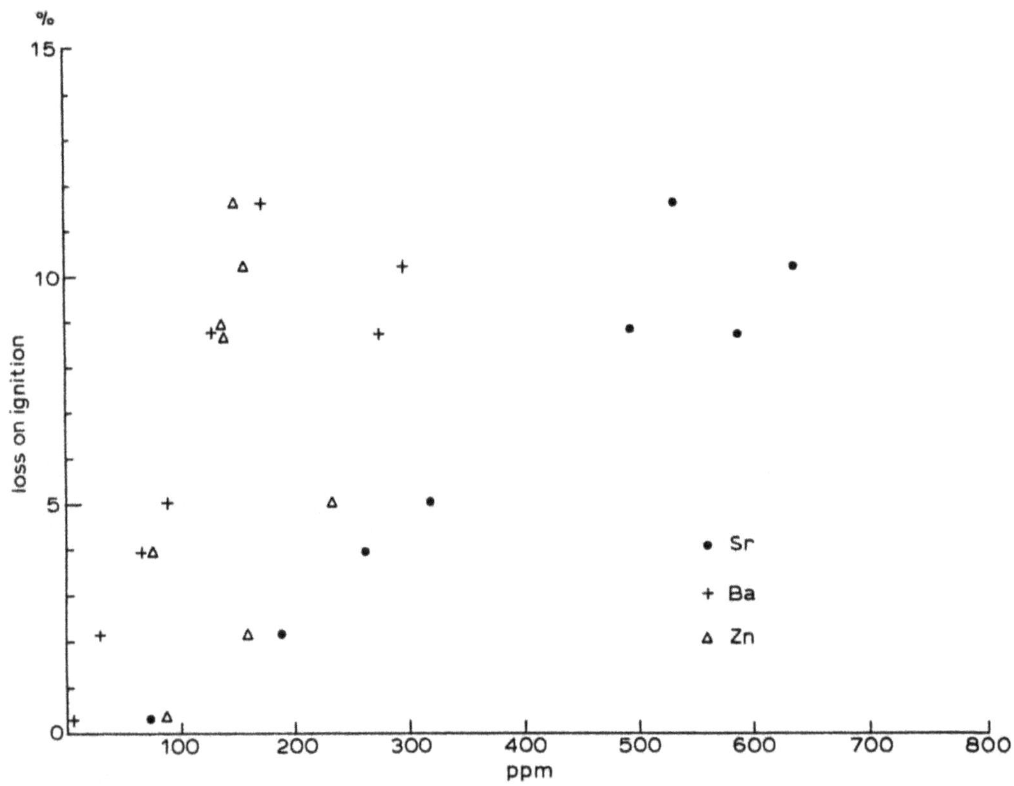

figure VIII.1 Correlation between trace element concentrations and organic matter content of 'cremated' bones from Grootebroek. Vertical axis: weight loss after heating to 750 °C; horizontal axis: concentration of trace elements in mg/kg bone ash.

Another indication for this process is the low relative mean concentration of trace elements in cremations from the Roman period. In the Valkenburg samples, due to 'explosion' of the samples in the furnace, no weight losses could be measured. The samples from Schagen-Muggenburg, upon heating to 750 °C lost a mean of 0.7 % weight, indicating that practically all organic matter had been burnt during the cremation. This, and the macroscopic appearance of the cremations suggest that they have been thoroughly burnt. The deviation from non-burnt bone trace element levels in these cremations is larger than in the cremations from the Bronze Age sites Grootebroek and Hoogkarspel (table VIII.4), which were not very well cremated, as indicated by the relatively large amount of organic matter still present.

E. CONCLUSION

Although only a small number of cremated bones were analysed, it is clear that cremated bones cannot be used to for dietary reconstruction with the present lack of knowledge concerning processes active during burning of bone and since the burial. The present-day concentrations of Sr and other trace elements in the cremations are probably the result of the processes acting on the bone during its burning and during the period of burial rather than a reflection of circumstances, including diet, before death. Because the hydroxyapatite fraction is still present in cremated bone although in altered form, this part of the study was started somewhat optimistically. Despite this first, negative result, it appears useful to investigate the effects of burning bone and of a long period of contact with soil on the trace element concentrations in the cremated bone. Experiments, for instance including leaching of freshly burnt bone, will be necessary.

IX
ANALYSIS OF SOIL AND PLANT MATERIAL

A. TRACE ELEMENTS IN THE SOIL

Analysis of soil samples in addition to the analysis of bone samples was considered necessary for a variety of reasons.

In the assessment of the diagenetic influences on bone trace and macro element levels, it appeared useful to (1) compare trace element levels in bones and surrounding soil; and (2) to compare the general levels of the ratios of trace elements and calcium in both bones and soils. Another reason for the analysis of soil samples was (3) the assessment of variations in trace element levels in various physiographic units. Furthermore, the contents of P and other elements in soil samples might give an indication as to possible manuring practices.

In the soil, Ca, Sr and Zn ions may be present in various states. Ions may be present in ionic form in solution, adsorbed on negatively charged soil particles or constituting part of a chemical/mineral compound. The state in which ions are present influences solubility, mobility and hence availability for plant roots. Between ions in various physico-chemical states, a dynamic thermodynamically determined equilibrium exists. After removal of ions, by leaching or by plant roots, the stock of easily available ions is re-supplied with ions from the stock of slowly soluble compounds.

In soil fertility studies, extraction techniques are commonly used to assess the ion quantities available to plants. In general, this amount comprises only a part of the total amount of ions in the soil, i.e. the fraction in solution and part of the adsorbed ions. Total element concentrations can be determined by using digestion techniques. The fraction determined by digestion techniques comprises all the ions present in the soil, including those in minerals and fixed on clay minerals.

For our study, total element concentrations were likely to be more useful than element concentrations in soil extracts. Bone, buried in the soil, is in fact part of the stock of phosphate minerals which are slowly soluble and not easily available to plants. Hence, concentrations in bone are better compared with total element concentrations. Furthermore, the relative concentrations in which Ca and Sr were avaliable for plants during the Bronze Age are a derivative of the then current total element concentrations in soil, which may in turn be derived from present-day total Sr/Ca ratios.

In soils, the concentrations of ions in solution, X_s and Y_s, are in equilibrium with the ions adsorbed at negatively charged sites of soil particles, X_a and Y_a, according to:

$$X_a / Y_a = k \times (X_s / Y_s)$$

The value of k depends on the radius of ions X and Y, and specific characteristics of the adsorbent and adsorbing environment (Bolt & Bruggenwert 1976). For the ion pair Sr and Ca the value of k is approximately 1.2 (Frissel et al. 1981), which indicates that Sr is adsorbed more strongly than Ca. For the ion pair Zn and Ca, the value may be slightly lower than 1, which would mean that Zn is somewhat less strongly adsorbed than Zn.

B. ANALYSIS OF SOIL SAMPLES

B.1. Experimental

Air-dry soil samples were dried at 105 °C and were ground and mixed in an agate mortar. Approximately 0.25-0.30 g of soil was weighed accurately into PTFE pressure vessels and digested with 7 ml of a mixture of concentrated HNO_3 - HF - $HClO_4$ (50:30:2.5) (6 hrs, 175 °C). After digestion, mixtures were transferred to PTFE evaporation dishes and on a hot plate evaporated to dryness. 3 ml of concentrated nitric acid was added and the mixture again evaporated to dryness. The residual 'soil cake' was resoluted in 7 ml of a 6:1 mixture of concentrated HNO_3 and HCl, transferred to polythene bottles and gravimetrically diluted to 100 ml.

Concentration measurements were carried out as with the bone ash solutions, i.e. Sr concentrations were measured using ICP-AES, Ca and Zn using AAS.

With the exception of five samples, no duplicates were analysed. Mean difference between concentrations in each of the five duplicates is, for Ca 3.4 %, for Sr 2.9 % and for Zn 4.7 %.

B.2. The soil samples

Soil samples were taken from two sites. Firstly, the 1984 excavation of Schagen-Muggenburg provided an opportunity to take soil samples near buried human and animal skeletons. Some soil around and below a dog skeleton was sampled. From a human skeleton (**59** Mug 4), soil in contact with skull and pelvis was collected. Besides this, samples from the light-grey clayey subsoil were taken some 0.2 m below the occupation layer.

Secondly, samples were collected from three physiographic units near the site Het Valkje. In the 'Archeological Monument' near Bovenkarspel, situated just south of the area excavated by the ROB (section II.C.2.6), the land has not been realloted. Here, soil samples from various horizons, e.g. the dark habitation layer and the subsoil, were collected using a hand operated soil auger.

B.3. Results

The results of the analysis of soil samples from Bovenkarspel- Monument are summarized in table IX.1. A preliminary discussion of some of these results is given in Runia (1987a).

Table IX.1. Results of analysis of soil samples from Bovenkarspel-Monument. Concentrations of Ca in mg/g dry soil, Zn and Sr as mg/kg dry soil. Units A, B and D correspond with fig. II.5.

soil unit	n	Ca	Sr	Zn	P
A. ridge: sand	4	37.7 ± 13.5	178 ± 60	41.6 ± 21.2	0.4 ± 0.2
B. ridge: sandy loam	8	60.1 ± 12.7	239 ± 41	40.0 ± 21.9	1.3 ± 0.9
D. basin: clay	5	62.4 ± 11.8	216 ± 17	74.6 ± 7.4	0.5 ± 0.2

The results of analysis of soil samples from Schagen-Muggenburg are presented in table IX.2. Soil samples from the 'occupation layer' were taken from the dark soil horizon in which the artifacts and habitation traces were found at some distance from interred skeletons. According to Therkorn (1985), this layer is the remnant of a thicker layer of peat that has been oxidized. Soil samples 'in contact with bone' were taken from a human skull and from underneath a human pelvis and a dogs' vertebral column. Calcium and Sr concentrations in Schagen are lower, Zn concentrations are higher than in the Monument samples.

Table IX.2. Results of analysis of soil samples from Schagen-Muggenburg. Concentrations of Ca and P in mg/g dry soil, Sr and Zn in mg/kg dry soil.

soil unit	n	Ca	Sr	Zn	P
occupation layer	3	9.5 ± 2.2	93.7 ± 5.3	93.0 ± 8.5	0.6 ± 0.1
soil next to bone	3	11.1 ± 0.9	131.3 ± 23.6	110.0 ± 13.4	2.5 ± 1.1
subsoil	4	4.6 ± 1.6	67.5 ± 5.5	65.8 ± 7.8	0.3 ± 0.1

B.4. Discussion

B.4.1. Bovenkarspel-Monument

In Runia (1987a) the analysis of soil samples was used in testing a hypothesis on herding practices in Het Valkje. Contrary to expectations, the sandy creek ridges appeared to have higher soil Sr/Ca ratios than the clayey basins (table IX.3). However, as a result of differential leaching of Sr and Ca, the present-day Sr/Ca ratios may differ from the ratios present during the Bronze Age occupation. Figure IX.1 was used to illustrate the relation between Ca content of the soil, the Cation Exchange Capacity (CEC) and Sr/Ca ratios. Soils with a low CEC, i.e. sandy soils, show a relatively strong decline in Sr/Ca ratio with decreasing Ca contents.

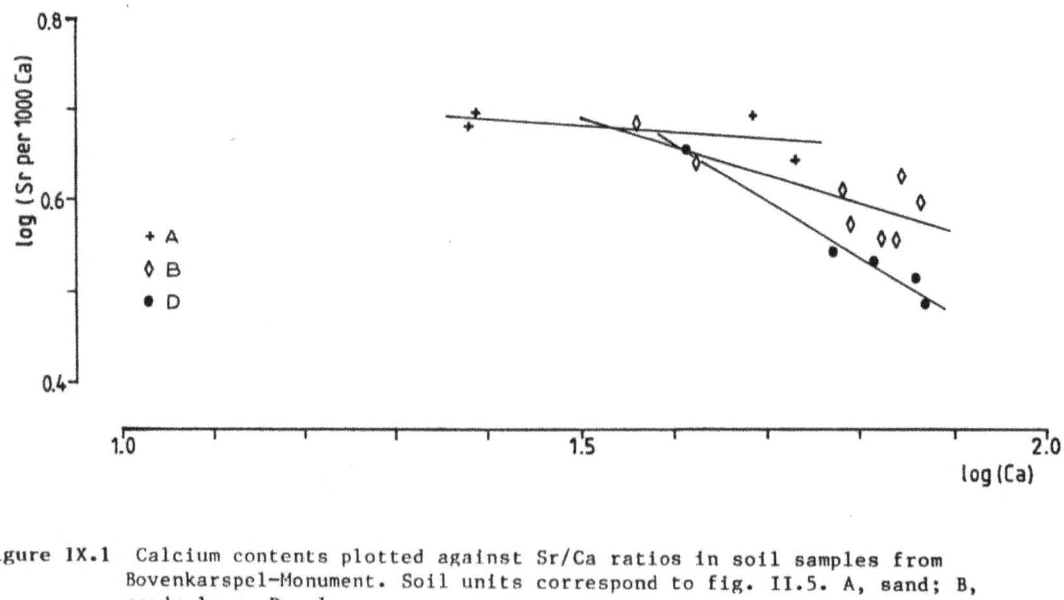

figure IX.1 Calcium contents plotted against Sr/Ca ratios in soil samples from Bovenkarspel-Monument. Soil units correspond to fig. II.5. A, sand; B, sandy loam; D, clay.

Interestingly, as far as Zn/Ca ratios are concerned, the relation between Ca contents and Zn/Ca ratios is different (figure IX.2). As stated above, contrary to Sr, Zn is probably somewhat less strongly adsorbed on negatively charged soil particles than Ca. This difference Zn and Ca may, however, be too small to explain the observed pattern.

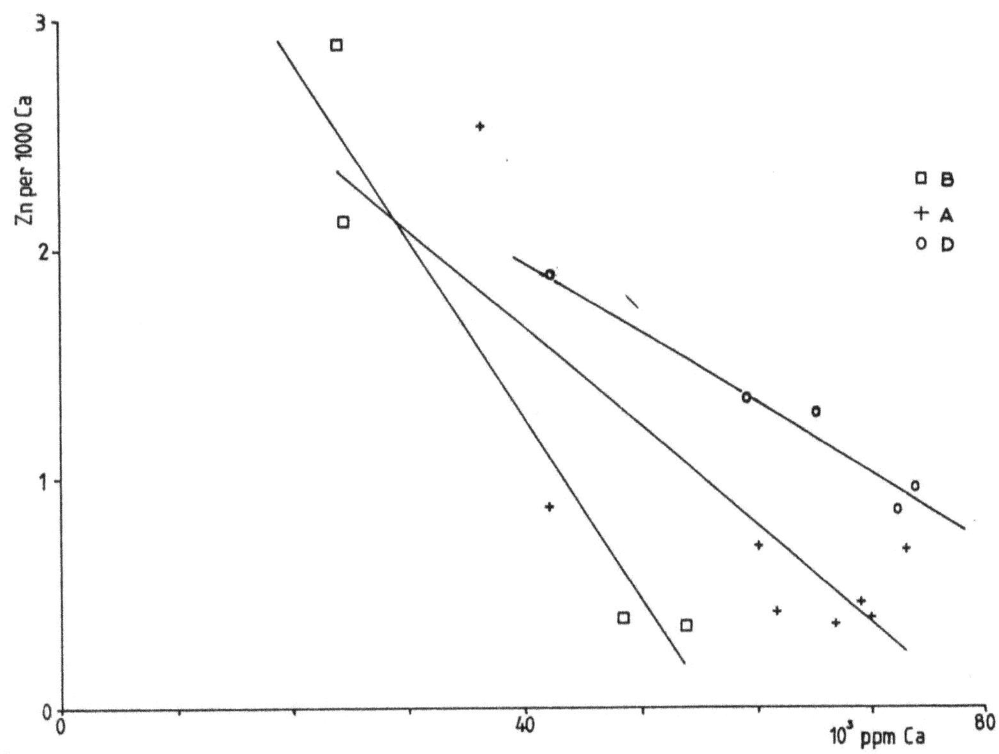

figure IX.2 Calcium contents plotted against Zn/Ca ratios in soil samples from Bovenkarspel-Monument. Soil units correspond to fig. II.5. A, sand; B, sandy loam; D, clay.

Table IX.3. Sr/Ca and Zn/Ca ratios (mg/g) and atomic ratio Ca/P in soil samples from Bovenkarspel-Monument. Units correspond to those in table IX.1. Means ± standard deviation.

soil unit	n	Sr/Ca	Zn/Ca	Ca/P
A. sand	4	4.8 ± 0.2	1.4 ± 1.1	118.4 ± 79.7
B. sandy loam	8	4.1 ± 0.4	0.8 ± 0.7	66.9 ± 50.9
D. clay	5	3.6 ± 0.5	1.3 ± 0.4	116.2 ± 47.1

As an alternative to the presented model, an option that should be discussed includes the effects of manuring practices on element concentrations in the soil. The relative concentrations of the elements in the occupation layer and the subsoil are given in table IX.4. The number of samples is very small, but still some differences between the clayey basins and the ridges appear to be present. In the basin, the occupation layer has low Zn and P contents and relatively high Ca and Sr contents. The high P contents of prehistoric habitation soils is well known (Arrhenius 1931). The data in table IX.4 suggest that P was removed from the pasture and meadow in the basins, and deposited on the ridges where the arable fields were located. The same effect is registered for Zn . The relative Ca and Sr concentrations, however, show opposite trends and remain puzzling in this model. The differences in Ca and Sr concentrations are, however, relatively small: the percentages in table IX.4 do not deviate much from 100%. For Zn and P, the effect is much stronger.

Table IX.4. Comparison of element concentrations in subsoil and occupation layer. Concentrations and ratios in the occupation layer as percentages of values for the subsoil. Units correspond to table IX.1.

	--- n samples ---		---occupation layer as % of subsoil---						
unit	subsoil	occ.layer	Ca	Sr	Zn	P	Sr/Ca	Zn/Ca	Ca/P
A+B	5	6	65	62	247	276	112	458	22
D	2	3	129	110	88	57	82	66	219

One or both of these processes may have been operative. In both cases, a gradual increase of Zn concentrations in the occupation layer on the ridges (units A and B) can be inferred. Zinc levels in the upper soil layers of the basin (unit D) would have been decreased. This may be of interest in relation to the observed differences between the Zn levels in bones from the Early and Late Period of Het Valkje. This aspect is discussed more extensively in chapter XI.

Theoretically, the ratio (Sr/Ca in herbivorous animal bone) / (Sr/Ca in the soil solution) has a value of approximately 0.25 (section V.A.2). This approximation is based on the Observed Ratios body-diet and plant-soil, which according to laboratory experiments have average values of 0.20-0.25 and 1, respectively (section V.A.2, IX.C), but to date has not been verified in actual field situations. As a consequence of the relatively strong adsorption of Sr, the Sr/Ca ratios in the soil solution are lower than overall soil Sr/Ca ratios. The ratio (Sr/Ca in herbivorous animal bone) / (overall Sr/Ca ratio in soil) is, therefore, less than 0.25 .
In the present situation, the cattle bone Sr/Ca ratios (mean 2.82 mg Sr/g Ca, n=32) and total soil Sr/Ca ratios (for the ridges, mean 4.29 $\pm$ 0.49 mg Sr/g Ca, n=12) differ by a factor 0.66, which is higher than the theoretical value of less than 0.25.

B.4.2. Schagen-Muggenburg

Concentrations of trace and macro elements in soil in contact with bone differ from the other settlement layer soil samples. Strontium and Zn concentrations are relatively high in the soil in contact with the bone. However, Sr/Ca and Zn/Ca ratios are no different from soil not in contact with bone.
Phosphorus concentrations in the soil in contact with bone are significantly higher, and Ca/P ratios significantly lower than in the other samples from the settlement layer. This might indicate that more P than Ca (and Sr) migrates from the bone to the soil. This corroborates the Ca/P ratios of the bones that are slightly higher than fresh bone Ca/P ratios (chapter IV).

Table IX.5. Sr/Ca and Zn/Ca ratios (mg/g) and atomic ratio Ca/P in soil samples from Schagen-Muggenburg. Means ± standard deviation.

sample from	n	Sr/Ca	Zn/Ca	Ca/P
occupation layer	3	10.4 ± 1.7	10.3 ± 2.3	11.4 ± 1.8
soil in contact with bone	3	11.8 ± 2.1	10.0 ± 2.0	4.7 ± 2.8
subsoil	4	16.2 ± 3.8	15.5 ± 3.3	14.2 ± 3.8

For Schagen-Muggenburg, mean Sr/Ca ratio in cattle bones is 3.37 ± 0.49 (n=32). For the occupation layer, this ratio is 10.4 ± 1.7 (n=3). These values differ by a factor 0.32, which is relatively close to the theoretical value of less than 0.25.

B.5. Conclusions

The number of soil samples was relatively small. Conclusions should therefore be considered tentative.

The macro and trace element contents of soil samples compared with the results of bone analysis suggest that diagenetic changes are small.

The differences between the physiographic units near Het Valkje are somewhat problematical. The mechanism responsible for the differences between subsoil and occupation layer remains obscure. The discussed mechanisms, i.e. a physico-chemical and an anthropogenous model cannot be rejected and may have been operative simultaneously. Still, the observed differences may be used in a discussion on herding practices (section XI.B).

C. STRONTIUM/CALCIUM RELATIONSHIPS IN PLANTS

Plants form the basis of terrestrial food chains. Herbivorous and to a lesser extent, omnivorous animals depend on plants as their source of minerals. In view of the elaborate and fastidious feeding habits of herbivorous animals (section V.A), differences in mineral contents between plants and plant parts will be reflected in the mineral intakes of the animals. The question of food choice in man and animals in connection with palaeodietary studies is treated in chapter XI. Here, Sr and Ca distribution patterns in plants will be discussed.

Different expressions may be used to describe the relationship between the Sr/Ca ratios in soil and various plants and plant parts. Comar et al. (1957) defined the Observed Ratio

OR = (Sr/Ca ratio in sample)/(Sr/Ca ratio in precursor), which is commonly used in Sr studies. In many cases in which it is used, the term 'Observed Ratio' fails to express its meaning: ORs often are not observed but are calculated from other data. For plant material, Menzel & Heald (1955, 1959) used the 'distribution factor' which is mathematically equal to the Observed Ratio. For plant material we are mainly concerned with differences in the distribution of Sr and Ca in plants and not, as in animals, with discrimination against Sr. When comparing Sr/Ca ratios in plant parts, there is no 'sample' and 'precursor' in the sense of the definition of the OR. Therefore, the term 'Distribution Ratio' ('DR') was proposed as an alternative for the term 'Observed Ratio' (Runia 1987b). The DR is, in fact, mathematically equal to the OR, but intended for use in the comparison of Sr/Ca ratios in any tissue or growth medium (Runia 1987b). Throughout the present work, the term DR is used for plant material.

In papers on the reconstruction of the diet of (pre)historic societies the differences in Sr/Ca ratios in plants species and plant parts are generally considered to be negligible (Sillen & Kavanagh 1982, Price et al. 1985b). However, the existence of considerable differences of Sr/Ca ratios have been convincingly established in numerous experiments as is recognized by various authors (Martin et al. 1958, Russell 1966b, Russell & Newbould 1966, Wallace & Romney 1971, Isermann 1981). Comar et al. (1957:486) state that 'the available evidence thus points to the conclusion that little discrimination between the dietary Ca and Sr of man and animals occurs in its passage through plants'. However, these authors also stress that little information on Sr/Ca relationships in storage organs of plants is available. For paleodietary studies, this information is essential, because many of the vegetable foodstuffs consumed by man are either storage organs such as roots and tubers, or seeds and fruits in which sugars, starch and other compounds are stored.

The variation in Sr/Ca ratios in plants is expressed in the range of the Distribution Ratios brought together in table XI.6, (Runia 1987b). The DR's in table XI.6 are calculated from numerous experiments reported in the literature. In considering these DR's, awareness of the inherent limitations of the experiments they are based on is essential. Extraction procedures to establish the amounts of available Sr and Ca in soils result in no more than an approximation of the amounts actually available to plant roots. In greenhouse experiments (for instance, Collander 1941), limited rooting space in pots, and the often limited growth period may lead to uptake and distribution of Sr and Ca in a manner that differs from real field situations. In experiments involving radioactive tracers, dilution effects may play a role (for instance, Martin et al. 1958). Despite the limitations of some of the experiments, ample evidence is available for the conclusion that, in a given vegetation, considerable differences in Sr/Ca ratios in plants and plant parts exist.

Table IX.6. Selection of Distribution Ratios, calculated from published data : DR= (Sr/Ca ratio in x)/(Sr/Ca ratio in y), x and y indicating plant parts or growth media as given in the first column. Numerals in the column 'type' refer to the experiments the DR is based on: 1=field, 2=greenhouse pots with soil, 3=nutrient solution. In the experiments with soil, Sr and Ca were usually measured in alkaline ammonium acetate soil extracts. From Runia (1987b)

Distribution Ratio	value	species	type	reference
plant-nutrient sol.	0.74	various	3	Menzel & Heald 1959
plant-soil	1.16	various	1	Bowen & Dymond 1955
plant-soil	ca. 1	various	1	Menzel & Heald 1959
plant-soil	1.1 ± 0.07	legumes	1	Russell & Newbould 1966
plant-soil	1.2 ± 0.17	grasses	1	Russell & Newbould 1966
shoot-soil	0.70 ± 0.41	lucerne	2	Bowen & Dymond 1956
shoot-soil	0.74 ± 0.63	barley	2	Bowen & Dymond 1956
leaves-soil	0.95	various	2	Sanzharova 1978
shoot-nutrient sol.	0.90 ± 0.09	tomato	3	Bowen & Dymond 1956
plant-nutrient sol.	ca. 1	various	3	Collander 1941
root-nutrient sol.	2.28 ± 1.59	tomato	3	Bowen & Dymond 1956
shoot-root	0.52 ± 0.21	tomato	3	Bowen & Dymond 1956
shoot-root	0.57	barley	3	Martin et al. 1958
leaves-roots	0.30	cowpeas	3	Menzel & Heald 1955
leaves-roots	0.36	sunflower	3	Menzel & Heald 1955
leaves-roots	0.1	tobacco	3	Menzel & Heald 1955
leaves-roots	0.34	*Lycium* sp.	3	Wallace & Romney 1971
leaves-roots	0.43	*Lycium* sp.	3	Wallace & Romney 1971
leavy veg.s-roots	0.65	various	1	Bryant et al.1958 *
leaves-roots	3.7 ± 1.8	Brazil Nut	1	Smith 1971a #
endosperm-leaves	3.65 ± 0.89	Brazil Nut	1	Smith 1971a
leaves-twigs & bark	0.54 ± 0.14	various	1	Price et al.1985a **
grain-straw	0.84 ± 0.22	*T. vulgare*	1	Smith 1971b
grain-straw	1.05 ± 0.12	various	1	this paper
ears-leaves	1.26	barley	3	Martin et al.1958
grain-weeds	1.55 ± 0.36	various	1	this paper
grain-grain	1.34	*Triticum* spp	1	this paper
grain-grain	1.97	*Triticum* var	2	Smith et al.1963 $
grain-grain	1.62 ± 0.47	*T. vulgare*	1	Smith 1971b
grain-grain	1.11	*Hordeum* var.	1	this paper
grain-grain	2.07	*Hordeum* var.	2	Smith et al.1963 $
flour-whole grain	0.76 ± 0.10	*T.vulgare*	1	Smith 1971b

mean value for roots of two trees from two depths
* calculated from App.1, data on vegetables (leafy and roots) from some shops selling local produce.
** calculated from data in table 4, n=8
$ DR for Sr/Ca ratio of highest and lowest of 20 varieties

In the Old World, consumption of cereals and the emergence of agriculture are inextricably connected, and grains form an essential part of human diet since the onset of agriculture. Therefore, when studying Sr concentrations in human and animal bones from societies with subsistence systems involving agriculture, the potential differences between Sr/Ca ratios in various grains and those in the other components of the vegetation involved must be recognized. In table IX.6, some DR grain-grain values are given. Grain varieties grown in identical media produced Sr/Ca ratios differing by a factor of about 2 at the most (Smith et al. 1963). Sr/Ca ratios in the bran of grains is about twice that in the endosperm (Bartlett & Gunn 1962, Russell 1966b). Our own experiments also yielded DR's for grains and other vegetable components; these will be discussed in section D and E.

A preliminary discussion on the effects of variations in Sr/Ca ratios in plant material is given in Runia (1987b). Data presented in the following sections of this chapter are used in a more extensive discussion on the Bronze Age diets (chapter XI).

D. ANALYSIS OF PLANT SAMPLES

D.1. Experimental

After harvesting, plant samples were air-dried for several weeks. Any soil adhering to the plant samples was removed manually. Cereal ears were separated from the straw and the grains were 'threshed' manually. The chaff of the hulled Hordeum varieties was removed from the sample after grinding.

Samples were dried at 105 °C for several hours and ground in an agate mortar or in a tungsten carbide disc mill. In the case of the cereals the entire grains, i.e. wholemeal flours, were used in analysis.

The plant samples were analysed in duplicate. Approximately 1 g of the sample was weighed accurately into PTFE pressure vessels. 10.5 ml of a 20:1 mixture of concentrated HNO_3 and $HClO_4$ was added and the samples were digested at 185 °C for 6 hours. After cooling, the digestion mixtures were transferred to polyethylene bottles and gravimetrically diluted to 50 ml. Concentration measurements were carried out in this solution as with the bone ash solutions: Sr concentrations were determined using ICP-AES and concentrations of Zn and Ca were determined using AAS.

D.2. Sampling strategy

The purpose of the analysis of plant material is to get some insight in differences in Sr/Ca ratios that may be present in plant species and in parts of one and the same plant (section IX.C). In settlements where the subsistence is based on agriculture and animal husbandry, it is of interest to know if there are any differences in the Sr/Ca ratios in the vegetable material consumed by man and animals, respectively. Man, in eating cereal grains and other selected plant parts, consumes only part of the available 'average plant material'. Herbivorous animals also feed selectively (compare Van de Veen 1979), but are more likely to ingest the 'average plant material'. Points of interest are, therefore, (1) differences between Sr/Ca ratios in cereal grain species and varieties, (2) the relation of the Sr/Ca ratio in grain to the ratio in 'average plant material' from the same site, and (3) the difference between Sr/Ca ratios in shoots and roots, and (4) variations in Sr/Ca ratio in plant material within the growing season. A number of plant samples was collected using a sampling strategy that was devised to give data on these problems.

During two growing seasons plant samples were collected at trial fields of the ROB (Rijksdienst voor het Oudheidkundig Bodemonderzoek, Drs. J. Buurman, Dr. G.F. IJzereef) located at 'De Schothorst' near Amersfoort. Some primitive grain species are grown here on small non-fertilized plots on sandy soil as part of an environmental education project. In one growing season, samples were collected at the IVP (Instituut voor Plantenveredeling, dr. A.C. Zeven) in Wageningen.

At the IVP, emmer (Triticum dicoccum) and einkorn (T. monococcum) are grown in mixed cultivation on two plots of circa 5x5 m^2. One plot is on fertilized coversand, the other on fertilized 'Nude clay', a river clay brown soil. These plots are part of a larger experimental field on which weeds are mechanically and chemically controlled. On the clay plot hardly any weeds were present, but on the sandy plot weeds growing between the Triticum could be collected in two instances. On June 25 1986, shoots of Triticum dicoccum and T. monococcum from the two plots were collected. Ears had already been formed but the grains were not yet filled. On August 18 1986, complete mature plants were harvested. Each grain sample consisted of some 10 shoots taken randomly from the plots. Besides these samples, grains of 'Gelderse Ris', a Triticum aestivum variety growing on the same soils were collected. An overview of the IVP samples is presented in table IX.7

Table IX.7. Samples of Triticum species and weeds from the IVP trial fields in Wageningen, growing season 1986. 'Gelderse ris' is a Triticum aestivum variety

date	soil	species	plant parts
June 25	coversand	T. monococcum	complete shoots
		T. dicoccum	complete shoots
		various weeds	complete plants (no roots)
	Nude clay	T. monococcum	complete shoots
		T. dicoccum	complete shoots
Aug. 18	coversand	T. monococcum	grains
		T. dicoccum	grains
		Geld. ris	grains
		various weeds	plants; roots
	Nude clay	T. monococcum	grains
		T. dicoccum	grains
		Geld. ris	grains
		various weeds	complete plants (no roots)

In the 1985 growing season, Triticum dicoccum and T. monococcum were grown at 'De Schothorst' in mixed cultivation on a circa 6x6 m^2 plot. In 1986, Triticum dicoccum and T. monococcum were grown on separate plots. In 1985, only cereals (three plots), vetch (Vicia sativa) and weeds were collected (table IX.8). Weeds were collected from 50x50 cm^2 squares in the V.sativa plot and in each of the three cereal plots, and pooled into one sample.

No weeds were collected at De Schothorst in 1986. Instead, some other plant species were harvested in addition to the cereals. Species with tap roots were selected: buckwheat (Fagopyrum esculentum), hemp (Cannabis sativa) and dandelion (Taraxacum sp.) (table IX.8). The Cannabis sativa

plants collected in september 1986 contained tough fibres that were removed after grinding for separate analysis.
Sampling of the grains was done similarly to the sampling in Wageningen. From De Schothorst, straw from the mature plants was analysed besides grains.
The soil at De Schothorst is a sandy soil in Coversand. The upper soil layer (Ap horizon) has been removed before the experimental plots were laid out. This was done to remove nutrients from the soil, which had been intensively exploited and fertilized in preceding years.

Table IX.8. Overview of samples of Triticum and Hordeum species and of other plant species from the experimental plots at 'De Schothorst' near Amersfoort, growing seasons 1985 and 1986. The Hordeum distichum is the hulled variety.

date	species	plant parts
Sept. 1985	einkorn *T. monococcum*	straw; grains
	emmer *T. dicoccum*	straw; grains
	vetch *Vicia sativa*	complete plants §
	4-rowed naked barley *H. vulgare*	straw; grains
	2-rowed barley *H. distichum*	straw; grains
	various weeds	complete plants §
June 25 1986	einkorn *T. monococcum*	shoots
	emmer *T. dicoccum*	shoots
	2-rowed barley *H. distichum*	shoots
	buckwheat *Fagopyrum esculentum*	shoots; roots
	hemp *Cannabis sativa*	shoots; roots
Sept. 1986	einkorn *T. monococcum*	straw; grains
	emmer *T. dicoccum*	straw; grains
	2-rowed barley *H. distichum*	straw; grains
	buckwheat *Fagopyrum esculentum*	grains; shoots
	hemp *Cannabis sativa*	shoots; roots
	dandelion *Taraxacum sp.*	leaves; roots

§ without roots

In total, there are four cases in which Sr/Ca ratios of *Triticum dicoccum*, *T. monococcum* and one or more other cereal grains can be compared. Root-shoot Distribution Ratios can be calculated for five cases.

D.3. Results

In 1985, samples from De Schothorst were analysed. A preliminary report on these analyses has already been published (Runia 1987b, table IX.9).

Table IX.9. Sr (mg/kg) and Ca (%) concentrations in dry plant material and Distribution Ratios in straw, grains and weeds from an experimental plot at Amersfoort. Means of duplicate analyses. Adapted from Runia (1987b).

species	part	Ca	Sr	mg Sr/g Ca	-- Distribution Ratio -- grain-straw	grain-weeds
V.sativa		0.81	25.7	3.16		
H. vulgare	straw	0.47	18.6	3.94		
	grain	0.07	2.3	3.48	0.88	1.18
H. distichum	straw	0.38	14.1	3.74		
	grain	0.03	1.2	3.88	1.04	1.32
T. dicoccum	straw	0.19	7.1	3.81		
	grain	0.03	1.4	4.67	1.23	1.58
T. monococcum	straw	0.24	14.2	5.99		
	grain	0.03	2.0	6.25	1.04	2.12
weeds		1.21	35.6	2.95	-	-
mean 4 sp.					1.05	1.55
SD					0.12	0.36

There are indications that Sr/Ca ratios in plants depend on a number of factors such as time, soil fertility and growth circumstances which includes amounts of available light and water (compare Isermann 1981). A simple and, in this case, the only available method for the assessment of growth is the weight of the grains. Good growing conditions will be reflected in high grain weights. In table IX.10, weights of the Triticum dicoccum and T. monococcum grains are presented. The Hordeum distichum is omitted from this table because the chaff was not separated from the grains.

Table IX.10. 100-grain weights of Triticum dicoccum and T. monococcum samples from Wageningen (IVP) and De Schothorst. Based on single determinations of the weight of 100 grains.

species	plot	soil	100-grain weight (g)
Triticum dicoccum	Wageningen	sand	4.22
		clay	4.29
	Schothorst 1985	sand	3.23
	1986	sand	2.12
Triticum monococcum	Wageningen	sand	3.15
		clay	3.11
	Schothorst 1985	sand	2.59
	1986	sand	2.27

The difference between the fertilized trial fields in Wageningen and the poor sandy soil in De Schothorst is clear. The data suggest that Triticum monococcum grain weight is less affected by the availability of nutrients than the T. dicoccum grain weight. The highest Triticum dicoccum grain weight is twice as high as the lowest weight, whereas the highest T. monococcum grain weight is a factor 1.4 higher than the lowest weight.

The lower concentrations of Ca, Sr and Zn at the Wageningen trial fields probably are the result of a diluting effect that results from better growing conditions.

The results of the chemical analysis of plant material are given in table IX.11 and IX.12.
Cereal and Fagopyrum esculentum grains have low concentrations of Ca and Sr. Zinc concentrations in the cereal and Fagoppyrum esculentum grains are relatively high. Concentrations in shoots and grains are lower in the samples from the fertilized trial fields at Wageningen. In the following section, Sr/Ca and Zn/Ca ratios are calculated as mg Sr/g Ca and mg Zn/g Ca.

Table IX.11. Results of analyses of plant material from De Schothorst, growing season 1986 (table IX.8). Results are means of duplicate analyses and expressed as mg/kg dry plant material for Sr and Zn, and as % for Ca. Sr/Ca and Zn/Ca in mg/g Ca.

sample		date	Ca	Sr	Sr/Ca	Zn	Zn/Ca
T. monococcum	shoots	June	0.77	22.3	2.90	226.7	29.5
	straw	Sept	0.43	16.5	3.85	89.9	21.0
	grains		0.03	1.8	5.28	188.6	553.1
T. dicoccum	shoots	June	0.71	21.7	3.06	173.6	24.5
	straw	Sept	0.48	15.9	3.31	132.2	27.5
	grains		0.06	1.9	3.15	100.7	166.7
H. distichum	shoots	June	0.48	14.9	3.10	63.2	13.1
	straw	Sept	0.51	18.4	3.62	66.9	13.2
	grains		0.03	1.0	3.69	56.6	208.9
F.esculentum	shoots	June	3.40	114.9	3.38	518.1	15.2
	roots *		0.99	38.1	3.84	88.1	8.9
	shoots	Sept	2.11	80.4	3.81	ND	-
	grains *		0.02	0.5	2.84	86.3	490.0
C.sativa	shoots	June	2.93	85.1	2.91	55.0	1.9
	roots *		0.53	23.3	4.43	42.8	8.1
	shoots	Sept	1.97	57.0	2.90	54.4	2.8
	fibres		0.62	22.5	3.61	31.0	5.0
	roots		0.40	20.4	5.07	45.6	11.3
Taraxacum sp.	leaves	Sept	1.48	36.3	2.46	319.8	21.7
	roots		0.17	10.6	6.08	54.5	31.3

* no duplicate

Mean Sr/Ca ratio in plant material sampled in June 1986 at De Schothorst was 3.07 ± 0.17 (n=5). From De Schothorst, the 1985 straw samples yielded a mean Sr/Ca ratio of 4.37 ± 0.94 (n=4), the 1986 straw samples 3.59 ± 0.22 (n=3).

Table IX.12. Results of analyses of plant material from Wageningen (IVP), growing season 1986 (table IX.7). Ca concentrations in %, Zn and Sr concentrations in mg/kg. Sr/Ca and Zn/Ca ratios are in mg/g Ca.

soil	sample		date	Ca	Sr	Sr/Ca	Zn	Zn/Ca
sand	*T. monococcum*	shoots	June	0.22	6.7	3.00	32.7	14.6
		grains	Sept	0.02	2.8	11.52	70.6	290.5
	T. dicoccum	shoots	June	0.24	4.8	2.01	39.5	16.6
		grains	Aug	0.03	1.0	3.28	66.4	217.7
	Geld.ris	grains	Aug	0.03	1.2	4.24	47.0	166.1
	weeds	shoots	June	1.55	27.5	1.78	50.3	3.3
		shoots	Aug	1.65	37.6	2.27	32.3	2.0
		roots *		0.33	11.8	3.58	20.7	6.3
clay	*T. monococcum*	shoots	June	0.41	9.9	2.40	20.5	5.0
		grains	Aug	0.03	3.2	11.39	47.6	169.4
	T. dicoccum	shoots	June	0.45	8.6	1.93	22.7	5.1
		grains	Aug	0.03	1.1	3.90	45.7	162.1
	Geld.ris	grains	Aug	0.03	1.1	4.33	28.7	113.0
	weeds	shoots	Aug	2.23	42.2	1.89	35.3	1.6

* no duplicate

No straw was analysed from the Wageningen fields. Weeds tend to have somewhat lower Sr/Ca than straw. This difference may be related to the ages of the plants. The weeds are generally younger and still have green leaves whereas straw is ripe and yellow.

D.4. Discussion

The difference between the concentrations of Sr and Zn is striking. Concentrations of Sr in the grains are low whereas Zn concentrations are high. Zinc is probably transported to the grains during the ripening of the grains by a mechanism involving phytohormones (Marschner 1983). The grain acts as a 'sink' for zinc. The grains are thus furnished with a Zn stock which is to be used in germination and during the early stages of growth. Such a stock is not necessary for Sr, which is not an essential element.

For the 1986 Schothorst samples, the Sr/Ca ratios in the straw and grains can be compared with the shoots. The Ca concentrations in straw are lower and Sr/Ca ratios are higher than in the shoots. Lower Ca concentrations may be the result of a diluting effect, but may also indicate that part of the Ca is transported to the grain. The higher Sr/Ca ratios in straw in comparison to shoots suggest that Sr is retained more strongly than Ca in leaves and stalks (compare Russell & Newbould 1966, Isermann 1981). This would cause the grain Sr/Ca ratios to be lower than those in the shoot and straw. This is, however, not the case. Mean DR grain-straw for De Schothorst is 1.08 ± 0.16 (n=7), mean DR grain-shoot is 1.35 ± 0.34 (n=3) for De Schothorst and 3.06 ± 1.28 (n=4) for the Wageningen samples. Thus, relatively more Sr than Ca is transported to the grains.

Different Sr/Ca ratios were registered within cereal grains, with the ratio in the bran being about twice as high as that in the endosperm (Bartlett & Gunn 1962, Russell & Newbould 1966). In the grains, both Sr and Zn are predominantly contained in the bran (Smith 1971b, Jonxis 1983).

A hypothetical mechanism causing the relatively high Sr/Ca ratios in the grains might be inferred from these data. Both Sr and Zn resemble Ca chemically, and thus Sr resembles Zn. In atomic weight, Sr is closer to Zn than Ca. In ionic radius, the difference between Zn and Sr is greater than between Zn and Ca (table I.1).

It is possible that some Sr is retained in the grains together with Zn. The mechanism causing the build-up of the Zn stock in the grains may act more selectively against the superabundant Ca than against the trace element Sr.

The possibility that some Sr is retained in the grains by the Zn retaining mechanism is not contradicted by the data in table IX.13. Grain-shoot DR's for Sr/Ca and Zn/Ca are correlated to some extent: the correlation coefficient is 0.69 (n=7).

Barium concentrations were also determined in the plant material but are not extensively reported here. In atomic weight and ionic diameter Ba differs more from Ca and Zn than Sr (table I.1). The consequence of the proposed hypothetical mechanism is that Ba concentrations will be less affected than Sr concentrations. The correlation coefficient for Ba/Ca and Zn/Ca grain-shoot DR's (table IX.13) is 0.54 (n=7), which is indeed lower than for Sr and Zn.

If Sr is transported in plants and retained in the grains to some extent by such a mechanism, this might also be the cause for the large differences in Sr/Ca ratios in grains of various cereal species and varieties (compare Smith et al. 1963).

Table IX.13. Grain-shoot Distribution Ratios for Sr/Ca, Zn/Ca and Ba/Ca ratios: DR = (ratio in grain)/(ratio in shoot)

sample		Distribution Ratio		
		Sr	Zn	Ba
Schothorst	Triticum dicoccum	1.03	6.80	3.48
Schothorst	Hordeum distichum	1.19	15.89	1.25
Wageningen sand	Triticum dicoccum	1.63	13.15	1.10
Schothorst	Triticum monococcum	1.82	18.74	3.02
Wageningen clay	Triticum dicoccum	2.02	31.83	2.64
Wageningen sand	Triticum monococcum	3.84	19.84	3.41
Wageningen clay	Triticum monococcum	4.73	34.08	6.20

One of the aims of the analysis of plant samples was to gain an insight into the differences in Sr/Ca ratios in cereals growing on the same soil. To facilitate comparison, grain-grain DR's have been calculated (table IX.14). The Sr/Ca ratio in Triticum dicoccum grains from the same plot was arbitrarily chosen as reference value.

A mean DR grain-T. dicoccum of 1.62 ± 0.90 can be calculated for the nine cases. The largest deviation from the Triticum dicoccum Sr/Ca ratio was found in the Wageningen Triticum monococcum samples. Compared to an Observed Ratio meat-diet of 0.20-0.25 (V.A.2), the DR of circa 3 in these samples cannot be ignored.

The DR grain-grain values apparently depend on a number of factors (Isermann 1981). Different cereal species react differently on variations in growing conditions (compare data in Smith 1971b, Smith et al. 1963). The Sr concentrations in the Wageningen Triticum monococcum samples are relatively high. No correlation with Zn concentrations is present.

The average DR Hordeum distichum-Triticum dicoccum is 1.0. The predominant cereal species in West-Friesland thus appear to have equal Sr/Ca ratios. This result is based on analysis of samples of De Schothorst. As is apparent from the Triticum monococcum samples, on other soils the DR's may have other values.

Table IX.14. Distribution Ratios (DR) of cereals from plots at De Schothorst and Wageningen (IVP). DR's are relative to Triticum dicoccum: (Sr/Ca in species)/(Sr/Ca in T. dicoccum).

species	sample from	value of DR
Hordeum distichum	Schothorst 1985	0.83
	1986	1.17
	mean (n=2)	1.00
Triticum monococcum	Schothorst 1985	1.34
	1986	1.68
	Wageningen sand	3.51
	clay	2.92
	mean (n=4)	2.36 ± 0.89
Hordeum vulgare var.nudum	Schothorst 1985	0.75
Gelderse ris	Wageningen sand	1.29
	Wageningen clay	1.11
	mean (n=2)	1.20
Fagopyrum esculentum	Schothorst 1986	0.90
mean, cereal grains (n=9)		1.62 ± 0.90

Sr/Ca ratios for 'average plant material' (APM) are difficult to establish because of the ambiguity of this term. The green plant material, i.e. shoots collected in June and weeds, whenever collected, may however be taken as representative material.

The Sr/Ca ratios for 'average plant material' can be calculated in three cases (table IX.15).

Table IX.15. Sr/Ca ratios (mg/g) in 'average plant material' (APM) from De Schothorst and IVP. Based on Sr/Ca ratios in shoots and weeds.

location	n	mean	SD
Schothorst	8	2.99	0.25
Wageningen sand	4	2.27	0.46
Wageningen clay	3	2.07	0.23

The 'average plant material' Sr/Ca ratios can be compared to the Sr/Ca ratios in cereal grains. This can again be carried out using a Distribution Ratio (table IX.16).

Table IX.16. Comparison between Sr/Ca ratios in cereal grains and in 'average plant material' (APM) for three experimental plots. Distribution Ratio = (Sr/Ca in cereal grain) / (Sr/Ca in APM).

location		cereal	DR
De Schothorst	1985	Triticum dicoccum	1.56
		Triticum monococcum	2.08
		Hordeum distichum	1.29
	1986	Triticum dicoccum	1.05
		Triticum monococcum	1.76
		Hordeum distichum	1.23
Wageningen IVP	sand	Triticum dicoccum	1.44
		Triticum monococcum	5.07
		Gelderse ris	1.87
	clay	Triticum dicoccum	1.88
		Triticum monococcum	5.50
		Gelderse ris	2.09

The data in table IX.16 yield mean values for the DR grain-APM of 2.24 ± 1.40 (n=12). In the Bronze Age of West-Friesland, only Hordeum distichum and Triticum dicoccum are of relevance. Triticum dicoccum yields a mean DR of 1.5 ± 0.30 (n=4). Triticum dicoccum and Hordeum distichum have a mean DR grain-APM of 1.4 ± 0.26 (n=6). These values can be used in calculations on the uptake of Sr and Ca by man and animal in Bronze Age West-Friesland (IX.E.2).

The data in table IX.16 and table IX.10 suggest a positive correlation between the DR grain-APM and the 100-grain weight for both Triticum dicoccum and T. monococcum. Coefficients of correlation are 0.82 (n=4) and 0.96 (n=4), respectively. High grain weights are combined with high Sr/Ca ratios.

A further point of interest is the relation between Sr/Ca ratios in plant shoots and roots. Values for DR shoot-root could be calculated in five cases (table IX.17). A mean value of 0.62 ± 0.15 was obtained. Roots thus have higher Sr/Ca ratios than shoots. This corroborates the shoot-root DR's calculated from published data (table IX.1). Values for DR roots-APM yield a mean of 1.61 (n=5), which equals the inverse of the DR shoot-root.

The mean Ca concentration in the roots is 0.48 ± 0.28 % (n=5). This is close to the mean value of 0.53 mg/g fresh weight (n=7, c. 10 % dry matter) for root crops calculated from data in on recent root crops (table V.1).

Table IX.17. Shoot-root Distribution Ratios (DR) in plant samples from Wageningen (IVP) and De Schothorst. DR= (Sr/Ca in shoot)/(Sr/Ca in root).

species	sample from	value of DR
Cannabis sativa	Schothorst June 1986	0.66
	Sept.1986	0.57
Fagopyrum esc.	Schothorst June 1986	0.88
Taraxacum sp.	Schothorst Sept.1986	0.40
various weeds	Wageningen sand Aug.1986	0.63
mean (n=5)		0.62 ± 0.15

In section V.A.2.5, the anatomical and physiological differences in the intestinal tracts of grazers and browsers have been discussed in relation to bone Sr levels. Unfortunately, no information is available on differences in Sr/Ca ratios within plant cells, but in relation to this the analysis of Cannabis sativa fibres and other C. sativa plant tissue is of interest. Cannabis sativa fibres contain relatively large amounts of cell wall material compared to the other C. sativa tissues. The difference between Sr/Ca ratio in the fibres and in the tissue (3.61 and 2.90 mg Sr/g Ca, respectively) suggests that the fraction of plants most resistant to digestion contains relatively more Sr than the better digestable fraction. This would result in higher Sr/Ca ratios in grazers than in browsers feeding on identical diets.

E. STRONTIUM AND CALCIUM IN THE VEGETABLE COMPONENT OF THE HUMAN DIET

E.1. General aspects

A reconstruction of the composition of prehistoric diets based on bone trace element levels for a part depends on knowledge of Sr and Ca relationships in vegetable food items. In section V.A, non-vegetable food items are discussed. In this section, relevant information on groups of vegetable food items is discussed.

In the assessment of Sr/Ca relationships in vegetable food items, a reference or 'baseline' vegetable material should be used. In the preceding sections, the term 'average plant material' (APM) was used. In essence, this APM consists of a representative sample of plant shoots: relatively young, above-ground, green, vegetative plant parts. Sr/Ca ratios in such material are likely to be close to Sr/Ca ratios in the soil solution (compare table IX.15). Sr/Ca ratios in vegetable food items may then be expressed in relation to the APM Sr/Ca ratio.

In present day vegetations, a Sr/Ca ratio for APM may be established by the analysis of suitable vegetable material. In prehistoric contexts, no such material is available. Although some prehistoric vegetable material survives in many instances, the wood, grains and seeds preserved under waterlogged conditions or in carbonized form are probably not suitable as 'baseline material', because Ca and Sr levels are low and, most likely, altered diagenetically. Besides, wood may have been transported to the site over a relatively long distance.
As an alternative, a baseline Sr/Ca ratio for plant material may be extrapolated from herbivorous animal bone Sr/Ca ratios using the OR bone-diet.

E.2. Cereals

Cereals are staple foods in the prehistoric agricultural societies in the Old World. Consumption of cereals by prehistoric cultures is documented by numerous finds of grain remains, impressions of grains in pottery and loaves of bread (Helbaek 1952, Brothwell & Brothwell 1969, Renfrew 1973). There are abundant indications for extensive cereal grain cultivation in the Bronze Age in West-Friesland (section II.C.1.4).
Cereals have low Sr and Ca contents (table V.1). Experiments indicate that grains have higher Sr/Ca ratios than green, leafy vegetable material from the same soil (section IX.D). A mean value of 1.4 was derived for the ratio (Sr/Ca in _Triticum dicoccum_ and _Hordeum distichum_)/(Sr/Ca in average plant material), _T. dicoccum_ and _H. distichum_ being the predominant grain species in Bronze Age West-Friesland.

We do not know how cereals were prepared for consumption in Bronze Age West-Friesland. The art of bread baking was certainly known in Bronze Age Switzerland (Renfrew 1973), and probably therefore also in West-Friesland. Shallow bowls and discs of pottery, found in excavations in the area (Bakker et al. 1977) might be interpreted as griddles used for baking small loaves or buns of bread (compare Renfrew 1973). For our purposes it is not essential to know whether cereals were baked to loaves or were eaten as a gruel, but any cleaning of milled grain, i.e. separation of bran and flour, which might be associated with the baking of loaves, will have an effect on the Sr/Ca ratio in the diet because of the different Sr/Ca ratios in bran and endosperm (IX.C). It appears, however, unlikely that flour was cleaned as the Bronze Age Swiss small loaves were composed of rather crudely milled grains (Renfrew 1973). Helbaek (1952) studied some small buns or cakes from an English Iron Age site. The buns were probably no more than portions of a stiff porridge that had been dried or baked, and contained coarsely ground cereals and seeds of weeds. Apparently, not much time was spent in cleaning the cereals. The abrasion of the teeth of the Bronze Age inhabitants of West-Friesland is another indication for coarseness of the food.

In other contexts, the difference in Sr/Ca ratios in endosperm and bran and, consequently, in coarse breads and in the finer white breads may be of some importance. Moritz (1958) discusses the various types of flours that were produced in the Roman Empire. The bread for the poor was baked of _secundarium_, a product that contained about twice as much bran as wholemeal flour. Other flours such as the more expensive as _pollen_ and _similago_ contained less bran. The army bread _panis militaris_ probably was a wholemeal bread. The consumption of different types of bread by the rich and poor in Imperial Rome may be reflected in bone Sr levels.

E.3. Pulses and other seeds

Pulses were important components of diets and essential in crop rotation schemes in North-Western Europe before the introduction of potatoes (Slicher van Bath 1960). Pulses were cultivated from Neolithic times onwards. Bakels (1978) summarizes finds of _Pisum sativum_ (pea) from LBK contexts and concludes that, at that time, it was a widely spread cultivated plant. However, no finds of pulses have yet been reported from West-Friesland.

No data on Sr/Ca relationships in pulses are available. In general, Sr/Ca ratios in green _Leguminosae_ in grass lands are comparable to grass Sr/Ca ratios (Russell & Newbould 1966). The Sr/Ca ratio in our _Vicia sativa_ sample is close to the Sr/Ca ratio in weeds (table IX.9). It appears likely that in the formation of the pulse seeds some discrimination against Sr or Ca occurs, but no data on this aspect are available.

Calcium concentrations in present-day pulses are some 8 mg/100 kJ (table V.1).

Seeds of various other plants were either consumed whole or as processed for oil. Flax or linseed has already been mentioned. The vegetable oil of this and other seeds consists of fatty acids and does not contain Ca. The cakes that remain after pressing may be consumed by man or animals and contain all the Ca and Sr of the seeds.

E.4. Nuts and fruits

In beechnuts, hazelnuts, acorns and other nuts high energy content is combined with high concentrations of trace elements. This implies that trace element concentrations per unit of energy are comparable to trace element levels in other plant material. Calcium concentrations of food items are presented in table V.1. Calcium concentrations per unit of energy in nuts are only slightly higher than in cereal grains. In a similar way Zn contents per unit of energy are not exceptionally high (section VI.A.2)

Archeological finds of nuts are frequent (Renfrew 1973, Jorgensen 1977). In temperate regions, nuts such as hazelnuts, acorns and beechnuts were almost certainly a component of many prehistoric diets. In West-Friesland, however, where woodlands were virtually absent, some nuts may have been imported from sandy regions, though it is unlikely that they constituted an appreciable part of the Bronze Age human diet. One hazelnut was found in Bronze Age Bovenkarspel, and some *Corylus* may have grown locally (J. Buurman, pers. comm.).

Few data exist on Sr/Ca discrimination in nuts. The high Sr levels in brazil nuts are probably exceptional (Smith 1971a, Runia 1987b).

Acorns from the Wisconsin Mount Horeb region have slightly different Sr/Ca ratios than grass and alfalfa: 1.16 $\pm$ 0.37 mg Sr/g Ca (n=3) and 1.24 $\pm$ 0.86 mg Sr/g Ca (n=7), respectively (items 40-49 in table 4 of Price et al. 1985a). This result is, however, of limited value considering the large variations in the alfalfa and grass Sr/Ca ratios, which are probably the result of the relatively large sampling area. More experimental data are needed.

Fruits, such as apples, brambles and berries most likely were probably all consumed in prehistoric times. As with nuts, woodlands form the principal suppliers of fruits. Except for some brambles, no finds of edible fruits such as apples are known from West-Friesland (J. Buurman, pers. comm.). Some *Rubus* may have grown locally.

Calcium concentrations per unit of energy in recent fruits are higher than in nuts and cereals (table V.1). In uncultivated wild fruits Ca concentrations may be slightly higher still. No data on Sr/Ca ratios in fruits relative to average plant material are available.

E.5. Roots and tubers

Roots and tubers are part of the diets of many modern hunter/gatherers (Hayden 1981, Eaton & Konner 1985). In tropical regions, cultivated roots and tubers such as yams, manihoc and sweet potatoes may be staple foods (compare Hawkes 1969). The present-day root and tuber crops in North-Western Europe, such as potatoes and carrots, were introduced in historic times and are archeologically of no interest.

The consumption of roots and tubers in prehistoric cultures is hardly traceable by archeological and botanical methods. There is, however, no reason why roots and tubers should not be eaten. In West-Friesland, wild plant species with edible roots occur, for example *Taraxacum* sp. (dandelion). Mention has been made of the roots of reeds and other plants that may have been gathered in the low-lying wet areas (section II.C.1.4).

In general, Ca concentrations in roots are relatively high. The mean Ca concentration per kJ in modern root crops is comparable to Ca concentrations in milk (table V.1). The Sr/Ca ratios in roots are higher than in plant shoots. A mean DR shoot-root of approximately 0.6 can be calculated from the experimental data (table IX.17).

E.6. Leafy vegetables

Green leaves of certain wild or cultivated plant species may have been consumed in prehistoric times. In the literature, this does not receive much attention because gathering or cultivation and consumption of leafy vegetables does not leave traces in the archeological record. Compared with other food items, leafy vegetables are rich sources of minerals and vitamins such as vitamin C. Calcium contents per unit of energy are very high, about four times higher than in milk (table V.1). A balanced human diet can hardly be composed without the inclusion of a certain amount of leafy vegetables. Though we have no archeological indications for the consumption of green plant material by humans, we may assume that a certain amount of it was indeed consumed. In the Bronze Age of West-Friesland, leaves of non-cultivated plants, such as species of Cruciferae and Chenopodiaceae, may have been eaten (J. Buurman, pers. comm.).

As stated above (section IX.E.1), green leafy plant material may be considered to represent the 'average plant material'. Thus, the Sr/Ca ratios of leafy vegetables and the Sr/Ca ratios in average plant material can be considered equal. As a consequence of its high Ca concentrations, leafy vegetables in the human diet will tend to depress the effects of other food items on the diet's Sr/Ca ratio.

E.7. Lower plants

In the preceding sections, edible products of Spermatophyta species have been discussed. There are, however, groups of lower plants that also produce edible material: the fungi (Mycophyta) and the algae (Phycophyta).

Fruit-bodies of a large number of species of fungi are edible and valued by humans and animals. Some species are cultivated today in and outside Europe, but until recently only gathered wild specimens were consumed. Even now, truffles and other species are gathered rather than cultivated.

Fungi may thrive in various ecosystems, such as meadows and woods. It is probable that in West-Friesland in the Bronze Age at least some species of edible toadstools were present, and presumably also eaten. There is no botanical evidence for these assumptions neither is it to be expected (Van Geel, pers. comm.). In the human diet, mushrooms can only have been of minor importance.

Modern edible mushrooms and chanterelles contain some 5-25 mg Ca per 100 kJ (table V.1), which is considerably less than the Ca contents of leafy vegetables. No data on Sr/Ca discrimination in fungi are available. Fungi live on many organic substrates, either as saprophytes or as parasites. In higher plants, distinct differences in Sr/Ca ratios are present (section IX.A). Consequently, the Sr/Ca ratio of the substrate of fungi may be different from APM Sr/Ca ratios. Any discrimination against Sr in fungi will thus be superimposed on the discrimination in the higher plants.

A second group of lower plants are the algae. Seaweeds in particular may be important as foodstuff and might be detected using carbon and nitrogen isotopes. In West-Friesland, proteins from marine sources were hardly consumed at all (chapter X).

Seaweeds contain relatively high amounts of trace elements (Luten 1983). We have no data on Ca levels and energy values.

Discrimination against Sr in algae is, most likely, small. Algae take up elements from the seawater, and lack a vascular system, which, in higher plants, is the main site of 'discrimination' against Sr (section IX.C). Two fresh water algae species had OR plant/water values of 0.6 and 1.5 (Isermann 1981). Thus, in algae as well as in other water plants discrimination against Sr or against Ca occurs (Isermann 1981). Considering the high Sr/Ca ratios in seawater, seaweeds will, irrespective of OR's, have Sr/Ca ratios that are high compared to Sr/Ca ratios in terrestrial plants.

X
STABLE ISOTOPES IN BONE COLLAGEN

A. INTRODUCTION

The potentials of the analyses of stable carbon and nitrogen isotopes in paleodietary studies have been outlined in section I.B.2. No C4 plants are indigenous in the area under review. Stable carbon and nitrogen ratios in human bones from this area can therefore be used to estimate the quantity of marine food in human diets.

Ratios of stable carbon and nitrogen in bone collagen reflect the ratios of these isotopes in the proteins consumed. Marine foods, such as fish and shellfish, in general contain relatively large amounts of protein (table X.1). In comparison to the terrestrial staple foods, meat and cereals, the protein content per unit of energy in marine fish and shellfish is about 4-4.5 times higher. The percentage of marine food in the diet calculated on protein basis is therefore roughly four times that calculated on energy basis.

Table X.1. Protein contents (g/100 g edible product and g/100 kJ) of some marine and terrestrial foods. Based on Paul & Southgate (1978)

food item	n	---- g protein per ---- 100 g	100 kJ
marine fish	7	17.5 ± 0.7	4.1 ± 1.4
marine shellfish	8	18.2 ± 5.4	4.7 ± 0.5
meats	4	14.3 ± 1.1	1.1 ± 0.2
wheat wholemeal flour	1*	13.2	1.0
leafy vegetables	13	2.5 ± 1.4	3.4 ± 1.3

* mean value for many analyses

Seafoods have high Sr/Ca ratios and will therefore have a marked effect on Sr/Ca ratios in diets. Knowledge of the marine component in diet is one of the essential factors in the discussion on concentrations of Sr and other trace elements in human bones. For this reason, the majority of human bones and a few animal bones from West-Friesland were selected for stable isotope analyses.

The collagen extraction and the determination of delta 13C and delta 15N were carried out at the Isotope Physics Laboratory of the Rijksuniversiteit Groningen.

B. EXPERIMENTAL

B.1. Extraction of collagen

B.1.1. Procedure

Bone powder and bone fragments were cleaned as described in section III.A. The collagen extraction procedure described by Bumsted (1984) was followed. In essence, this procedure is identical to the Longin (1971) procedure.

Bone mineral was dissolved in centrifuge tubes in 0.5 N hydrochloric acid during 1 hour at 3 ^{o}C, c. 0.5 g bone powder in c. 40 ml acid. Subsequently, the solution was centrifuged at 1200 rpm for 10 minutes. Supernatant was discarded and the residue washed with acidified (pH=3) demineralized water. After centrifugation, the supernatant was again discarded. This step was repeated twice. The residue was then transferred to small glass bottles with 10-15 ml of demineralized water (pH=3). The closed glass bottles were placed in a stove at 90 ^{o}C. After 24 hours, the supernatant,i.e. the collagen solution, was transferred to clean glass vials using a pasteur pipette. The collagen solution was placed in a stove at circa 75 ^{o}C and evaporated to dryness. Prior to combustion for carbondioxide, collagen samples were dried at 105 ^{o}C for 1 hour.
For small bone fragments, the first step in the extraction was different. Some 0.5-1.0 g of bone fragments were placed in centrifuge tubes. Some 40 ml of 0.5 hydrochloric acid was added. Tubes were closed with Parafilm and placed in a refrigerator at 3 ^{o}C for 5 days.

Some experiments including cleaning of the collagen using ion exchange resins were carried out, but without success.
Though the material extracted from the bones probably is, strictly speaking, not collagen but a product of the chemical and microbiological alterations of the original collagen that took place in the soil, the term 'collagen' is still used in this text. Most likely, this collagen is largely composed of fragments of the original collagen. The assumption underlying this statement is discussed in section X.C.1.

B.1.2. Assessment of purity

The collagen prepared from the bones appeared to be fairly pure. Colours of the extracted collagen fractions varied from dark brown to clear yellow. Most of the collagen samples showed clear 'crystallic' features. Some 'collagen' samples were 'dusty' rather than 'crystal-like' in appearance. These samples yielded delta 13C values (c. -26 per mil) which were too negative, and most likely were not collagen.
Soil particles that for some reason are present in the bone samples do not seem to bias delta 13C measurements. Tests with soil samples show that the extraction procedure employed extracts no more than a very small fraction of soil organic matter.

Various techniques may be employed to purify extracted 'collagen'. These include chemical techniques using acid and alkaline solutions (Schoeninger & DeNiro 1984), and techniques using adsorbing media (Bumsted 1984). It may, however, be doubted whether further purification of the collagen is justified by any improved reliability of delta 13C measurements. Every step in the treatment of collagen is accompagnied by isotopic fractionation to a greater or lesser degree. Another aspect of these techniques is that they implicitely assume that collagen and 'dirt' are present as separate compounds. It is, however, likely that fragments of collagen, resulting from microbiological degradation processes, form new macromolecular compounds with fragments of soil organic matter. Chemical and physico-chemical purifying techniques would appear to be rather futile for the removal of such impurities. In fact, the exchange column treatments used by Bumsted (1984), had only minor effects on the delta 13C values of the resulting collagen.

B.2. Carbon isotopes

Collagen was burned in a standard carbon dioxide system. Some 10 mg of collagen is placed in a quartz boat and placed in the vacuum system. Under a continuous flow of pure oxygen, the collagen is heated to 900 ^{o}C. For purification of the CO_2, the combustion gasses are led through CuO (900 ^{o}C) and Ag (400 ^{o}C) furnaces. Water is trapped in a acetone/dry ice mixture. Carbon dioxide is collected in a liquid air trap during the combustion period. After complete combustion is achieved in c. 10 minutes, the combustion furnace and the oxygen flow are turned off. Subsequently, the system is evacuated and the carbon dioxyde is allowed to evaporate and is led over a Cu furnace (600 ^{o}C) to a second liquid air trap. Here, the carbondioxyde yield is measured manometrically. Finally, the CO_2 is collected in a glass tube fitted with a vacuum valve.

Delta 13C values were determined in a VG Micromass 903 or SIRA 9 mass spectrometer and are, as customary, expressed as per mils relative to Pee Dee Belemnite.

Accuracy of the delta 13C determinations is checked by analysing ANU sucrose reference material.

The reproducebility of delta 13C determinations was determined by multiple analysis of a standard sample. Collagen extracted from a fresh cattle bone yielded a mean delta 13C of -21.56 per mil, SD= 0.06 per mil, CV=0.3 %, n=7.

B.3. Nitrogen isotopes

Unfortunately, attempts to get pure nitrogen from the collagen samples have not (yet) been successful.

The Kjeldahl method of producing N_2 from the collagen has been tried. Cryogenic purification of the gas was, however, not successful, so the measured delta 15N values were useless. A combustion system designed for the collection of N_2 is being made operational at present.

C. RESULTS AND DISCUSSION

C.1. General

According to DeNiro (1985), the C/N ratio of the collagen fraction of prehistoric human bones is an indication for the reliability of its stable carbon and nitrogen isotope ratios. Collagen samples possessing atomic C/N ratios outside the range 2.9-3.6 yielded delta 13C and delta 15N values that did not agree with the expected values. Unfortunately, determinations of the C/N ratio were not possible in the present research due to problems in the purification of nitrogen from the collagen (section IV.B.3). The C/N ratio can therefore not be used here.

Collagen with a 'dusty' look yielded too negative delta 13C values (c. -25 per mil) and have been omitted from the results discussed here.

The recorded delta 13C values are discussed in the following sections, and are presented in the figures X.1-X.4 together with published reference data.

C.2. Fish

In total, nine fish bone samples were analysed. The fish bones were obtained from the excavated material from some sites outside West-Friesland. One sample of fresh water fish from West-Friesland could be analysed, but no sea fish was present at all. Though not from the same area as the human bones, the bones of sea fish were buried under comparable circumstances. The bones from Vlaardingen date from the late Neolithic (Van Regteren Altena et al. 1962), the Velsen bones are of the Bronze Age (Woltering 1979).

The analyses of the fish bones are of interest in relation to the assessment of the reliability of the delta 13C values in the extracted collagen. According to published data, bones of marine fish have delta 13C values of circa -10 to -14 per mil (Schoeninger & DeNiro 1984). Any incorporation of soil carbon, which has delta 13C values of circa -26 per mil (compare Calderoni & Schnitzer 1984), in the fish bone collagen would result in delta 13C values which are too negative.

Delta 13C values of the fish bones are summarized in table X.2 and presented in fig X.1. Specimen of the marine fish species mullet (Mugil sp.) and cod (Gadus morrhua) have 'marine' delta 13C values. The only fresh water fish analysed, common eel (Anguilla anguilla), has a 'terrestrial' value. Dissolved inorganic carbon in fresh water generally has a delta 13C value of -12 per mil as compared to + 1 per mil for seawater; brackish water values are intermediate (Mook 1968). The delta 13C values of the anadromous sturgeon (Acipenser sturio) are intermediate between the terrestrial and marine delta 13C values. This is comparable with the observation on anadromous salmon by Schoeninger & DeNiro (1984).

The collagen exctracted from the fish bones was dark-brown in colour and showed a 'crystal-like' structure. The material causing the brown stain of the collagen apparently has little effect on its delta 13C value.

Table X.2. Delta 13C values (per mil to PDB) in some fish bones. Bones were taken from the excavations at Vlaardingen (Van Regteren Altena et al. 1962), Velsen (Woltering 1979) and Het Valkje (section II.C.2)

species	n	ecology	delta 13C PDB	sites
Mugil sp.	3	marine	-13.58 ± 0.73	Vlaardingen, Velsen
Gadus morrhua	3	marine	-14.06 ± 0.21	Velsen
Acipenser sturio	2	anadromous	-17.05	Vlaardingen
Anguilla anguilla	1	fresh	-21.64	Bovenkarspel Valkje

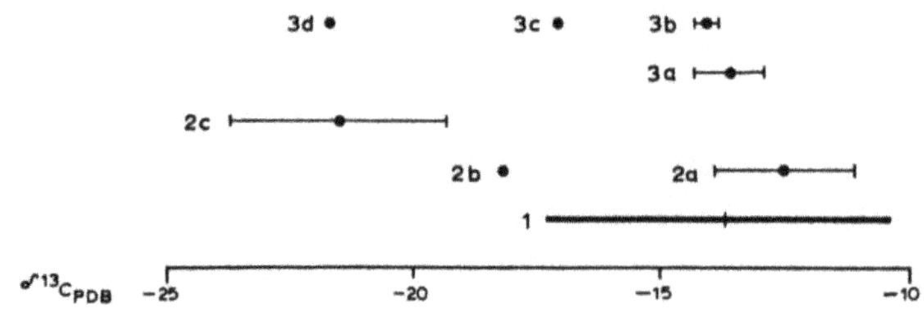

figure X.1 Delta 13C values of fish bones. 1 marine mammals (n=16), range and mean (Tauber 1983); 2 (Schoeninger & DeNiro 1984, mean and standard deviation) a: marine fish (n=10), b: anadromous fish (n=2), c: freshwater fish (n=4); 3 (table X.2, mean and standard deviation) a: cod (Mugil sp.), b: cod (Gadus morrhua), c: sturgeon (Acipenser sturio), d: common eel (Anguilla anguilla).

C.3. Animal delta 13C values

A limited number of animal bone delta 13C values was determined (table X.3). The mean delta 13C value for cattle in Hoogkarspel and for four domestic animals (two cows, one pig, one dog) from Het Valkje are within the range for terrestrial animals supplied by Schoeninger & DeNiro (1984) and others (fig. X.2).

In regions without C4 plants, herbivorous animal bone delta 13C values are of interest solely in relation to the assessment of the reliability of delta 13C determinations. The delta 13 C values of herbivorous animals in regions without C4 plants will lie in a rather narrow range around -19 to -21 per mil . Tauber (1983) gives a mean value of -20.1 per mil for collagen in bones of 40 terrestrial herbivores from Denmark and Greenland. Other data for terrestrial herbivores, as supplied by Schoeninger & DeNiro (1984) and Schoeninger (1985) include data from regions with C4 plants which causes the mean value to be less negative.

The fresh bovine bone reference material (section X.B.2) yielded a delta 13 C of -21.56 per mil The delta 13C values for fresh and prehistoric cattle bones indicate that the analytical procedures employed are capable of producing delta 13C values comparable to those registered by other researchers.

Table X.3. Delta 13C values (per mil to PDB) in animal bones.

sample		n	mean	SD	CV(%)
Het Valkje	cattle	2	-21.67		
	pig	1	-22.80		
	dog	1	-21.23		
	total	4	-21.84	0.62	2.9
cattle Hoogkarspel		3	-21.11	0.47	2.2
cattle Grootebroek		1	-20.52		

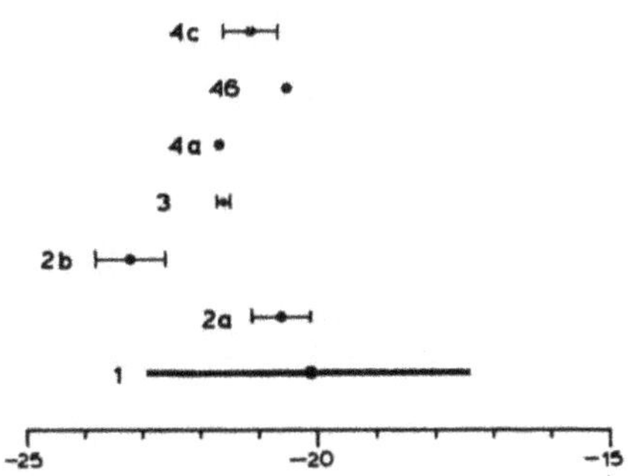

figure X.2 Delta 13C values in terrestrial animals. 1 terrestrial animals (n=40), range and mean (Tauber 1983); 2 (Hobson & Schwarcz 1986, mean and standard deviation) a: deer (n=55), b: vole (n=22); 3 fresh cattle bone reference sample, mean and standard deviation (n=7); 4 (table X.3, mean and standard deviation) a: cattle Het Valkje, b: cattle Grootebroek, c: cattle Hoogkarspel.

C.4. Human delta 13C values

C.4.1. Results

The delta 13C values for 62 human individuals are summarized in table X.4 and figure X.3. The mean value is -20.86 ± 0.60 per mil , which is close to the mean value of -21.4 ± 0.78 per mil for 31 pre-maize North American inland humans (Van der Merwe & Vogel 1978, compare fig X.4).

Table X.4. Delta 13C values (per mil to PDB) in human bones.

site	n	mean	SD	CV(%)
Zwaagdijk				
barrows	4	-20.89	0.36	1.7
flat graves	4	-20.34	0.29	1.4
Grootebroek	4	-20.93	0.46	2.2
Oostwoud	11	-20.79	0.72	3.5
Andijk	10	-21.04	0.61	2.9
Het Valkje				
Early Period	8	-20.73	0.30	1.5
Late Period	5	-21.18	0.72	3.4
Hoogkarspel				
settlement	8	-20.56	0.38	1.8
barrows	2	-20.96		
Schagen-Muggenburg *	-			
Velsen	5	-21.52	0.34	1.6
Valkenburg (S-H)	1	-20.24		
total humans	62	-20.86	0.60	2.9

* no collagen could be extracted from the individuals from this site

There are no significant differences between the mean delta 13C values. Ranges of the delta 13C values per site overlap to a greater or lesser extent, except for the ranges for the inhumations from the barrows at Hoogkarspel and Zwaagdijk. The delta 13C values for bones from the Zwaagdijk flat graves are slightly but not significantly less negative than those of the other samples.

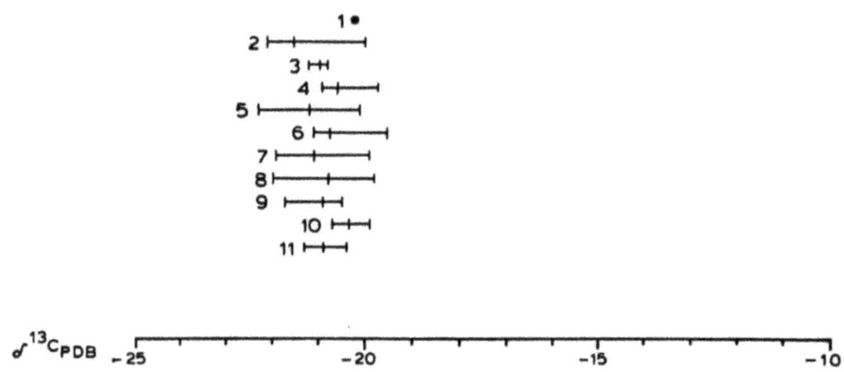

figure X.3 Delta 13C values in human bones (mean and range, table X.4). 1 Valkenburg; 2 Velsen; 3 Hoogkarspel barrows; 4 Hoogkarspel isolated finds; 5 Het Valkje Late Period; 6 Het Valkje Early Period; 7 Andijk; 8 Oostwoud; 9 Grootebroek; 10 Zwaagdijk flat graves; 11 Zwaagdijk barrows.

Differences in delta 13C values within the skeleton of one and the same individual could be established in three cases. In prehistoric bones, such differences are the result of ante-mortem variation and post-mortem diagenetic influences upon the isotopic compostion in different bones. As is the case for trace element concentrations, the isotopic composition in the more porous bones, such as ribs and vertebrae, will probably be affected more readily than in the compact bones of the femur and other long bones.

In three cases, delta 13C values in collagen from one of the long bones and in collagen from ribs or vertebrae from the same individual were determined. In these cases, long bone delta 13C values (mean -19.98 per mil) are less negative than rib/vertebra delta 13C values (mean -21.46 per mil). This difference might be the result of the incorporation of some soil carbon, with its rather negative delta 13C values, in the bone organic matter. However, the difference may also reflect ante-mortem variations in carbon isotopic ratios which may exist within skeletons. There are no data available on this aspect.

Collagen from a tibia and a femur of the Oostwoud skeleton **35/38** (section II.C.2.3) were analysed, giving delta 13C values -19.83 per mil and -19.79 per mil, respectively.

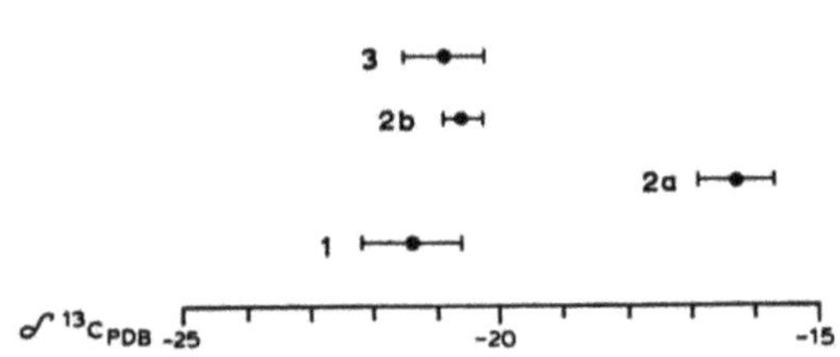

figure X.4 Delta 13C values in human bones from regions without C4 plants. Means and standard deviation. 1 (Van der Merwe & Vogel 1978) pre-maize North American Indians n=31; 2 (Johansen et al. 1986) Scandinavia a: coastal sites, n=4, b: inland site, n=20; 3 (this study) n=62.

C.4.2. Dietary implications

The data suggest that the dietary protein of all the individuals concerned was predominantly derived from terrestrial sources. Marine fish and other seafoods were probably of little or no importance as protein sources. In the system suggested by Johansen et al. (1986), humans with delta 13C values lower than -19.5 per mil are consuming predominantly terrestrial proteins, with marine proteins accounting for less than 10 % of the dietary proteins. This value can then be taken as a maximum for the amount of protein from marine foods in human diets in Bronze Age West-Friesland.

We have already seen that the protein content of marine fish and shellfish is about 4-4.5 times higher than that of the terrestrial staple foods such as meat and cereals (table X.1). A maximum of 10 % marine protein in the diet in West-Friesland implies that at most some 2.5 % of the energy in the human diet was supplied by marine foods.

The impact of marine food on the Sr/Ca ratio of the total diet depends on its Ca content (section V.A), and thus on the question which marine food was consumed. The mean Ca contents per unit of energy of marine fish and terrestrial staple foods are comparable (table X.5). In a diet consisting of meat, cereals, some leafy vegetables and marine fish, the terrestrial component has a Ca concentration which is as it is in the marine component, i.e. fish. In the case of West-Friesland, this would imply that at the very most about 2.5 % of the Ca in the diet is derived from marine fish.

Marine shellfish, however, have Ca concentrations which are about 10 times higher than those in diet consisting of meat, cereal grains and some leafy vegetables. This implies that Sr/Ca ratios in diets will be relatively strongly affected if the marine component in a diet consists of shellfish. For West-Friesland, the maximum share in diet of 2.5 % of energy from marine foods would imply that some 25 % of the Ca in the diet derived from marine shellfish. Considering the high Sr/Ca ratios in marine shellfish (section V.A.5), this would have a pronounced effect on the Sr/Ca ratio of the diet as a whole. Fortunately, the consumption of shellfish is well documented in the archeological record by means of shell refuse. In Bronze Age West-Friesland the consumption of shellfish was negligible (section V.A.5)

Table X.5. Mean protein and Ca contents in some groups of foods. Based on data from Paul & Southgate (1978) as assembled in tables X.1 and V.1.

food item	g protein/100 kJ	mg Ca/100 kJ
marine fish	4.1	4.9
marine shellfish	4.8	41
meats	1.1	0.5
wheat wholemeal flour	1.1	3
leafy vegetables	3.4	142

A special problem in relation to marine foods is formed by edible seaweeds. It is to be expected that seaweeds contain considerable quantities of Ca, Zn and other trace elements in comparison to their protein levels (Luten 1983, compare also values for terrestrial leafy vegetables). This implies that where seaweeds are the chief marine food component, these may supply a large proportion of the dietary Ca even if the proportion of marine protein in the diet is so small that the delta 13C shows a terrestrial value. Unfortunately, consumption of seaweeds is hardly traceable with archeological methods. It appears, however, likely that seaweeds were of negligible importance in Bronze Age diets in West-Friesland. The sites lie a fair distance from the sea, and the collection of seaweeds probably took more time and energy than the production and/or collection of other foods.

D. Conclusion

The carbon isotope data suggest that marine foods played a minor role in the diet of Bronze Age humans in West-Friesland. This corroborates the conclusion of IJzereef (1981). At the very most, some 10% of protein might have been derived from marine sources, which corresponds to about 2.5% of the amounts of energy and Ca.

The differences in protein and Ca contents of various marine foods may cause problems when relative amounts of marine foods in diets, as based on isotopic ratios in bone collagen, are converted to relative amounts of energy or Ca. It is therefore essential that ecoarcheological information on the potential food items is available, just as it is when Sr and Zn levels in bone are interpreted.

XI
DISCUSSION: AGRICULTURAL AND DIETARY IMPLICATIONS

A. INTRODUCTION

The more or less scattered pieces of information and the preliminary conclusions that are presented in the preceding chapters remain to be fitted into a single ecoarcheological and paleodietary model of the prehistory of West-Friesland. In this chapter, an attempt at such an integration of evidence will be made.

It appears useful to subdivide the discussion in two parts. The first part of the discussion deals with general ecological problems, the second part more specifically deals with dietary reconstruction.

B. TRACE ELEMENTS IN DOMESTIC ANIMALS

B.1 Discussion

In a preliminary report on the analysis of bones from Het Valkje in West-Friesland, the Sr concentrations in domestic animal species were discussed and tentatively explained (Runia 1987a). Theoretically, bone Sr levels decrease with an increasing proportion of meat in the diet, i.e. herbivores are expected to have higher Sr levels than omnivores and carnivores. The pattern of mean Sr levels in animal species from Het Valkje is, however, at variance with the pattern that would be expected on theoretical grounds. The herbivores, cattle and sheep/goat, have significantly different Sr concentrations. Sheep/goat and bones of the omnivorous dog have quite high Sr levels (compare table V.6, V.7, fig. V.3). The discrepancy between the expected and the observed pattern was tentatively explained by a model involving different herding practices for cattle and sheep/goat in combination with differences in Sr/Ca ratios in soils of various physiographic units. Cattle and pigs would have been kept close to the farms whereas sheep/goat flocks, guarded by dogs, would have been grazed in the basins or even farther away (Runia 1987a). Plant remains in dung found in an Iron Age house situated in an area with peat and salt marshes suggest that here too the cattle and goats were grazed on different meadows (Therkorn et al. 1984).

The pattern found in the Sr levels of animals in Het Valkje is also visible in the Sr levels of bones of animals from other sites (fig. V.3). Dogs and sheep/goat have fairly high Sr levels compared with the Sr concentrations in cattle and pigs.

A fairly consistent pattern is also visible for the relative Zn levels in bone of animals from the sites (table VI.4, VI.5, fig. VI.2). The omnivorous pig and dog have higher Zn levels than the cattle, but the caprovids also have high Zn levels compared to cattle.

In reviewing the animal bone trace element levels, it should be kept in mind that only a limited number of samples was analysed from some sites. In this discussion, Ba levels are not referred to because it is suspected that these have suffered from diagenetical influences (compare section VII.A).

As stated above (section V.C.3, VI.C.3), the interpretation of relative trace element levels in groups of animals is hampered by the lack of a good set of reference data. Though some studies on trophic level effects exist

(Schoeninger 1985, Rheingold et al. 1983), no detailed field studies have been published. The expected patterns in relative Sr levels in herbivores, omnivores and carnivores are based on Observed Ratio studies. From the evidence presented previously (chapter V, IX, Runia 1987b) it may be concluded that in actual field situations the reactions are far more complicated. The differences in Sr/Ca ratios in various plants and parts thereof in combination with the food selection by animals and the differential digestion and utilization of food in intestinal tracts of animals result in a divergence between the actual field situation and the theoretical models.

The actual field situation for relative Zn levels is similarily more complex than theoretical models. The active treatment of Zn in animal bodies which takes place under optimal circumstances, but also in times of food shortage or disease, is still another factor that might result in a divergence of field situations compared to the values expected theoretically. Conclusions based on these patterns should be viewed cautiously because of the obvious lack of reference material.

Returning to the relative Sr levels in humans and animals from the various sites, the following general picture emerges (fig. V.3). The most important observation is that the ranking of the mean Sr levels of the domestic animals species always follows in the same order. The Sr concentration in dogs ranks below that of sheep/goat in all sites. Thus, the theoretical rule that omnivores have lower Sr levels than herbivores appears to be valid for this pair of species. This is an interesting observation in the light of the supposed 'functional' relationship between the caprovids and the herding dog.

At all sites except Andijk the combination dog-sheep/goat has higher Sr levels than cattle. Both sheep and cattle are herbivores of the grazer type, which makes differential digestion of plant material of minor importance. This corroborates the suggestion that sheep/goat and cattle were grazed in different areas (Runia 1987a). Zoological evidence for goat, which is a browser, among the West-Frisian livestock is so scanty that this species probably did not contribute appreciably to the sheep/goat Sr concentrations. The mean relative levels of Zn in the bones again corroborate the evidence: sheep/goat have higher Zn levels than cattle. The relation between mean Zn levels in sheep/goat and dogs is, however, somewhat less clear.

A difference in Observed Ratios for sheep/goat and cattle should be considered as an alternative explanation for the observed pattern in their relative Sr levels. Though it may be possible to explain the differences between cattle and sheep/goat in this way, it fails to explain the high Sr levels in dogs. Moreover, the data for Andijk suggest no difference in OR values in cattle and sheep/goat, for which there are also no experimental indications.

The remaining pair of animal species is formed by pigs and cattle. These animals were supposedly kept on the ridges near the farms (section II.C.1.4). The omnivorous pigs generally have Sr levels that are higher than the herbivorous cattle, whereas theoretically the opposite would be expected. For Zn, the observed pattern agrees with theoretical considerations: pigs have higher Zn contents than cattle. The high Sr levels in pigs may be explained as the consequence of the effects of a combination of food selection and differences in Sr/Ca ratios in plants and parts thereof. Pigs feed on all kinds of vegetable and non-vegetable matter which they root up from the soil. The stomachs of many recent wild boars were found to contain plant roots (Groot Bruinderink 1976). One would expect similar feeding habits in prehistoric domestic pigs. Roots which have high Sr/Ca ratios (section IX.D.4) may thus be responsible for the high Sr levels in the West-Frisian pigs.

At only one site, Velsen, do pigs have lower Sr levels than cattle. This suggests that at this site the pigs were fed differently. It should be noted that Velsen is the only site where some forests may have been present in the neighbourhood (section II.C.2.10); this might explain the observed difference.
The low Sr concentration for pig at Oostwoud is of dubious value, as from this site only a single pig bone was analysed.

The site of Andijk is the only one that does not conform to the general pattern where Sr levels in sheep/goat rank first, followed by dog, pig and cattle. In fact, the pattern for mean Sr and Zn levels of the Andijk samples agrees best with the theoretical model. Here, cattle and sheep/goat have approximately equal Sr levels, pigs somewhat higher levels and dogs and humans lower levels. The omnivorous pigs and dogs have relatively high Zn levels whereas cattle and sheep/goat have lower Zn levels. This raises the question of what the reason for the observed difference between Andijk and the other sites could be. The model explaining the general pattern for the other sites would gain in credibility if it allows the different pattern for Andijk to be fitted in. In this case, an explanation which takes the environment of the site into account should be sought: one possibility is that cattle and sheep/goat were herded in the same area and thus on the same soils.

A second possibility is that no differences in soil Sr/Ca ratios were present near Andijk. As mentioned previously (section V.C.3.3), Andijk is situated in an area where the main creek ridge branches into a number of smaller ridges. The area of sandy and sandy loamy soils near the site Andijk appears rather more extensive than that around Het Valkje. As suggested in section II.C.1.4. there is some difference in the relative quantities of animal bones from Andijk and from Het Valkje (table II.4). Andijk has low percentages of pigs (3.5 %) and sheep/goat (8.9 %) and a high percentage of cattle (86.2 %). This suggests that the conditions for animal husbandry at Andijk differed from those at Het Valkje.

The relative numbers of bones from the various domestic animal species in relation to the environment of sites has been discussed by Prummel (1979). The availability of woodland appears to be an important factor in relation to the proportion of pig bones in a site. For sheep/goat the quality of pasture may be important. In wet and non-saline grasslands the sheep/goat may suffer from the liver fluke parasite *Fasciola hepatica* (Prummel 1979, Barker 1985). The snail *Galba truncatula* which may act as the intermediate host for the liver fluke has been found in Hoogkarspel (Kuyper 1977, Prummel 1979). The liver fluke may therefore have been a threat to Bronze Age sheep grazing in the clay basins, and it can also be seen as a threat for the proposed model on livestock management. However, 'unenclosed grazing in prehistoric times, as with cattle and pigs, would have effectively forestalled the worst attacks of the parasites' (Barker 1985:41-42), which in turn can be seen as a reason for sheep/goat grazing away from the farms.

The site of Zwaagdijk differs from the other sites in the relatively large differences between the trace element concentrations in cattle bones and in bones from the other species. For Sr, Zn and Ba concentrations, the difference between cattle and pig is very large in comparison to the other sites. The Ba concentrations for cattle bones are low compared with the those of pig, dog and sheep/goat (fig. VII.2). The data suggest that the cattle bones have trace element concentrations that are too low compared to with the other bones. The somewhat deviant pattern of Zwaagdijk might be the result of taphonomic processes. A possible explanation is that the cattle bones from the Zwaagdijk site are of a more recent date than the other bones from the site. The low mean Fe content in these cattle bones (0.50 ± 0.08 %, n=6) compared with the mean Fe content of all cattle bone samples of 1.94 ± 0.72 % (n=145, difference sign. at 99% level, Student's t=4.87, 149 DF) corroborates this idea. The absolute Sr concentration in the Zwaagdijk cattle bones (964 ± 69 mg/kg, n=6) is also significantly lower than in the other cattle bones from Bronze Age West-Friesland (1181 ± 119 mg/kg, n=97; t=4.38, 101 DF). The concentrations of Fe and trace elements for the other animal species from Zwaagdijk are no different from the levels in the other sites. Thus, it can be concluded that it is unlikely that the cattle bones analysed date from the same occupation period as the other bones from Zwaagdijk. In this case, the bones must all represent a cow buried at the site before the 13th century (Modderman 1964, Clason 1964). Though Modderman found no archeological reasons against an association with the prehistoric occupation, Clason suspected this skeleton to be of more recent date.

This is, of course, unfortunate, in that the analysed cattle bones of Zwaagdijk are useless as reference material for the trace element levels in human bones from this site. On the other hand, this case illustrates the potential of bone chemistry in ecoarcheological studies. In subsistence agriculture, trace element levels of all animal bones found in a site should, within certain limits, be of fixed proportions. Animal bones which do not fit into the pattern of chemical data are to be viewed with suspicion. One should try to determine whether they have a different taphonomy or represent animals that were imported to the site, or, as discussed above, animals that were grazed in a different area. However, field studies to establish the 'normal' pattern for trace element levels in animals from a restricted area remain to be carried out.

Still another example for the use of chemical analysis of animal bones is formed by the material from Schagen-Muggenburg. In this site, some exceptionally large cattle specimen were found (shoulder height 148 cm compared with 100-110 cm for average Roman Age cattle, Therkorn, pers. comm., IJzereef 1981). The chemical composition of these and the other cattle bones was compared. The interesting feature of this material is, however, a distinction observed in the chemical data from the normal sized cattle. A group with low Zn and low Sr concentrations (cattle I), and a group with somewhat higher Sr levels and distinctly higher Zn levels (cattle II) can be distinguished. Bones of the 'giant' cattle are found to contain low Zn levels comparable to the levels found in the cattle I grouping, while their Sr levels are even lower than those of this group (table XI.1).

The comparison with other animal species and the pattern for Zn levels in other sites (fig. VI.2) suggests that the cattle II Zn concentrations are abnormally high. The cause of this phenomenon is not clear, but the possibility of cattle trade comes to mind. Trade of cattle in native-Roman contexts is documented by at least one literary source: the contract for the purchase of a cow found in Tolsum (Friesland, Van Es 1981). This problem will be further discussed in connection with the excavation report for Schagen-Muggenburg (Therkorn & Runia, in prep.).

Table XI.1. Comparison between Sr and Zn concentrations (mg/kg bone ash) in bones from three groups of cattle and in other animal species from Schagen-Muggenburg. Identical letters in columns 'sign.' indicate that mean values do not differ at the 95% level of significance (Student's t test).

group	n	Sr	sign.			Zn	sign.		
cattle I	16	1257 ± 203		B		157 ± 50	A		
cattle II	10	1296 ± 133		B		539 ± 153			C
'giant' cattle	6	1128 ± 59	A			168 ± 42	A		
pig	9	1550 ± 275			C	309 ± 136		B	
dog	7	1633 ± 242			C	478 ± 240		B	C
sheep/goat	11	1649 ± 253			C	454 ± 183		B	C

B.2. Conclusion

Though the first 'paleodietary' study focussed on Sr levels in animal bones and on animal diets (Toots & Voorhies 1965), in later studies the analysis of animal bones has been carried out as an appendix to the analysis of human bones. Analysis of animal bones is generally motivated by the indications for diagenetic influences and relative levels of trace elements in the paleoenvironments it may yield (Sillen 1981, Price 1985, compare section I.B.1.3). In fact, the motives in this study were no different.

The material presented here does, moreover, indicate that the chemical analysis of prehistoric animal bones is of interest in its own right. With the aid of chemical data, far-reaching paleo-economic conclusions may drawn that are not possible using the conventional paleoenvironmental data. Both intra- and inter-site comparisons can be used to further our understanding of the relationship between man and the domestic animals within a spatial framework.

C. DIETARY IMPLICATIONS OF TRACE ELEMENT LEVELS IN HUMAN BONES

C.1. A quantitative assessment of prehistoric human diets: the agricultural and nutritional background

C.1.1. General aspects

The data presented in the preceding chapters and collected elsewhere prove that the 'vegetable versus animal food' approach in Sr studies is an oversimplification of the actual complex situation (chapter V, IX, Runia 1985a, b). The levels of Sr and other trace elements in human bones are the result of numerous discrimination processes active both within the human body, and outside it during the formation of trace element concentrations in food items. These processes include the physico-chemical discrimination between Ca and other divalent cations such as Sr and Zn. Furthermore, the food selection by animals and humans can also be seen as a discrimination process affecting trace element levels in human bones (Runia, in prep.). The interpretation of trace element levels in human bones in terms of diet is, therefore, not a simple matter and can only be attempted with the aid of adequate ecoarcheological information. Results of chemical analysis of human and animal bones have been presented and discussed in the preceding chapters. In the present chapter an attempt is made to combine the results and to extrapolate, in terms of dietary composition, from the combined results. The agricultural and nutritional feasiblity of diets will also be discussed.

A discussion of the diet and nutrition of the West-Frisian farmers may be structured around the five basic questions formulated by Dennell (1979:122): '(i) what foods are eaten? (ii) how much of each is eaten? (iii) what is the value of each food in terms of energy-production (fat, protein and carbohydrate) and of maintaining and regulating the body (minerals and vitamins)? (iv) how is the diet of an individual affected by his/her age, sex and status? and (v) how does it vary in composition and quantity throughout the year?'.

Integration of information from all kinds of (eco)archeological sources is required in order to answer these basic questions. The information extracted from the bones can be seen as a specialized source of ecoarcheological information. In addition, data on the nutritive value of modern foods are needed and the nutritional requirements of the human body must be known.

The range of potential food items that may have been consumed in the area under scrutiny has been outlined in the chapters V and IX. As stated before, the (eco)archeological record gives an incomplete and biased picture of the range of food items. It may be inferred from human nutritional requirements that at least some foods which are not archeologically traceable, such as leafy vegetables and milk, were also consumed.

There is no direct information available on the precise composition of prehistoric foods. Some vegetable and animal foods or remains of foods have been preserved in exceptional circumstances, but diagenetic changes obstruct reliable analysis of this material. We have, therefore, to rely on the composition of modern foods as source of information on prehistoric foods. It is likely that differences in the nutritive value of prehistoric and modern foods will be small, provided that suitable, similar modern foods are selected as reference material.

A further aspect in the assessment of the nutritive value of prehistoric foods encompasses the effects of food storage and food preparation. Boiling, smoking, roasting, salting, storage, and other treatments are likely to affect the composition of foods. These changes probably have relatively small effects on the gross composition of foods, i.e. on protein, carbohydrate and fat contents. Vitamins, however, are susceptible to treatment with or exposure to, for example, air, temperature, high or low pH and light (Den Hartog et al. 1978, Wing & Brown 1979, De Wijn & Van Staveren 1980).

A discussion on the nutritive value of the foods must, therefore, comprise a review of the treatments to which the foods were exposed. Some treatments, such as smoking of meat, boiling of gruels, storage, roasting and milling of cereal grains, may be inferred from artifacts, ecoarcheological sources and plain common sense, but the essential cooking finesses in relation to loss of nutrients remain largely unknown. The vitamin C contents of foods are, for instance, influenced by height of temperature and the duration of treatment. Another vitamin, thiamine, is relatively stable at high pH values, but degrades at low values of pH (Den Hartog et al. 1978, Wing & Brown 1979, De Wijn & Van Staveren 1980).

It can be concluded that Dennell's basic questions (i) on the range of food items, and (iii) on their relative nutritive value can be answered within certain limits. There remain, however, uncertainties, especially in relation to the nutritive losses that occur during the processing of vegetable foods.

Basic question (v) on the variation in the composition of the diet throughout the year is in fact of little interest in the present study. Bone chemistry based paleodietary studies deal with long-term average diets, because these are reflected in the composition of the bones. The storage of food in agricultural societies is one of the basic aspects in the discussion on variations in dietary composition throughout the year. In comparison with hunter/gatherers, agriculturalists probably have less seasonal variation in diets.

The trace element concentrations in human and animal bones are essential in answering the basic questions (ii) and (iv), i.e., how much of each food item was eaten by individuals of various sex, age and status. The 'how much' can be viewed absolutely, in kilograms of food items, or relatively, in percentages. The use of trace element data in answering these questions is inherently restricted to the relative aspect. The conversion of relative to absolute amounts of food requires additional agricultural and nutritional data.

In paleodietary research in general but also in studies using bone trace element levels, few attempts have been made towards a quantitative approach. As pointed out, the normal paleoecological methods are not suitable for a quantitative reconstruction of paleodiets, though in many cases a semi-quantitative 'ranking' of the relative importance of food items may be inferred (Dennell 1979).

Bone chemistry has only rarely been used in quantitative reconstructions due to the lack of basic information (Price et al. 1985b, Bumsted 1985, Schoeninger, in manuscript). Paleodiets may be studied using quantitative, mathematical methods (Keene 1981, 1985, Boyle 1986, Belovsky 1986).

Besides economic, paleoecological and archeological data on food items and diets, the chemistry of bones is an independent source of information which may be treated mathematically.

There are a number studies on the economics of prehistoric people that incorporate dietary data. The agro-economics of our study area have been discussed by IJzereef and Brandt (section II.C.1.4). These and similar studies (for instance, Bakels 1978, Dennell 1978) deal with the 'supply side' of diets, whereas the 'demand side', i.e. apart from energy, the nutritional requirements of the consumers, is not taken into consideration. The linear programming studies of Keene (Keene 1981, 1985) are of interest not only from a methodological point of view (section XI.C.3), but also because they pay attention to human nutritional requirements.

C.1.2. Nutritional requirements

The diet, i.e. the total amount of food that is consumed within a certain timespan, must contain a variety of components to fulfill the nutrional requirements of the consumer. It is thus necessary to know what the human nutritional requirements when the feasibility of a reconstructed human diet is judged. Obviously, these requirements cannot be outlined precisely. Nutritional requirements vary between individuals and depend on individual intrinsic factors such as age, physiological efficiency and body weight, and on a number of external factors, such as climate, work load and working conditions. The quantification of the minimum amounts of essential components needed to keep a human body 'running' is, therefore, not easy, and is further hampered by the vague boundaries between being well nourished, under nourished or malnourished. This problem has been discussed by various authors (Clark & Haswell 1964, Den Hartog et al. 1978, Wing & Brown 1979, Dennell 1979, Caselitz 1986).

In the assessment of agricultural and nutritional feasibility of potential prehistoric diets it is useful to work with a 'standard family', which exploits one farmstead and which in fact, is a largely self-supporting economic unit. Each family produces and consumes its own food, and a (small) surplus for purchasing non-food commodities. An average family of six persons, two to three adults and three to four children of various ages appears to be commonly used (Brandt 1976, Bloemers 1978, IJzereef 1981). The nutritional requirements in the form of energy, proteins, and some minerals and vitamins will here be discussed briefly.

Energy

The amount of energy required by humans depends on a number of factors. The basic amount of energy which is needed for the essential body functions depends on sex, and weight and composition of the body. In addition, energy is needed to perform all kinds of activities. The advised daily amount of energy for males aged 20-35 years and a body weight of 70 kg ranges from 9.6 MJ at a low level of activities to 15.9 MJ per day at a high level of activities, for females of the same age and a body weight of 60 kg the values are 7.6 to 10.9 MJ per day, respectively (NVT 1983). Children between 1 and 10 years of age need some 5-9 MJ per day. Girls aged 10-19 need some 9.5-10 MJ per day whereas boys in that age group need some 12.5 MJ per day. These data appear relevant for the present study because the skeletal material suggests that the Bronze Age inhabitants of West-Friesland do not differ much from present day Dutchmen in height and weight of their bodies.

For the 'standard family' it can be estimated that a mean of some 10 MJ per person per day is needed. This estimate is close to the mean value of 9.9 MJ per person per day given by the FAO for a population of 50 children, 25 adult males and 25 adult females (quoted in Bakels 1978). IJzereef (1981) reckons with two values, 2000 and 3000 kcal, the mean of which, 2500 kcal, equals 10.5 MJ. Keene (1981) arrived at a somewhat lower average minimum of 9 MJ per person per day. Clark & Haswell (1964) stress that energy requirements are related to body weights, and their data on energy contents in diets from tropical regions are lower in consequence of the lower body weights of the people involved.

Proteins

Proteins, or rather the amino acids present in proteins, are needed for the growth and maintenance of the human body. A number of aminoacids cannot be synthetised by humans and have to be supplied by the food. Because not all the aminoacids in proteins are present in quantities desired by the body dietary proteins usually are utilized incompletely.

Advised daily doses of proteins are some 65 to 95 g for adult males and 55 to 70 g for adult females (NVT, 1983). The amount of protein required by children is only little less than the adult requirements. Daily doses as advised by other authorities are considerably lower than the Dutch values (Den Hartog et al. 1978). According to De Wijn & Van Staveren (1980), protein requirements for adult males are 0.8 g and for adult females 0.75 g per kg body weight. Keene (1981) arrived at a minimum of 32.6 g protein per person per day. Actual amounts of proteins consumed are, however, higher than the advised doses. Den Hartog et al. (1978) quote FAO reports in which for 1961 a world average of 65.2 g protein consumption per person per day is calculated. For third world countries the mean value is 54.9 g and for the industrial countries 87.0 g protein per person per day.

For the standard family a mean consumption of at least 50-60 g protein per person per day appears a reasonable estimate, which equals a total of some 300-360 g of protein per day per standard family.

Calcium

Calcium is needed for the build-up of the skeleton and in a number of physiological processes. Advised daily doses of Ca vary considerably. In countries where milk and dairy products are important food items the advised daily doses tend to be relatively high while in other countries the advised amounts are lower. An amount of 500 mg in food per person per day is generally considered necessary for the maintenance of the skeleton and of adequate Ca levels in the body (De Wijn & Van Staveren 1980). Pregnant and lactating women need a supplementary amount of some 500 mg Ca per day. Keene (1981) arrived at an average minimum of 511 mg Ca per person per day. The standard family would need a minimum amount of about 3 g Ca per day.

In the discussion on Bronze Age diets, in which Ca contents of food items are used as reference material for trace element concentrations, the amount of Ca in the diet may be a useful independent parameter in judging its feasibility. Diets containing less than 500 mg Ca per day are not considered to be realistic.

Vitamins

In prehistoric cultures where a relatively broad spectrum of foods is consumed in unrefined form vitamin shortage in the food is not very likely. As an example, the thiamine contents of diets are discussed below. In his linear programming study, Keene (1981) found that in general vitamins were present in sufficient quantities in diets of hunter/gatherers.

A discussion of all vitamins that have to be present in diets would not appear to be useful here. Only those nutrients that cause deficiency features in the skeleton are useful. For the discussion on the feasibility of diets, it should be known from the skeletal material whether a vitamin was present in a quantity sufficient to prevent deficiency features. For this reason the discussion on vitamin requirements is restricted to the vitamins B1, C and D.

Thiamine, vitamin B1

Thiamine plays a role in the biochemical conversion of carbohydrates, and the amounts needed are therefore correlated to the amount of carbohydrates in the diet. The minimum amount of thiamine necessary to prevent beri-beri is 0.06 mg per MJ of carbohydrate, protein and alcohol energy, but the advised daily doses are higher: 0.14 mg/MJ (Den Hartog et al. 1978, De Wijn & Van Staveren 1980). Thiamine is stable at pH values below 5, but detoriates at higher pH values and at temperatures higher than 100 ^{o}C.

The figures in table XI.2 indicate that in prehistoric, non-refined foods usually enough thiamine is present, even if some of it is lost in food processing. Thiamine deficiency may occur when sugars (honey) and refined cereal products, which includes beer, supply a considerable part of the energy in the diet. It appears likely that in the Bronze Age diets in West-Friesland thiamine was present in sufficient quantities. Thiamine contents can therefore not be used as constraining factors in the discussion on the feasibility of diets. Thiamine deficiency is also not apparent from skeletal material.

Table XI.2. Mean contents of thiamine and ascorbic acid in groups of modern food items, in mg per 100 g edible product and mg per MJ. Calculated from Paul & Southgate (1978).

		----per 100 g----		------per MJ------	
item	n	thiamine	asc.ac.	thiamine	asc.ac.
meat	4	0.28±0.22	0	0.21±0.01	0
organs	8	0.35±0.10	12±6	0.77±0.35	23±9
cows'milk	1	0.04	1.5	0.15	5.5
eggs	1	0.09	0	0.15	0
wholemeal	1	0.46	0	0.30	0
nuts	5	0.25±0.10	tr.	0.16±0.09	tr.
leafy vegetables	13	0.07±0.03	45±38	1.0±0.4	560±40
root crops	7	0.05±0.02	29±38	0.46±0.16	200±170
fruits	11	0.04±0.02	19±16	0.31±0.16	190±197

Ascorbic acid, vitamin C

Ascorbic acid is a nutrient only marginally present in the calculated diets in the model study by Keene (1981). It appears justified to assess the dietary compositions based on bone trace element levels for their ascorbic acid contents. Diets deficient in vitamin C cause pathological changes which may be recognized in (prehistoric) skeletons (Maat 1986).

Ascorbic acid plays a role in a number of physiological processes. Advised minimum daily doses of ascorbic acid range from 30 mg per day in the UK and Canada to 100 mg in Russia (Den Hartog et al. 1978). Doses of 20 to 30 mg per day suffice to prevent scurvy (Den Hartog et al. 1978, De Wijn & Van Staveren 1980). Keene (1981) reckons with an average minimum daily dose of

27 mg per person per day. For the present study, a minimum of 25 mg per person per day has been chosen. Per standard family therefore, 150 mg would be required each day.

Ascorbic acid is present in fruits, leafy vegetables, root crops and animal organs (table XI.2). Considerable portions, up to 50 % or more, of vitamin C are lost upon heating. Taking this into account, diets should therefore contain at least 300 mg ascorbic acid per family per day.

Vitamin D

Vitamin D is essential in Ca metabolism and can be synthetised in the human skin under the influence of direct sunlight. The effects of severe vitamin D shortage can be easily diagnosed in prehistoric skeletal material (Brothwell 1981, Caselitz 1986, Maat 1986).

Food is the source of extra vitamin D in the winter period in temperate regions. The amount of vitamin D which should be supplied by the diet is difficult to estimate, because it supplements an unknown quantity of vitamin D synthetised in the skin. In comparison with modern people the West-Frisian farmers probably spent more time out of doors, and thus synthetised relatively more vitamin D. As pointed out by Keene (1981), lack of reference data hamper the estimation of the amount of vitamin D that must be supplied by the food.

Fish livers have high vitamin D contents. Other dietary vitamin D sources are milk, dairy products and egg yolks. For the present study it is assumed that these products were consumed in sufficient quantities to prevent rickets.

Conclusion

For the discussion on Bronze Age diets, the nutrient requirements of an average or standard family of six persons can be summarized as follows. The food must supply an average of at least 60 MJ of energy, 300 to 360 g protein, 3 g Ca, and 300 mg ascorbic acid per day. The dietary requirements of thiamine and vitamin D have not been quantified.

C.1.3. The nutritional status of Bronze Age West-Frisian farmers

It is obvious that prehistoric people were not guided in their eating habits by the advice of nutritionists and dieticians . The minimum amount of nutrients, as advised by modern nutritionists, may therefore not have been present in prehistoric diets. The skeletal material from the Bronze Age people of West-Friesland may, however, be used for the assessment of their over-all nutritional status, since malnutrition and/or a diet deficient in specific components may affect the skeleton (Wing & Brown 1979, Brothwell 1981, Caselitz 1986, Maat 1986).

Few features indicating mal- or undernutrition are encountered in the skeletal material (Appendix 1). One individual (**48** 320) showed osteoporosis, which may be the result of a diet deficient in Ca and/or vitamin D. One other individual (**36(1)**) had suffered from rickets as may be concluded from the bowed L tibia. A number of Harris' lines can also be seen on radiographs of this tibia.

Radiographs of tibias from some other individuals were made in order to detect whether undernourishment during formation of the bones was a common feature (for Harris' lines see Caselitz 1986, Maat 1986). Harris' lines were virtually absent in these specimens. This suggests that severe food shortage did occur not often, and certainly not on a yearly base. This is substantiated by the absence of hypoplasic features in the tooth enamel of the individuals involved.

Scurvy, which is caused by vitamin C deficiency, leaves less clear traces in the skeleton than vitamin D deficiency. Scurvy may result in infractions of the bone cortex in the long bones of the legs, and in the loss of teeth (Maat 1986). The skeletal material (Appendix 1) does not suggest that the Bronze Age inhabitants of West-Friesland suffered from chronic scurvy.

The absence of features indicating malnutrition corrobarates the general impression of the skeletal material, i.e. robust bones and mean body heights of about 175 cm for males and 163 cm for females, which suggests that the people under study were fairly well nourished.

C.1.4. Agricultural possibilities

'Land classification'

The soils which in Bronze Age West-Friesland were used in cereal cultivation and animal husbandry may be subjected to what in present day soil science is called land classification or evaluation. In this method the characteristics of soil and land are classified in relation to their agricultural potential. It is likely that prehistoric farmers employed their own empirical and straightforward system of judging agricultural possibilities of soils.

Soils

In West-Friesland the low-lying clayey soils and the higher, sandy to loamy soils of the ridges are distinct in that the former are suitable for pasture and meadow and the latter for use as arable.

The sandy to loamy soils in (peri)marine sediments were probably rather fertile and relatively easy to till. The dimensions of Triticum dicoccum and Hordeum vulgare grains suggest that growing conditions were good (Buurman 1979). Archeological finds suggest that arable fields were manured (IJzereef 1981), which is corroborated by the analysis of soil samples which suggest that material was brought from the basins to the arable fields on the ridges (section IX.B).

Climate

The weather was found to be an important factor for cereal yields at Butser Ancient farm (Reynolds 1981). This may be the case for all (subsistence) agriculture and the climate is therefore of interest. Dry summers probably did not result in decreased yields in Bronze Age West-Friesland. The water table was comparatively high, and the soils could probably contain adequate moisture reserves. The climate was temperate-oceanic, i.e. extremely cold winters and hot, dry summers were exceptional.

Infrastructure

Agricultural settlements are generally situated at points not far from water, arable land and grazing grounds (Bakels 1978, Dennell 1978, Barker 1985). These resources were all closely spaced in West-Friesland. In modern terminology, the infrastructure was suitable for subsistence agriculture in the form of mixed farming.

Though the high water table, especially in the later habitation period, may have caused some agricultural problems, such as a late start to spring growth, the West-Frisian Bronze Age landscape does appear to be well suited for intensive, mixed farming. The technological level of the period would only allow small scale farming. IJzereef (1981) estimated that at Het Valkje each farm had at maximum an area of 3.0 to 8.8 ha of arable.

Cereal yields

Estimates for cereal yields in prehistoric West-Friesland are difficult to give. Both absolute yields, in kg grains per hectare, and relative yields, in seed/yield ratios, are of interest. Yield estimates have been discussed by various authors (Bakels 1978, Dennell 1978, Rowley-Conwy 1981, IJzereef 1981, Mercer 1981, Barker 1985, Pals in press).

Estimates can be based on experimental data for yields on non fertilized fields and on published data regarding yields in primitive agricultural systems. Both sources of information are to be used with caution. Present-day yields on non fertilized fields may be increased as a consequence of air pollution, i.e. deposition of nitrogen and by other factors such as better weed control. Data from medieval and more recent written sources should be seen in the light of the 'raison d'etre' of these sources: often the yield figures were to be used in connection with tithing and taxes. Yields were probably underestimated in many cases (Slicher van Bath 1960, 1963a, b).

A large body of seed/yield ratios was collected from published and written sources by Slicher van Bath (1963a, b). Seed/yield ratios in general were in the range 1:3 to 1:6 before the 19th century. The majority of these seed/yield ratios stem from large estates, such as those owned by churches and nobility. Individual farmers, however, probably achieved lower seed/yield ratios, i.e. higher yields per amount of sowing seed. Mean gross yields range from some 600 kg/ha in German demesnes to over 2000 kg/ha of Frisian farmers (calculated from the yields in hectoliters (Slicher van Bath 1962), using Mercer's (1981) estimate that 1000 kg equals 1.15 m3).

Experimental data from trial fields at Butser Ancient Farm and Rothamsted Experimental Station indicate that over 800 kg of wheat may be produced per hectare on unmanured fields each year (Rowley-Conwy 1981, Reynolds 1981). At Butser the average seed/yield ratio was 1:30 at a mean yearly yield of 1850 kg of Triticum dicoccum/ha in 8 years of continuous cultivation without manuring. The yields were found to depend largely on the weather during the growing season. Cold springs and dry summers cause low yields. The Butser trial fields are situated on former grazing ground. The soil, a rendzina on chalk, has a high organic matter content, which, as other rendzinas, probably has a low C/N ratio (compare de Bakker 1979). The decomposition of the organic matter that took place under arable conditions, as can be inferred from the decrease in organic matter content (Reynolds 1981: table 2) may have supplied the wheat with some nitrogen.

Yields at Rothamsted were lower than at Butser, with a mean of 900-1000 kg wheat/ha from continuous cultivation on unmanured fields (Rowley-Conwy 1981). This may be the result of soil factors and of the Triticum species used. T.dicoccum, grown at Butser, is better adapted to low N levels than modern T.aestivum varieties (Reynolds 1981). At Rothamsted, the introduction of a fallow year was followed by a considerable increase of yields. The gradual increase of mean yields in the four-year cycles since 1930 may, however, in part result from increasing deposition of N from the air.

Though absolute quantities of experimental yields, especially at Butser, may be somewhat suspect, the experiments clearly show the effects of manuring and fallow periods on the yields. The arable fields of Bronze Age West-Friesland were most likely manured in one form or the other. The farm buildings were designed for keeping animals indoors and dung produced in the stables was probably brought out onto the fields.

Shortage of land may have caused continuous cultivation of cereals. However, periods of use as arable probably were alternated with years during which animals, most likely cattle and pigs, were kept on fallow fields on the sandy ridges. Such a system would result in a smaller area under cereal crops, but total yields would not be lower, and might even be higher than with continuous wheat cultivation. The fallow year would result in higher yields per hectare, as well as enabling tillage, weed and predator control and harvesting to be carried out more efficiently. These considerations might have been a strong stimulus to concentrate on high yields per hectare in a system where harvesting time was an important limiting factor in cereal production.

A system like this 'husbandry with high cereal yields' (Slicher van Bath 1962) is feasible for small-scale farming, such as was, most likely, practiced in Bronze Age West-Friesland. Farm accounts of two 16th-17th century farmers who used such a system contained mean seed/yield ratios of approximately 1:12 for wheat and 1:7.5 for barley. Both farmers manured their fields and reached mean wheat yields of 2040 and 2270 kg/ha (Slicher van Bath 1962). Yields in Bronze Age West-Friesland probably amounted to 1000 kg/ha or more in view of the favorable circumstances for cereal grain cultivation. This is twice the amount estimated by Dennell (1978) for Bulgarian sites. Pals (in press) envisages yields of some 800-1000 kg/ha for 9th-10th century Kootwijk on poor sandy soils in a system using sheep and cattle dung.

Table XI.3. Gross yields and amounts of seed necessary for net yields of 1630 kg cereal grains at various seed/yield ratios and storage losses

seed/yield ratio	loss (%)	seed (kg)	gross yield(kg)
1:2	10	2038	4075
	20	2717	5433
1:3	10	958	2875
	20	1162	3490
1:5	10	466	2329
	20	543	2717
1:10	10	204	2038
	20	466	2329
1:20	10	96	1918
	20	109	2173
1:30	10	63	1881
	20	71	2126

The discrepancy between the average seed/yield ratios in experiments and in written sources remains puzzling. This is, however, not a serious problem in relation to a quantitative approach. The average family on a 100% grain diet would consume 1630 kg grain each year. The gross yield necessary to supply this amount can be calculated for various seed/yield ratios. Furthermore, storage losses have to be accounted for. Mercer (1981) counts with 20% loss. This figure is probably too high, so 10% loss was considered as another possibility (table XI.3).

It is evident that changes in gross yields needed per family are relatively small at seed/yield ratios of 1:10 and lower (i.e. higher yields per amount of seed), though there are relatively large differences in the amounts of sowing seed necessary. At seed/yield ratios smaller than 1:10 a family on a pure cereal diet would need a total amount of about 2000 kg of grain each year for consumption, losses and sowing seed.

The time needed to harvest cereals is generally considered to be the limiting factor in North-West European subsistence agriculture (IJzereef 1981, Pals in press). Under the assumption that yields amounted to 1000 kg/ha and that the maximum amounts needed per family were 2000 kg, the amount needed by a family could be harvested without problems. IJzereef (1981) and Pals (in press) arrive at estimates of some 4 ha which could be harvested by a single family.

According to Brandt (1976, 1977, 1980) the arable fields in West-Friesland appeared to have had a standard area of some 40x40 to 50x50 square meters, i.e. 0.16 to 0.20 ha. In the area the dimensions of the fields also depended on the physiography. The number of fields needed by each family can be calculated using the estimates for total yields (table XI.4). The values in table XI.4 are for cultivated fields and should be multiplied by 2 or 1.5 if fields were left fallow every second or third year. Some 8 to 15 fields should have been available per farm if the yields amounted 1000 kg/ha and the diet contained 50-75% cereals.

Table XI.4. Number of fields of 50x50 square meter needed for the production of cereal grains and various yields/ha and percentages of cereals in diet (100% equals 2000 kg)

	yield kg/ha			
% cereals in diet	750	1000	1500	2000
100	13.3	10	6.7	5
75	10	7.5	5	3.8
50	6.7	5	3.3	2.5
25	3.3	2.5	1.7	1.3

Production of meat

Numbers of cattle and other animals per unit of grazing area are difficult to estimate. The dimensions of the farm houses probably offer a better basis for the estimation of the numbers of animals that were kept per family while the kill-off pattern can be derived from the age profile of the recovered animal bones. IJzereef (1981) used these data in an estimation of the amount of meat, fat and offal available per farm at Het Valkje using an elaborate method which included various caloric values for meat and fat content depending on the age of the animals. This resulted in estimates of amounts of animal food calories available per farm per year. A mean energy value of

15.5 MJ/kg cattle tissue and 15.9 MJ/kg pig and sheep/goat tissue can be calculated from IJzereef's tables. This is somewhat higher than the mean value for 'dressed carcasses' tabulated by Paul & Southgate (1978, see table V.1.). The total amount of animal tissue energy for the Early Period of Het Valkje was estimated at some 6300 MJ and for the Late Period some 4100 MJ per family per year. Within the Early Period, available animal food ranged from 3800 to 8900 MJ per year per family.

These figures are based on the assumption that all places in the stables were occupied. It remains, however, possible that some animals, for instance, the yearling cows, were kept out of doors all the year. This would result in the availability of a greater quantity of animal calories and there is, therefore, some justification for accepting a somewhat higher upper limit for the amount of animal food available each year. In addition, some game may have been consumed. It can be concluded that a maximum amount of some 10000 MJ from animal tissue food may have been available per family per year. The amount actually consumed may, however, have been lower. Some of the animals may have been exchanged for flint, bronze or other materials.

The dimensions of the farm houses in other sites in West-Friesland appear to be no different from those at Het Valkje, and a similar upper limit for the amount of available meat may be accepted.

Milk yields

The amount of milk available for human consumption in Het Valkje has been estimated by IJzereef (1981). His estimate is based on the numbers of milch cows and a milk surplus per animal per year of 100 l. The number of milch cows is derived from the dimensions of the farm houses and the kill-off pattern. If, however, the young cows and bulls were kept out of door, the number of animals and, in consequence, the number of milch cows may have been higher than in IJzereef's estimate. Milk yields per animal of some 100 l per lactation period appear reasonable. Estimates for the amounts of milk range from some 1400 to 2500 MJ per farm per year, with a mean of some 1900 MJ for the Early Period while for the Late Period the estimate is 1400 MJ per farm per year.

It appears reasonable to set the maximum available amount of milk per family per year at some 3000 MJ. A similar upper limit may be accepted for the other sites.

Leafy vegetables and roots

No data on yields of leafy vegetables and root crops are available. It may be supposed that only limited amounts of these food items were consumed. The data in table V.1 and XI.5 show that leafy vegetables and roots have relatively low energy contents. It is, therefore, unlikely that these vegetables supplied more than a few percent of the energy in diets.

Small garden plots, field boundaries, fallow arable land and the low-lying area probably could supply leafy and root vegetables in amounts up to a few percent of the diet.

Conclusion

The estimated maximum outputs of agricultural products for Bronze Age West-Friesland can be summarized as follows. Cereal grain yields probably ammounted 1000 kg/ha or more with seed/yield ratios of 1:10 or lower, which would allow a standard family of six persons to grow enough cereals for a 100% grain diet. The maximum amounts of meat and milk that may have been produced each year are estimated at 10,000 MJ and 3000 MJ, respectively. Leafy vegetables and roots were probably of minor importance as energy sources in the human diet.

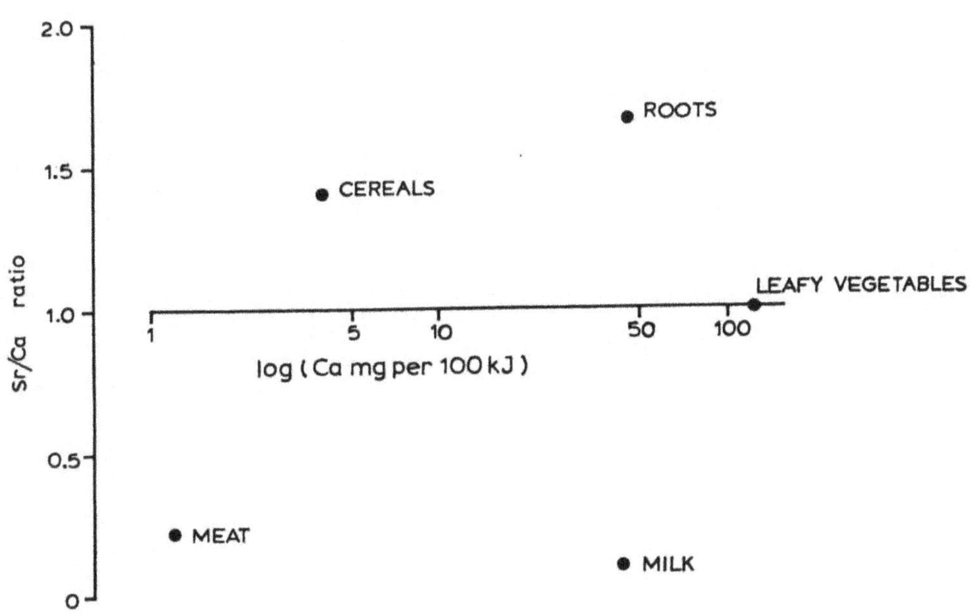

figure XI.1 Calcium contents and Sr/Ca ratios relative to Sr/Ca ratios in average plant material in some important components of human diets. Based on data in section V.A and IX.C.

C.2. Calculating diets: some examples

C.2.1. Calculations: framework

The trace element concentrations in the reference or baseline animal species and in the human bones may be used in calculations on the human dietary compositions. The actual calculations are based on the Sr and Ca concentrations in human and animal bones. The concentrations of other trace elements may enter the discussion in a later stage as a kind of additional constraint.

Prior to entering upon the calculations, a basic assumption has to be made, namely that bone Sr/Ca ratios now measured deviate only slightly from the original, in vivo Sr/Ca ratios. Furthermore, the principle of 'actuality' is adopted, i.e. that there are no differences in prehistoric physiological processes compared with present day situations.

Cattle bones are useful as reference material for various reasons. Firstly, in many sites in North-Western Europe, they are present in fairly large numbers (Barker 1985, Randsborg 1985). Cattle produce meat and milk, which for many sites were probably important food items quantitatively. Secondly, the cow is a strict herbivore of the grazer type, which means that large amounts of vegetable material are ingested and subsequently effectively digested (section V.A.2.5). Thus, cattle may ingest and digest vegetable material with Sr/Ca ratios close to the Sr/Ca ratio in 'average plant material' (APM, section IX.D.4). The relation between dietary and bone Sr/Ca ratios is well known (Comar et al. 1961, Comar 1963, section V.A.2). A third aspect of cattle is that they are often kept close to, or even in, the farm buildings, and thus, in West-Friesland, probably also close to or on the arable fields where cereals are grown for human consumption (compare section II.C.1.4, XI.A).

In the following calculations, cattle bone Sr/Ca ratios are used as the 'standard' from which the Sr/Ca ratios in various terrestrial food items are derived. Non-terrestrial animal foods (fish, shellfish, seaweeds) are for the moment omitted from the potential menu.

The relations between Sr/Ca ratios in various food items have been discussed in chapter V and IX. In figure XI.1, these relations have been expressed schematically with reference to APM Sr/Ca ratios and mean Ca concentrations.

The following steps have been taken: first of all, the Sr/Ca ratio in 'average plant material' (APM) is derived from cattle bone Sr/Ca ratios (termed Rc, section V.C.4.3), using the OR bone-diet for cattle. The Sr/Ca ratio in APM is subsequently used in calculating the Sr/Ca ratios in the vegetable food items, cereals, roots and leafy vegetables, and the Sr/Ca ratio in milk. The Sr/Ca ratio in beef equals the Sr/Ca ratio in cattle bones. Other meats (mutton, pork) are not taken into consideration because these supplied only a limited part of the energy in the diets under scrutiny.

Calcium concentrations in prehistoric foods are not known, but mean values for groups of prehistoric food items probably do not deviate substantially from mean Ca concentrations in recent foods (section XI.C.1.1, table V.1). Values for recent foods are, therefore, used in the calculations.

Strontium concentrations in the different groups of food items can be calculated by combining the Sr/Ca ratios derived from the cattle bone Sr/Ca ratios with the Ca concentrations. The result of this action is a table with Sr concentrations S1, S2, ..., Sn and Ca concentrations C1, C2, ..., Cn, per unit of energy, in the components 1, 2, ..., n that potentially made up the diet of the people involved.

The Sr/Ca ratio of the diet under scrutiny (termed Rd) can be calculated using the human bone Sr/Ca ratio and the human OR bone-diet. The final step in the calculation comprises the solution of two equations with many variables, i.e. the relative proportion p1, p2, ..., pn of the components in the diet:

$$Rd = (p1xS1 + p2xS2 + ... + pnxSn)/(p1xC1 + p2xC2 + ... pnxCn)$$

and

$$p1 + p2 + ... + pn = 100\ \%$$

Obviously, there is an indefinite number of possible solutions. These possible solutions to the equations may be visualised in two or three dimensions by choosing fixed percentages for a number of components. A simple iterative computer programme was used for the calculations.

Calculations were carried for three of the sites in West-Friesland because, in fact, three possible relationships between Sr/Ca ratios in human bone and in cattle bones can be distinguished: Sr/Ca ratios in human bones (Rh) may be smaller than, equal to, or larger than cattle bone Sr/Ca ratios (Rc). If OR bone-diet values for cattle and humans are equal, this grouping corresponds to the grouping on the basis of relative Sr/Ca ratios in diets. Examples of all three cases have been observed in the database from West-Friesland. In the following sections, one example of each of the possible cases are presented.

C.2.2. The models

In each of the three cases, the number of dietary components is restricted to five: meat (beef), milk, and the vegetable products cereal grains, roots and leafy vegetables. Other vegetable products such as nuts and fruits may have been part of the diet (section IX.E). They have, however, been omitted from the model, because the relative amounts of these items in diets probably were small, and because no data on Sr/Ca ratios are available. The data in chapter X indicate that the amount of seafood in the diet was very small. Seafood was therefore not incorporated in the model.

All percentages in this sections are based on energy values, and may be converted to kilograms of edible products with the aid of table XI.5. In the discussion on the calculated diets, two additional constraints are used, the first of which, the assumption that diets comprising less than 30 % cereal are not feasible, was arbitrarily chosen. The second constraint is that a diet of 10 MJ should contain no less than 500 mg Ca. This constraint is based on the discussion in section XI.C.1.2.

In short, the basic assumptions in the models are:

(1) Rc and Rh reflect the Sr/Ca ratios of diets of cattle and humans,

(2) cattle ingested and digested 'average plant material',

(3) human diets contained a maximum of five components: beef, milk, roots, leafy vegetables and cereal grains,

(4) human diets contained 10 MJ of energy and 500 mg Ca per person per day,

(5) at least 30 % of the energy in diets derived from cereals

(6) average compositions of groups of recent and prehistoric foods are equavalent.

Table XI.5. Reference values for the discussion on the agricultural feasibility of calculations on dietary composition. Values are in kg edible product for families of 6 persons each consuming an average of 10 MJ/day, total 22000 MJ/annum. Mean energy values of food items taken from Paul & Southgate (1978) in table V.1.

food item	MJ/kg	---- 1 % of diet equals ---- kg per day	kg per year
meat	13.50	0.04	16.30
milk	2.72	0.22	80.88
cereals	13.50	0.04	16.30
leafy vegetables	0.75	0.80	293.33
roots	1.31	0.46	167.94
fruits	1.44	0.42	152.78
nuts	18.86	0.03	11.66

Case 1: Rh < Rc : Oostwoud

The Late Neolithic and Bronze Age barrows near Oostwoud yielded a series of more or less complete human skeletons (section II.C.2.3).

In the majority of sites, Sr/Ca ratios in human bones are lower than in herbivorous bones (table V.13). Generally, this is explained by the incorporation of meat in the human diet. From the sites of West-Friesland, Oostwoud may be taken as an example. The Oostwoud cattle bones had a mean of 3.32 mg Sr/g Ca, the human bones had 2.50 mg Sr/g Ca.

Calculations were made for two situations: firstly, with a DR grain-APM of 1, i.e. the 'traditional' concept of no variations in plant Sr/Ca ratios. In a diet without root crops, the solutions of the set of two equations (section XI.C.2.1), which represent the theoretically possible compositions of diets, are points on a plane (fig. XI.2). A diet without milk, roots and vegetables would consist of 30 % grain and 70 % meat. Figure XI.2 shows that the 'solution plane' is almost parallel to the 'cereal' axis. This indicates that small changes the relative proportion of milk and leafy vegetables in the diet result in large changes in the relative proportion of cereals. The high Ca levels in milk and vegetables are the cause of this phenomenon (compare Runia 1987a).

If root crops enter the potential menus and a DR roots-APM of 1.6 is adopted (section IX.D.4), the possible solutions for the composition of diets are represented by points in planes which are parallel behind and below the solution plane of fig. XI.2. All possible solutions are represented by the points in the space body in fig. XI.3. The tetrahedron (fig. XI.2), in which the solution planes stand, 'shrinks' with increasing percentages of roots in the diet, because the endpoints of the axes represent 100% minus the percentage of roots.

Figure XI.3 shows that there are limits to the relative proportions of the food components in diets. Approximate maximum percentages are, for milk, 55-60 %, for leafy vegetables, 45-50 %, for cereals and meat almost 100 %, and for roots 40-45 %. Obviously, these limits are only arithmetically determined. Nutritional and agricultural factors will result in other, lower limits, which are discussed in section C.3.

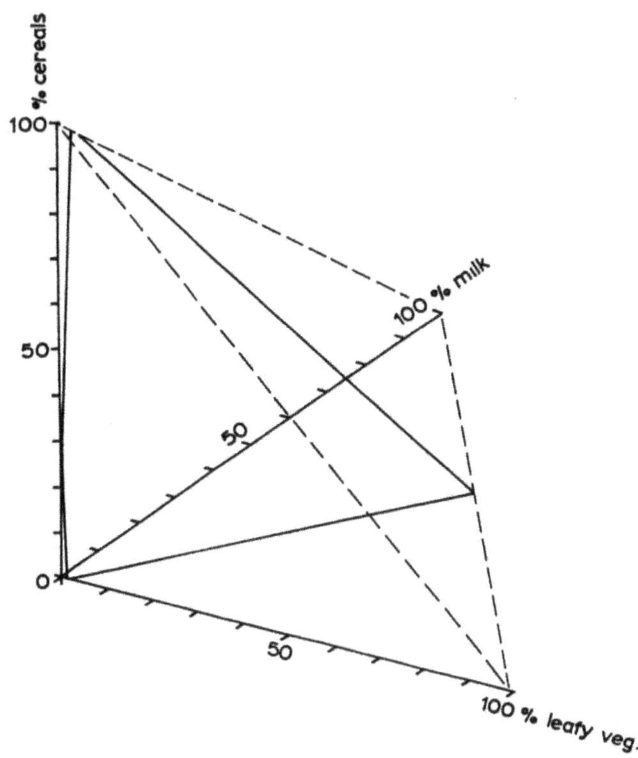

figure XI.2 'Solution plane' for a diet consisting of cereals, milk, leafy vegetables and meat, for human diets of Oostwoud, Rc=3.3 mg Sr/g Ca, Rh=2.5 mg Sr/g Ca (table V.13). DR grain-APM =1. Axes show percentages based on energy contents. Discussion in the text.

The second series of calculations involved a DR grain-APM of 1.4, i.e. the value established for the grain species cultivated in West-Friesland (section IX.D.4). For diets without roots, this results in a solution plane (fig. XI.4) that is tilted backwards in comparison with the plane in fig. XI.2. Lower percentages of cereals suffice to bring the Sr/Ca ratio of the diet at the desired level. A pure meat-cereal diet would have to consist of approximately 15 % cereals and 85 % meat.

The shaded area in fig. XI.4 represents the projection on the plane through the milk and the cereal axes of that part of the solution plane that represents diets which contain at least 30 % cereals and 500 mg Ca/10 MJ. All solutions (still for a diet without roots) for milk and leafy vegetable percentages are represented by points in this area. Amounts of milk and leafy vegetables in diets thus appear positively correlated.

The solutions for all diets again form a tetrahedron-like body, the basal plane of which is identical to that in fig. XI.3. The top of the body is displaced slightly in the plane through the milk and grain axes. Maximum percentages for meat, roots, milk and leafy vegetables are the same as in fig. XI.3. The maximum percentage for cereal grains is somewhat lower, i.e. some 95 %. It appears that changes in DR grain-APM have only minimal effects on the range of possible diets, but a clear effect on the relative proportions of cereals in relation to specific combinations of roots, milk and leafy vegetables.

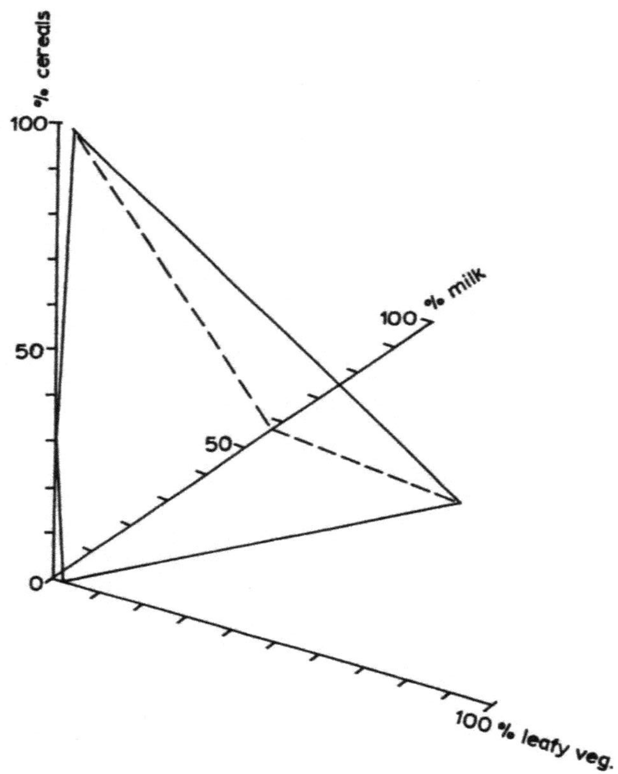

figure XI.3 As fig. XI.2, but with roots as additional component of diet. The three dimensional body contains all points which represent the possible compositions of human diets consisting of cereals, milk, leafy vegetables, meat and roots for Oostwoud.

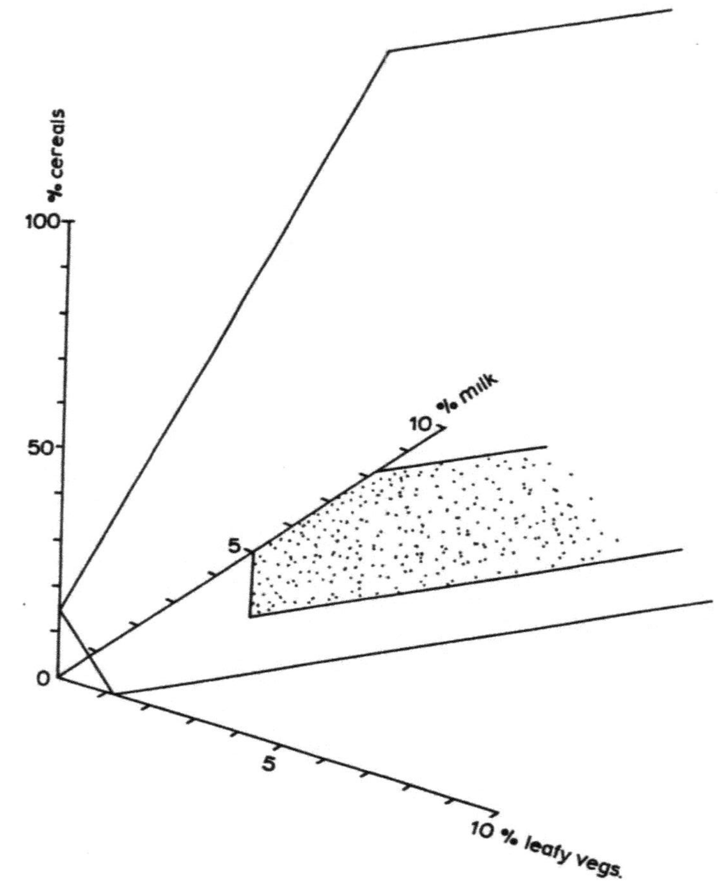

figure XI.4 As fig. XI.2, but with different scaling of basal plane axes. Diets of cereals, milk, leafy vegetables and meat for Oostwoud, Rc=3.3, Rh=2.5 mg Sr/g Ca, DR grain-APM=1.4 (section IX.C). The shaded area of the basal plane represents possible combinations of percentages of milk and leafy vegetables of diets containing more than 500 mg Ca/10 MJ and at least 30 % cereals.

Case 2: Rh=Rc : Het Valkje, Late Period

The occupation traces of the site Het Valkje consisted of numerous farm houses and house terps. The subsistance of this site was probably relative intensive, small scale mixed farming (section II.C.2.6).

In West-Friesland, there is one site in which the Sr/Ca ratios of cattle and humans are equal: the Late Period of het Valkje. Calculations for this site resulted in fig. XI.5. For a DR grain-APM value of 1, all diets without roots consist of cereals and leafy vegetables. Diets with roots (DR roots-grain=1.6) may contain some milk and meat.
A value of 1.4 for DR grain-APM results in a plane parallel to the leafy vegetable axis. The shaded area in fig XI.5 is the projection on the basal plane of that part of the solution plane that represents diets with more than 30% cereals and more than 500 mg Ca/10 MJ. This area suggests that the relative proportion of milk in diets lies within certain limits and is not correlated with the relative amount of leafy vegetables.

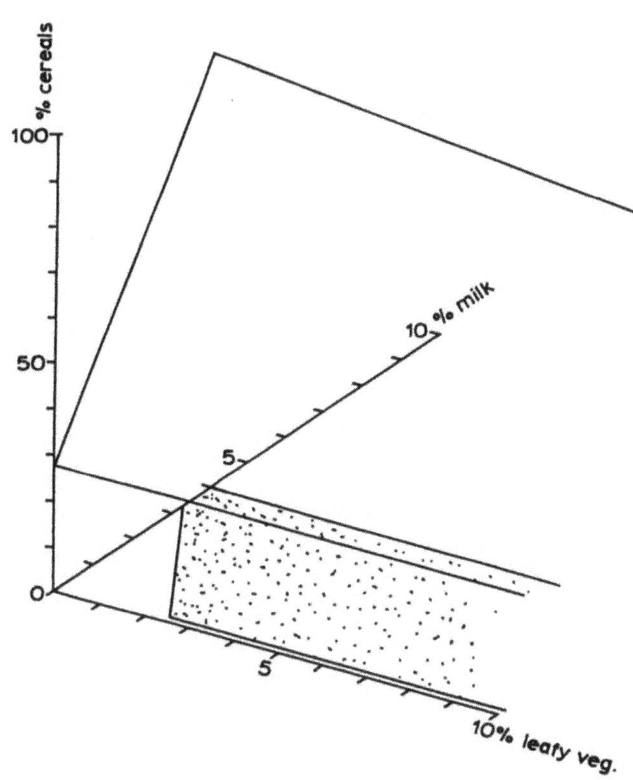

figure XI.5 As fig. XI.3 for Het Valkje Late Period, Rc=2.8, Rh=2.8 mg Sr/g Ca (table V.13), DR grain-APM=1.4.

Case 3: Rh > Rc : Schagen-Muggenburg

The occupation traces of Schagen-Muggenburg date from the Roman Period. The site is described in section II.C.2.9. The analysed human bones are part of some inhumations that were found in the settlement.

Schagen-Muggenburg is the only site in the database in which the human Sr/Ca ratios are higher than the cattle Sr/Ca ratios.

It is obvious that in this case no diet can be constructed without food items which have Sr/Ca ratios higher than APM Sr/Ca ratios. Thus, if DR grain-APM = 1, a certain amount of roots (DR roots-APM = 1.6) has to be incorporated in the diet in order to get solutions for the set of two equations.

Possible solutions for the set of two equations and a value of 1.4 for the DR grain-APM are represented by points on the plane in fig. XI.6. The shaded area is the projection of that part of the solution plane on the basal plane that represents the diets with more than 30 % cereals and more than 500 mg Ca/10MJ.

In this case, the relative proportions of of milk and leafy vegetables in the diets appear to be correlated negatively.

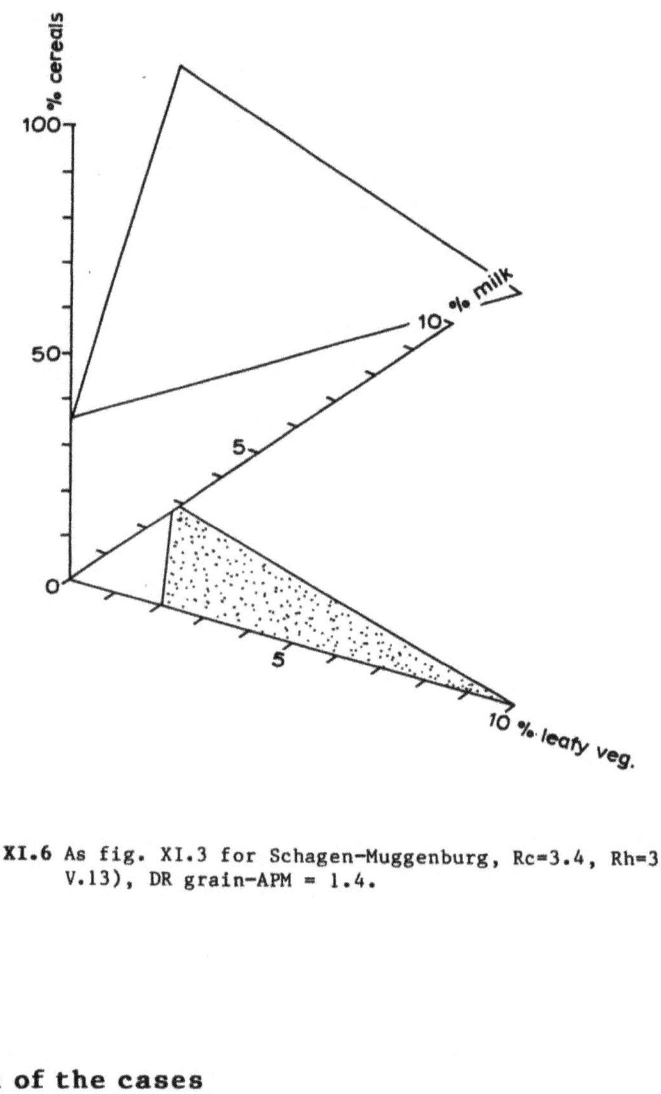

figure XI.6 As fig. XI.3 for Schagen-Muggenburg, Rc=3.4, Rh=3.6 mg Sr/g Ca (table V.13), DR grain-APM = 1.4.

Comparison of the cases

It is obvious that the solution planes contain a large number of points that do not represent realistic diets. The calculations show, however, that basic differences between the three cases exist. These differences are visualised by the orientation of the solution plane in the three cases. The result of the differences in orientation of the solution planes is the difference in the relation between relative proportions of milk and leafy vegetables in diets. In case 1, the correlation is positive, which means that in diets a higher proportion of milk in the diet has to be accompanied by a higher proportion of cereals. In case 2 no correlation between proportions of milk and leafy vegetables is present: the relative proportion of milk is within fairly narrow limits, whereas the amount of leafy vegetables can be varied without consequences for the relative proportion of milk. In case 3, the correlation between relative proportions of milk and leafy vegetables is negative, which means that higher proportions of milk imply lower proportions of leafy vegetables.

C.3. Discussion

C.3.1. Feasible and realistic diets

The example calculations show that changes in relative levels of the Sr/Ca ratios in cattle and human bones are reflected by changes in the orientation of the 'solution planes'. Variations in the Observed Ratios for cattle and humans will have a similar effect. In the calculations it is assumed that the discrimination against Sr in cattle and human organisms is equal. There may, however, be some differences in OR values, but these would not bring essential changes to the model.
It is evident that, because of their high Ca contents, milk, leafy vegetables and root crops exert a major influence on the Sr/Ca ratios of diets. In the diagrams, the 'solution planes' are almost parallel to the cereal grain axis.

A second aspect is the effect of variations in Distribution Ratios grain-APM. In comparison to the effects that food components with high Ca concentrations will have on the overall Sr/Ca ratio of diet (fig.XI.1) the effect of discrimination in grains appears to be minor. However, in cases with low proportions of other food items, the effect of introducing high cereal Sr/Ca ratios in the model (for instance, the experimentally determined DR grain-APM of 1.4), the relative proportion of cereals in a diet may change many percent. It is obvious that such differences would have considerable agricultural implications. Moreover, if differences in Sr/Ca ratios in vegetable foods are ignored, cases where herbivores have lower Sr concentrations than humans (as, for example, in Schagen-Muggenburg), may be prematurely put aside under the suspicion of being diagenetically biased .

So far, the diets have been approached in a purely mathemathical sense. The feasible solutions for the two equations of section XI.C.2.1 have been established. For each component of diet the minimum and maximum values for the relative proportions can be estimated. Many of the calculated dietary compositions are, however, not realistic from practical, nutritional or agricultural points of view. Additional external conditions, based on practical, nutritional and agricultural aspects must therefore be imposed on the model. Moreover, the concentrations of Zn in bones should be taken into consideration.

In section C.1.2 the nutritional requirements for an average household of six persons have been outlined. In table XI.5, the energy requirements of a household are correlated to quantities of different foodstuffs, which allows rough limits to be established within which the relative importance of food items in the diet lie. Each day some 800 g of leafy vegetables are required for a 1 % contribution to the family's diet. Diets with more than a few percent of leafy vegetables are therefore unlikely. Leafy vegetables are, however, essential as sources of ascorbic acid and other nutrients. With a mimimum daily dose of 50 mg ascorbic acid per day, leafy vegetables with a mean ascorbic acid content of 560 mg/MJ (table XI.2) must comprise at least 1% of a diet of 10 MJ if no other vitamin C sources are present. For root crops (200 mg asc.acid/MJ) as sole ascorbic acid source in the diet this amount equals 2.5 % of the energy in the diet or 1150 g roots per family per day . With no other ascorbic acid sources this can be formulated as: $2.5 * p(\text{leafy vegetables}) + p(\text{roots}) \geq 2.5\ \%$.

The maximum amounts of root crops and leafy vegetables that were consumed may be roughly estimated at 5% of the energy value of diets each, i.e. a mean maximum of some 4000 g of leafy vegetables and some 2300 g of roots per family per day. It is unlikely that in the West-Frisian agrarian setting larger quantities of these food items could have been collected and consumed each day.

Agricultural practice probably does not pose strict limitations to the cereal contents of diets. The maximum amount of grain needed under the assumptions outlined in C.1.4 (2000 kg) could have been produced on some 2 ha of arable. According to IJzereef (1981), at Het Valkje in the Late Period some 3 ha, and in the Early Period some 3.6 to 8.8 ha arable land was available per farm. In the marginal situation (3 ha arable per farm), with one-third fallow and under the present assumptions, just enough cereals for a 100% cereal grain diet could have been produced.

The maximum amount of meat that could have been produced per farm was estimated at some 10000 MJ per year. This amount is some 45% of the 22000 MJ that are required. Similarily, the maximum amount of 3000 MJ of milk corresponds with some 14 % of the energy needed.
In total, the amount of energy derived from dietary components other than cereals, i.e. meat plus milk plus vegetables, is at maximum some (100 % - 45 % (meat) - 14 % (milk) - 10 % (roots and vegetables) =) 70 % of the energy needed. Thus, diets containing less than 30 % cereal grains should be considered as unrealistic. A lower limit for the amount of meat in the diet can be derived from data on diets of recent subsistence farmers. Proteins in meat account for some 25 % of total protein intake in industrial countries, some 8 % in third world countries and about 22 % in Europe (Den Hartog 1976). Protein/energy ratios in meat and cereals are approximately equal (table X.5). A relative proportion of about 20 % animal proteins in diets appears to be a reasonable lower limit. This value corresponds to a minimum of some 20 % of energy from meat. Thus, the maximum proportion of grain in the diet is about (100 % - 20 % (meat) - 5 % (vegetables, milk, roots) =) 75 %.

The absolute quantitative approach may supply solutions for theoretically feasible diets. However, in the comparison of material from various sites, the wide margins make the absolute amounts less suitable. Even if additional nutritional and agricultural constraints are imposed on the models, the 'bodies' of points representing possible dietary compositions (section XI.C.2.2) become smaller but numerous diets still remain feasible. In reality the situation is even more complex because in the models mutton and pork, which may have Sr and Zn contents different from beef, as well as seafood have been ignored. Besides this, it should be remembered that the basic assumption underlying the model, i.e. that Sr/Ca ratios in bones have not been altered or only slightly so, may prove not quite correct. In the following sections a number of sites are therefore compared in a semiquantitative sense.

C.3.2. Isochronic and diachronic aspects

Uptil now, no extrapolations of the available data towards variations in the composition of human diets in time and space, which is the aspect of paleodietary studies most interesting for archeologists, and the reason why this kind of studies are carried out, have been presented. The data and discussions in the preceding sections in fact seem to frustrate any comparison between human diets in different sites. As stated above, the margins in the possible proportions of components in diets are wide, and the solutions for the equations of section XI.C.2.1 for various combinations of Rc and Rh largely overlap. It is tempting and worthwile to try to overcome the methodological problems in order to compare the compositions of average human diets in the sites under scrutiny. The study of the bones was, after all, undertaken to effectuate such a comparison.

The majority of the material analysed dates from a rather limited time span, dated by radiocarbon to between c. 3300-2600 BP. Still, some isochronic and diachronic aspects can be discussed.

Apart from differences between age and status groups within sites (section XI.C.3.3), the isochronous aspects of paleodiets comprise the effects of different environments and agricultural potentials of the sites on the average diets of their inhabitants. Within West-Friesland, the differences in environments of the sites may be relatively small, but they appear to be sufficient as to leave traces in the ecoarcheological material, as discussed in section XI.B. A comparison between the diets of particular sites is impaired by the lack of a 'complete' spectrum of chemical analysis of bones of the domestic animals from the sites concerned. The material from Het Valkje is therefore used as reference in the discussions on human diets because it consists of complete spectra of trace element contents in domestic animals for two occupation phases, the economic background to which has already been extensively discussed (IJzereef 1981).

Relatively large differences in environment are present between the sites in West-Friesland and Velsen, which is situated in the dune area.

The diachronic aspects of paleodiets to some extent represent similar problems as the isochronic aspects, because there is a variation of subsistence potentials of environments not only in space, but also in time. For Het Valkje, the isolated human bones from settlement features can be related to occupation chronology, which in the present study is condensed to an Early and a Late Period. On a larger scale there is the difference between the Bronze Age sites in West-Friesland and the Iron Age / Roman Period site Schagen-Muggenburg.

In the comparison of human diets at various sites reference, is regulary made to the histograms which show the Sr and Zn concentrations in human and animal bones relative to the concentrations in cattle bones (fig. V.3, VI.2). The Sr and Zn concentrations in the cattle bones within each site are used as reference basis to which the levels of trace element concentrations in other species are compared. In fact, cattle are used as a 'baseline' species.

In the discussions it is assumed that meat from animals whose bones show high Zn levels also contains high concentrations of Zn. At present, this assumption lacks experimental proof. Zinc levels in bones react relatively slowly to changes in Zn concentrations in plasma. Zinc is actively treated in the body (section VI.A), but organisms apparently do not maintain their plasma Zn levels at a more or less fixed level. High environmental Zn levels may therefore result in high Zn levels in tissue.

Het Valkje: Early and Late Period

There are no archeological indications for status differences within the skeletal material from the two periods of Het Valkje, so that it may be assumed that the comparison of the periods is not biased by status effects.

Cattle bone Sr levels in the Early and Late Period do not differ. In the Late Period, Sr/Ca ratios in the human bones are almost equivalent to cattle bone Sr/Ca ratios while in the Early Period they are lower. A difference between the two periods is to be found in the absolute and relative Zn concentrations. In the Late Period, Zn levels in the bones are quite high (table XI.6). Zinc levels in human and sheep/goat bones from the Late Period are twice as high as those in the Early Period. Differences in pig and cattle bones are smaller, and the dogs are intermediate. Thus, Sr levels suggest that no major changes in human diets occurred during the occupation period, whereas Zn levels suggest the opposite.

Table XI.6. Comparison between mean concentrations of Sr and Zn in human and animal bones from the Early and Late Period of Het Valkje: (mean concentrations of Late Period)/(mean concentrations of Early Period). Calculated from table V.6, V.10, VI.4 and VI.7

element	human	cattle	pig	dog	sheep/goat
Sr	1.0	1.0	1.1	1.0	1.1
Zn	2.0	1.3	1.2	1.5	2.3

The high Zn levels in the humans from the Late Period may indicate that in this period meat was a more important constituent of the diet than in the Early Period. An alternative explanation is, however, that Zn levels in Late Period dietary components were higher than in Early Period foods. Similar diets would then contain different amounts of Zn.

Tentative indications for the latter option can be found in the analysis of soil samples. In section IX.B, it has been suggested that during the habitation period the Zn levels in the upper soil layers on the ridges, where the arable fields were situated, gradually increased. In the basins, the Zn levels in the upper soil layers decreased.

If the observed pattern in the bone Zn concentrations is related to a change in concentrations of Zn in the soil, it might be tentatively explained by a model which comprises a change in both human dietary composition and in animal husbandry practices. The Zn levels in sheep/goat are comparatively strongly affected, which may indicate that changes in herding practices are involved in addition to the changes in soil Zn levels. The Zn levels in dogs also show reveal a difference between the Early and Late Period but less marked than that for sheep/goat. By the Late Period the lower parts of the basins had become too wet for grazing, and the sheep/goat woudl have had to graze on other grounds, perhaps including the fallow arable on the ridges.

The changes in cattle and pig bone Zn levels may reflect the changes in soil Zn which may have occurred in the ridges (section IX.B.4). The products from the arable fields, such as cereals, in the Late Period would have had higher Zn contents than in the Early Period. The increase in human bone Zn levels, which is more marked than the change in cattle and pigs, might be the result of an increased portion of sheep/goat meat in the diet. This is also suggested by the zooarcheological data which show an increase in the relative proportion of sheep/goat in the Late Period (section II.C.2.6). Sheep/goat have higher Zn levels than cattle (compare table VI.4). The higher Sr levels in the sheep/goat bones compared with cattle bones would then also have caused higher Sr levels in Late Period human diets. This is, however, not visible in the human bone Sr levels. The higher Sr levels were probably to some extent compensated by a higher milk consumption in the Late Period (compare IJzereef 1981 and section II.C.2.6).

In this model, the average Late Period diet would have contained more sheep/goat meat, less beef and more milk than the Early Period diet. The tentative differences between Early and Late Period diets are schematically indicated in table XI.7.

Table XI.7. Tentative comparison of average human diets in the Early and Late Period of Het Valkje.

item	Late relative to Early
Sr/Ca ratio	equal
Zn/Ca ratio	strong increase
beef content	decrease
mutton content	increase
milk content	increase
total meat content	approximately equal
cereals and vegetables	approximately equal

Oostwoud and Het Valkje

The comparison between the diet the humans from Oostwoud with that of the inhabitants of Het Valkje is problematical because of the possibility of distortion by status differences. No status differences can be established amongst the scattered human remains from Het Valkje. It is, however, possible that the material from Oostwoud represents a specific (high ranking ?) segment of the population whereas the material from Het Valkje would be representative of the average population.

In addition to the possible differences in status, the sites also represent different periods of occupation. The material from Oostwoud dates from the Late Neolithic whereas the material from Het Valkje dates from the Bronze Age.

As shown above, differences in relative Sr concentrations in human bones can be the result of various factors. Unfortunately, only one pig bone from Oostwoud was analysed besides human and cattle bones. It is evident that adequate chemical and zooarcheological data are needed in a discussion on the composition of diets (XI.C.1.1).

The relative Sr levels are low in the Oostwoud samples and higher in the samples from the settlement (table V.13). These lower Sr levels are, however, not correlated with relatively higher Zn levels, as might be expected if the lower Sr levels were caused by the proportion of meat in the diet. Though the amount of meat in the diets in Oostwoud may have been slightly higher than in Het Valkje, another possible cause for the low dietary Sr levels is the consumption of milk. The calculations (C.2.2) show that for Oostwoud, high proportions of milk in the diet are theoretically possible. Considering the relatively high Sr/Ca ratios in cereals, it appears likely that at Oostwoud the amount of cereal in the human diet was lower than in Het Valkje. The tentative differences in the human diets shown in table XI.8 agrees with the general picture for differences between, on the one hand, the Oostwoud 'pastoralists', with emphasis on optimal exploitation of domestic animals, and the other hand the settled farmers from Het Valkje, who probably employed an agricultural system in which grain cultivation was relatively important. The relatively high consumption of milk in Oostwoud is somewhat unexpected in the light of the 'secondary products revolution' the effects of which are not supposed to be visible until a slightly later period (Sherratt 1981). The inhabitants of Oostwoud may, however, have kept relatively large numbers of animals.

Table XI.8. Tentative comparison of average human diets in Oostwoud and Het Valkje. Within each site, cattle bones are used as reference material.

item	Oostwoud relative to Het Valkje
Sr/Ca ratio in human diet	lower
Zn/Ca ratio in human diet	lower
% of milk in human diet	higher
% of cereals in human diet	lower
% of meat in diet	lower

Het Valkje and Andijk

As pointed out in section XI.B, the data for the domestic animals suggest that differences in agricultural practices existed between Het Valkje and Andijk. The question is whether these differences are reflected in the human trace element levels and in the average diets at Het Valkje and Andijk.

A conspicious feature in Andijk is the relatively low mean Zn concentration in the human bones, which is almost equal to the mean Zn concentration in cattle bones (fig. VI.2). This differs from a theoretically expected pattern (section VI.C).

In Andijk, beef and mutton will have had approximately equal Sr/Ca ratios whereas in Het Valkje mutton Sr/Ca ratios were higher than those in beef (compare fig.V.3). The relative number of cattle in Andijk is higher than in Het Valkje. As a consequence of these two factors, the meat total, i.e. beef and mutton, in Andijk will have had a lower Sr/Ca ratio than in Het Valkje. This implies that, if Sr levels in human bones relative to cattle bone Sr levels in Andijk and Het Valkje were equal, the proportion of plant material, i.e. cereals, in the diet at Andijk would have been correspondingly higher. Relative human Sr/Ca ratios in Andijk are however lower than in Het Valkje. It is unclear whether this difference results solely from the lower Sr/Ca ratio in the meat component of diet or if the proportion of cereals in Andijk diets was also higher.

Though cereals have high Zn levels, the amount of Zn that can be absorbed from meat is probably much larger (section VI.A.2). Higher proportions of cereals in diet may therefore result in lower Zn levels in bone. It is, however, more likely that the low Zn levels in the Andijk diets result from a relatively large proportion of milk in the diet. The data thus suggest that the relative amounts of milk and cereals in Andijk diets may have been higher than in diets of Het Valkje.

A considerable area of sandy to sandy loamy soils is present around the site Andijk. Thus, more arable, and hence a higher amount of grain might have been available.

A tentative comparison between diets in Het Valkje and Andijk can be based on the avialable material (table XI.9). It must be stressed that certain components of diets, such as roots and vegetables, are not taken into account. Moreover, all Sr and Zn values are mean values for limited numbers of bones, sometimes with relatively large standard deviations. No data on male/female ratios in the Andijk cattle are available. In any case, the differences in diet were probably small.

Table XI.9. Tentative comparison between average diets in Andijk and Het Valkje. Cattle bones are the reference material within both sites.

item	Andijk relative to Het Valkje
Sr/Ca in mutton	lower
Sr/Ca in beef + mutton	lower
ratio beef/mutton in diet	higher
Sr/Ca in human bones	lower
Zn content in diet	lower
amount of cereals in diet	higher ?
amount of milk in diet	higher ?

Bronze Age and Iron Age/Roman Period

One site from a native Roman context was studied. To date, no ecoarcheological report for this site has been published. Preliminary results of the study of animal bones were given by L.L. Therkorn (IPP, pers. comm.). The site can be viewed in comparison with the Bronze Age sites in the broader context of North-West European agriculture as outlined by Randsborg (1985) and Barker (1985).

The occupation at Schagen-Muggenburg was situated on peat (section II.C.2.9). Salt marshes were present near the site, and though cereals were probably cultivated locally, the potential for cereal cultivation appears to be less favourable than in the surroundings of Het Valkje.

The zoological assemblage of Schagen-Muggenburg differs from the earlier sites in that some abnormally large cattle specimens were present and horse forms some 6% of the domestic animal bone (table II.4). It is likely that the inhabitants of Schagen-Muggenburg were in contact with the Roman Empire (section VII.C) which may have influenced the composition of the zoological assemblage from the site. Some of the animals that were raised near the site may have been exported, either on the hoof or slaughtered, i.e. in preserved form. The age of slaughter could be estimated from a small number of cattle mandibles (n=32). Half of the animals were slaughtered between 4 and 5 years (Therkorn, pers. comm.). In comparison with Het Valkje, rather more animals reached the age of four, which may suggest the export of younger beasts.

A consequence of cattle trade (i.e. import) may be that trace element levels in some of the animals which were consumed differed from the levels which would be present in animals in or near the site. As pointed out in section XI.A, two groups of cattle bones can be distinguished at Schagen-Muggenburg on the basis of Zn levels. Though Zn levels in bones probably change relatively slowly in comparison with changes in plasma, it may be assumed that the beef that was consumed showed variations in Zn levels comparable to the variations in the bones. For the discussion on diets, the mean Zn levels of the cattle bones are therefore used as an indication of mean Zn levels in beef.

As far as the chemical composition of the bones are concerned, Schagen-Muggenburg is distinct from the other sites in that it is the only site in which the human bones have Sr/Ca ratios higher than cattle bones (fig. V.3). In comparison to Het Valkje, the pigs of Schagen also have relatively high Sr contents, but low Zn concentrations.

Horses were rather more frequent at Schagen-Muggenburg than at the earlier sites (table II.4). Horse meat probably had Sr/Ca ratios approximately equal to Sr/Ca ratios in mutton (table V.6). If horse meat was eaten, the Sr/Ca ratio in the meat component of the diet, i.e. beef, mutton, pork and horse meat taken together, must have been higher in Schagen-Muggenburg than in Het Valkje. The mean Zn content in human bones relative to mean cattle bone Zn concentrations of Schagen- Muggenburg is slightly higher than the Early period of Het Valkje, but lower than the Late period (fig. VI.2).

The comparatively high Sr concentrations in human bones at Schagen-Muggenburg may be the result of a greater role of cereals in the diet. It is, however, also possible that the high dietary Sr levels result from a lower amount of milk consumed or from the comparatively high levels of Sr in the non-beef meat, which at Schagen-Muggenburg formed a rather larger part of the diet. The calculations (section XI.C.2.2) suggest that the upper limit for the percentage of milk in the diet was fairly low.

Table XI.10. Tentative comparison of average human diets at Het Valkje and Schagen-Muggenburg. Cattle bones are used as reference material within each site.

item	Schagen relative to Het Valkje
ratio of beef/non-beef meat	lower
Sr/Ca ratio in meat*	higher
Sr/Ca ratio in human diet	higher
Zn/Ca ratio in human diet	approximately equal
amount of cereals in human diet	higher?
amount of milk in human diet	lower

* beef + mutton + pork + horse meat

Velsen and Het Valkje

Velsen is the only site under scrutiny that was situated in the dune area. Velsen and Het Valkje are roughly contemporaneous. The human bones from Velsen were found in a barrow and differ from the isolated bones from Het

Valkje. A 'complete' spectrum of Sr and Zn concentrations in animal bones is available (fig. V.3, VI.2) for both sites.

The Sr content in human bones from Velsen is relatively low and the Zn content relatively high. Though Velsen was fairly close to the sea the amount of seafood in the human diet was probably just as low as at Het Valkje (section X.C.4, table X.4). The low Sr levels also point to low proportions of seafood in diets at Velsen. The low concentrations of Sr in the human bones from Velsen might be regarded as indicative for milk consumption. The high Zn concentrations suggest, however, that meat consumption was the cause of the low Sr levels. The combination of high Zn levels and low Sr levels in human bone from Velsen may therefore be the result of a comparatively large proportion of meat in the diet. In addition to domestic animals some game may have been eaten. In consequence, the proportion of cereals in the diet was probably depressed.

The different environments of Velsen and Het Valkje appear to be reflected in the chemical data. The fairly low Sr levels in pigs from Velsen have already been discussed (section XI.A). The woods in the dune area may have supplied the inhabitants of Velsen with nuts and fruits. It is, however, not likely that the high Zn levels result from a high proportion of nuts in the diets because Zn levels per unit of energy are not high (section VI.A).

Ard scratches indicate that arable was situated on the sandy soils (Beemster & Brandt 1986), which were probably less favourable for the cultivation of cereals than the creek ridges at Het Valkje.

A tentative comparison of human diets in Velsen and Het Valkje is presented in table XI.11. In this case, the theoretical concept of low Sr-much meat and high Zn-much meat appears to be applicable.

Table XI.11. Tentative comparison of average human diets at Het Valkje and Velsen. Cattle bones are used as reference material within each site.

item	Velsen relative to Het Valkje
Sr/Ca ratio in human diet	lower
Zn/Ca ratio in human diet	higher
amount of sea food in diet	equally low
amount of meat in diet	higher
amount of cereals in diet	lower
amount of milk in diet	equal?
amount of nuts & fruits in diet	higher?

C.3.3. Sex and status differences

Though sex and status differences in bone trace element levels appear to be present in the skeletons from West-Friesland, it is evident from the material presented in the preceding section that these differences do not necessarily reflect differences in relative proportions of meat and vegetable foods in the diets. Actual diets, obviously, are more complex because they consist of a number of components each with Sr and Zn levels that depend on environmental factors. It is, therefore, hardly, if at all, possible to interpret the observed differences (section V.C.4, VI.C.4) in terms of differences in relative proportions of dietary components.

The question of what might be the cause for the observed difference between the inhumations and the isolated human bones, possibly representing a status difference, remains to be answered. Low Sr levels in diets may be caused by higher amounts of milk and/or meat, high Zn levels by high amounts of meat. As stated before, the chemical composition of human bones is the result of a number of factors. The discussions in section C.3.2. show that for each site the dietary relevance of high or low Sr and Zn levels in human bones may be differently explained once they are discussed in relation to other ecoarcheological information, for instance regarding Sr and Zn levels in animal bones. The discussion on the diets in section C.3.2 regards average diets for the sites. Any discussion of individual diets or diets of higher ranking persons would appear to be hazardous in the light of the great number of variables involved.

A special problem in the Sr and Zn levels in age/sex groups of the inhumed individuals is formed by the low Sr levels in the males over 35 years of age (table V.11). The three individuals concerned suffered from arthritis. It is thus possible that disease rather than diet was the cause for the low Sr levels. There are no other arthritic individuals present in the material from the area nor are there old males without arthritic features, and it is thus not possible to check the relationship, if any.

A diet with high amounts of meat and/or milk might be responsible for the low Sr levels. The Zn content of the bones is avarage and does not suggest that the old males consumed large amounts of meat. A high proportion of milk in the diet of these individuals is, however, not contradicted by the Zn data. Though consumption of meat rather than milk is usually associated with high ranking, the data thus suggest that the older males consumed comparatively more milk or dairy products. The poor state of the dentition of the individuals involved may, however, also have played a role in their food choice. This assumption is not contradicted by the data in table V.16 and VI.13 which show the low mean Sr and Zn concentrations in individuals with dental pathologies. Though it is unclear if a causal relationship is present between the bone trace element levels and the condition of the dentition, it is obvious that dental pathologies affect the masticating capacities and the choice of food. The dentition of the old females is, however, in possibly an even worse state than that of the old males.

To conclude, the data suggest that the older males were fed differently than the older females. Males at higher ages possibly received a higher proportion of milk in their diets whereas females remained more or less on the same diet.

D. ECONOMIC ASPECTS: SURPLUS AND TRADE

D.1. Introduction

The analysis of bones from domestic animals may yield suggestions on trade and other economic aspects of animal husbandry (section XI.A), and the analysis of human bones may provide additional information. The Pb content of human bone may, for instance, be used as a source of information on trade links between native settlements and Imperial Rome (section VII.C.3). There is also a possibility that chemical analysis of bone may add to solving problems on trade in still another way. This (still theoretical) aspect of trace element analysis of human bones is discussed in this chapter.

In section XI.C.1 mention has been made of the two sides of human diet, loosely using the economic terms 'supply side' and 'demand side'. The supply side of the diet comprises the agricultural system and its output of agricultural products, which in subsistence agriculture for a major part consists of edible products. The amounts of food actually consumed may in turn be viewed as the demand side of diet. In a situation where it is possible to study both sides of the diet indepedently, the comparison of these could be interesting. A descrepancy between supply and demand would suggest a surplus of products which could have been traded. In the following section, both sides of the diet are discussed.

D.2. The 'supply side'

In the present case, we are dealing with an agricultural system which in essence produced for home consumption, though a surplus in the production was probably present. The agricultural system of Bronze Age West-Friesland has been described as being rather productive (section XI.C.1.4). The material culture is, however, poor. Grave gifts are scarce and poor in comparison with other regions (Butler 1979, Coles & Harding 1979) but this may also have had non-economic ritual causes. West-Friesland is situated at the fringe of the continent and is devoid of any natural (mineral) resources except for the agricultural potential of the soils. Despite this, the inhabitants of Bronze Age West-Friesland must have been able to purchase bronze and flint objects, a number of which have been found (Woltering 1985). The economic value of imported material is unknown, as is the system by which the material was purchased, but agricultural produce was one of the possible comodities which the West-Frisian farmers could have offered in exchange.

The discussion of the agricultural system of the area (section XI.C.1.4) suggests that cereals rather than meat may have been produced in surplus. Under the adopted assumptions, the farmers could have produced enough cereals for an entirely vegetarian way of life whereas the animal products meat and milk could only have supplied a maximum of some 60% of the energy needed (section XI.C.3.1). There are, of course, other factors which, in addition to production potentials, influence the possible role of agricultural products as merchandise. The technical and logistic problems in temporary storage of a cereal surplus and the transport thereof may have been considerable in prehistoric contexts, though in later periods these problems were probably solved, as may be concluded from fortified complexes of grain storage buildings which have been found in the eastern part of the Netherlands (Waterbolk 1977).

The products of animal husbandry, i.e. living animals, can be transported relatively easily 'on the hoof' and may therefore predate cereals as a trading comodity. The ease with which animals can be moved from one area to another can be illustrated with many present-day, historic and prehistoric cultures which make use of transhumance systems. Exchange of living animals may also have taken place in order to prevent inbreeding. Animals exported on the hoof do not leave traces in the archeological record of a site and may therefore bias estimates of the animal husbandry system. The estimates of the productivity of stock raising in West-Friesland were based on the dimensions of stables, which may be less susceptible for such bias.

The supply of agricultural products may be estimated by using straightforward estimates for the (maximum) output of cereals, meat, milk and other agricultural products irrespective of costs. There may, however, be more sophisticated methods which can be employed in estimating productivity of subsistence agriculture.

Linear programming has been used in estimates on diets of hunter-gatherers (Keene 1981, 1985, Belovsky 1987) and the potentials of this technique in modelling subsistence farming should be investigated. Linear programming is a technique used in economics to calculate optimal solutions for production, consumption or transportation problems (Van de Panne 1976). For instance, diet problems, that is, the fulfilling of nutritional demands at minimal costs using various food items of various prices and nutritional values, may be solved (for instance, Gould & Sparks 1969). In the present case linear programming would have to produce a production scheme which would optimally use the available resources, land and labour, in the production of sufficient food.

Application of linear programming in case of the West-Frisian Bronze Age agriculture and, basically, in all agricultural systems poses a number of problems which differ from those for the subsistence of hunter-gatherers. Linear programming invokes quantitative data on the costs of procurement of various components of diet. In subsistence agriculture the cost factors are the amounts of land and labour needed in the production. A difference with hunter-gatherer subsistence is that in subsistence farming a more stringent year-round planning of production (and consumption) of food is needed. Keene (1981) reckons food storage, but in the estimated diet stored foods are of minor importance for most of the year. In agriculture much work done during the growing season of cereals does not immediately result in food that can be eaten. Thus, in an agricultural system much of the labour has 'delayed productivity'. Another aspect of agriculture is that there are distinct peaks in activity. Mention has been made of the harvest which generally is thought a bottleneck in grain production (section XI.C.1.4). For animal husbandry similar phenomena are present.
The input of land and labour in grain, meat and milk production may somewhat roughly be estimated using ethnographic and experimental data.

It is questionable whether or not the Bronze Age farmers were free to produce either food item A or food item B. The maximalization of cereal production implies manuring, which in turn implies animal husbandry.
In an attempt to model the use of arable and pasture, a new production cost factor, next to land and labour, could therefore be introduced: the amount of manure. This production factor in turn depends on other costs, i.e. labour and the area of pasture and meadow. In such a model, the additional output of the production of manure are meat, milk and traction power. Such a model assumes a predominancy of cereal cultivation, a premise which may

not be *a priori* just for the West-Frisian Bronze Age. In this area, it is also possible that animal husbandry was predominant, cereal cultivation being an attractive extra to the farmers.

A more fundamental criticism of modelling prehistoric subsistence by mathematicel methods is illustrated by a remark of R.W. Brandt (IPP) that 'people may walk tens of kilometers just for one little special feather they want to put on their hats', or more plainly, the conduct of people can be quite strange and unexpected from an economic point of view.
It can be concluded that the development of a sophisticated model of West-Frisian agrarian production is beyond the scope of the present study, but despite the fundamental and practical pitfalls in linear programming of subsistence farming it might be rewarding to try to develop a model for a (prehistoric) agricultural system.

D.3. The 'demand side'

Attempts to assess what has been termed the 'demand' side of human diet in quantitative terms have been presented in section XI.C.2 and XI.C.3. If certain assumptions are accepted, it is possible to estimate the minimum and maximum proportions of components in human diets. As has been pointed out previously, a more detailed approximation of the composition of human diet cannot be made on the basis of the available chemical and ecoarcheological data. No ecological data on the consumption of leafy vegetables, roots and milk, which all exert a marked influence on the chemical composition of the diet, are available.

D.4. Conclusion

The preceding sections show that the present knowledge of both agricultural production and composition of human diet lacks the detail which is needed in order to draw conclusions on surplus and trade of agricultural products. The comparison between the possible dietary compositions and the agricultural potentials of the area shows, on the other hand, no discrepancies. The dietary compositions calculated in section XI.C.2.2 turn out to be feasible in the context of the agricultural system as discussed in section XI.C.1.4. This suggests that the procedures which have been used in estimating the Bronze Age diets yield results that are realistic.
Despite the negative result of the comparison between the two sides of diet, it might be rewarding to further explore this aspect of trace element analysis of human bones.

REFERENCES

Abbreviations

BAR : British Archaeological Reports
BROB : Berichten van de Rijksdienst voor het Oudheidkundig Bodemonderzoek
JAS : Journal of Archaeological Science
WFON : West-Frieslands Oud en Nieuw (in Dutch)

AeA, 1979. Arbeitsgruppe europäischer Anthropologen: Empfehlungen für die Alters- und Geschlechtsdiagnose am Skelett. Homo XXX, Anhang 1-32

Alexander, G.V. & Nusbaum, R.E., 1962. Zinc in bone. Nature 195, 903

Alexander, G.V., Nusbaum, R.E. & McDonald, N.S., 1956. The relative retention of strontium and calcium in bone tissue. Journal of Biological Chemistry 218, 911-919

Allen, L.H., 1982. Calcium bioavailability and absorption: a review. American Journal of Clinical Nutrition 35, 783-808

Ambrose, S.H. & DeNiro, M.J., 1986. Reconstruction of African human diet using bone collagen carbon and nitrogen isotope ratios. Nature 319, 321-324

Andersson, H., Nävert, B., Bingham, S.A., Englyst, H.N. & Cummings, J.H., 1983. The effects of breads containing similar amounts of phytate but different amounts of wheat bran on calcium, zinc and iron balance in man. British Journal of Nutrition 50, 503-510

Arrhenius, O., 1931. Die Bodenanalyse im Dienst der Archaeologie. Zeitschrift für Pflanzenernährung Dungung und Bodenkunde 10 (serie B), 427-439

Aufderheide, A.C., Neiman, F.D., Wittmers, L.E. & Rapp, G., 1981. Lead in bone II: Skeletal-lead content as an indicator of lifetime lead ingestion and the social correlates in an archaeological population. American Journal of Physical Anthropology 55, 285-291

Bakels, C.C., 1978. Four Linearbandkeramik settlements and their environments: a paleoecological study of Sittard, Stein, Elsloo and Hienheim. Analecta Praehistorica Leidensia XI 1-245

Bakker, H. de, 1979, Major soils and soil regions in the Netherlands. Wageningen: Pudoc

Bakker, J.A., 1959. Opgravingen te Hoogkarspel I. Het onderzoek van tumulus I en naaste omgeving. WFON 26, 158-191

Bakker, J.A., 1966. Opgravingen te Hoogkarspel II. Grafheuvelresten bij tumulus I achter de Watertoren. WFON 33, 168-175

Bakker, J.A., 1974. Prehistorische mensenresten uit Westfriesland, volgens de archeologische berichtgeving. IPP internal report, IPP publication 165.

Bakker, J.A., 1979. in (P.J. Woltering) Archeologische kroniek van Noord-Holland over 1978. Holland 11, 242-274

Bakker, J.A., & Brandt, R.W., 1966. Opgravingen te Hoogkarspel III. Grafheuvels en een terp uit de Late Bronstijd ten ZW van het Medemblikker Tolhuis. WFON 33, 176-224

Bakker, J.A., Brandt, R.W., Geel, B. van, Jansma, M.J., Kuijper, W.J., Mensch, P.J.A. van, Pals, J.P. & IJzereef, G.F., 1977. Hoogkarspel-Watertoren: towards a reconstruction of ecology and archaeology of an agrarian settlement of 1000 BC. in (B.L. van Beek, R.W. Brandt & W. Groenman- van Waateringe, eds) Ex Horreo. Cingula IV. Amsterdam: IPP, 187-225

Bakker, J.A. & Metz, W.H., 1967. Opgravingen te Hoogkarspel IV. Het onderzoek in 1966 van vindplaats F ten ZW van het Medemblikker Tolhuis (voorlopige mededeling). WFON 34, 202-228

Bakker, J.A., Woltering, P.J. & Manssen, W.J., 1968. Opgravingen te Hoogkarspel V. Het onderzoek van vindplaats F in 1967 (voorlopige mededeling). WFON 35, 193-199

Barker, G., 1985. Prehistoric farming in Europe. Cambridge: Cambridge University Press

Barneveld, A.A. van, 1983. De invloed van fytaat in de voeding: een overzicht. Voeding 44, 51-58

Bartlett, B.O. & Gunn, K.B., 1962. Discrimination between stable strontium and calcium in cereal grain. Agricultural Research Council Radiobiological Laboratory Annual Report 1961-62, 77-78

Beck, L.A., 1985. Bivariate analysis of trace elements in bone. Journal of Human Evolution 14, 493-502

Becker, R.O., Spadaro, J.A. & Berg, E.W., 1968. The trace elements of human bone. The Journal of Bone and Joint Surgery 50A, 326-334

Beemster, D.C.M. & Brandt, R.W., 1986. Velserbroekpolder-Rugbyveld Hofgeesterweg HOG I. in (P.J. Woltering, ed) Archeologische Kroniek over 1985. Holland 18, 273-303

Bender, M.M., 1968. Mass spectrometric studies of carbon 13 variations in corn and other grasses. Radiocarbon 10, 468-472

Bellow, S., 1982. The Deans December. New York: Harper & Row

Belovsky, G.E., 1987. Hunter-gathering foraging: a linear programming approach. Journal of Anthropological Archaeology 6, 29-76

Bloemers, J.H.F., 1978. Rijswijk (Z.H.), 'De Bult', Eine Siedlung der Cananefaten. Nederlandse Oudheden 8. Amersfoort

Bohman, V.R., Blincoe, C., Wade, M.A., Lesperance, A.L. & Fountain, E.L., 1966. Accumulation of strontium in bovine bones. Journal of Agriculture and Food Chememistry 14, 413-415

Borgognini Tarli, S., Paoli, G. & Francalacci, P., 1986. Problems and perspectives in palaeoserology. in (B. Herrmann, ed) Innovative Trends in der prähistorischen Anthropologie Mitteilungen der Berliner Gesellschaft für Anthropologie, Ethnologie und Urgeschichte 7, 107-115

Bolt, G.H. & Bruggenwert, M.G.M., 1976. Soil Chemistry. A. Basic elements. Amsterdam: Elsevier

Bowen, H.J.M. & Dymond, J.A., 1955. Strontium and barium in plants and soils. Proceedings of the Royal Society (London) B 144, 355-368

Bowen, H.J.M. & Dymond, J.A., 1956. The Uptake of Calcium and Strontium by Plants from Soils and Nutrient Solutions. Journal of Experimental Botany 7, 264-272

Boyle, K.V., 1986. Mathematics and the archaeologist: return to basics. Science and Archaeology 28, 32-37

Brandt, R.W., 1976. Landbouw en veeteelt in de Late Bronstijd van West-Friesland. Westerheem 25, 58-66

Brandt, R.W., 1977. Ditches and fields. in (Bakker, J.A., Brandt, R.W., Geel, B. van, Jansma, M.J., Kuijper, W.J., Mensch, P.J.A. van, Pals, J.P. & IJzereef, G.F.) Hoogkarspel-Watertoren: towards a reconstruction of ecology and archaeology of an agrarian settlement of 1000 BC. in (B.L. van Beek, R.W. Brandt & W. Groenman- van Waateringe, eds) Ex Horreo. Cingula IV. Amsterdam: IPP, 214-222

Brandt, R.W., 1980. De kolonisatie van West-Friesland in de Bronstijd. Westerheem 29, 137-151

Brandt, R.W. & IJzereef, G.F., 1980. West-Friesland in de Bronstijd. Leven en sterven 'binnen de grenzen van een model'. in (M. Chamaloun & H.T. Waterbolk, eds) Voltooid verleden tijd? Amsterdam: Backhuys

Brandt, R.W., Leeuw, S.E. van der, & Wijngaarden-Bakker, L.H. van, 1984. Transformations in a Dutch estuary: research in a wet landscape. World Archaeology 16, 1-17

Brothwell, D.R., 1981. Digging up bones. London: British Museum (3rd edition)

Brothwell, D., & Brothwell, P., 1969. Food in antiquity. London: Thames and Hudson

Bryant, F.J., Chamberlain, A.C., Spicer, G.S. & Webb, M.S.W., 1958. Strontium in Diet. British Medical Journal June 14, 1371-1375

Bryant, F.J. & Loutit, J.F., 1964. The entry of strontium-90 into human bone. Proceedings of the Royal Society of London B 159, 449-465

Bult, E.J. & Hallewas, D.P., 1986. Graven bij Valkenburg. Het archeologisch onderzoek in 1985. Delft: Eburon

Bumsted, M.P., 1984. Human variation: delta carbon-13 in adult bone collagen and the relation to diet in an isochronous C(4) (Maize) archaeological population. Ph.D. dissertation, Univ. of Massachusetts

Bumsted, M.P., 1985. Past human behavior from bone chemical analysis-respects and prospects. Journal of Human Evolution 14, 539-551

Burleigh, R., Matthews, K. & Leese, M., 1984. Consensus delta 13C values. Radiocarbon 26, 46-53

Butler, J.J., 1964. The bronze rapier from Zwaagdijk, gemeente Wervershoof, Prov. North Holland. BROB 14, 37-43

Butler, J.J., 1979. Nederland in de bronstijd. Haarlem: Fibula- Van Dishoeck

Butter, J., 1935. Zandwerven. WFON 9, 66-69

Buurman, J., 1979. Cereals in circles-Crop processing activities in Bronze Age Bovenkarspel (the Netherlands). in Festschrift Maria Hopf zum 65. Geburtstag. Archaeo-Physica 8, 21-37

Buurman, J. & Pals, J.P., 1974. Some remarks on prehistoric flax in the Netherlands. BROB 24, 107-111

Calderoni, G. & Schnitzer, M., 1984. Effects of age on the chemical structure of paleosol humic acids and fulvic acids. Geochimica et Cosmochimica Acta 48, 2045-2051

Caselitz, P., 1986. Ernährungsmöglichkeiten und Ernährungsgewohnheiten prähistorischer Bevölkerungen. BAR International Series 314

Cate, C.L. ten, 1972. Wan god mast gift..., Bilder aus der Geschichte der Schweinezucht in Walde. Wageningen:Pudoc

Chipman, W.A., 1966. Food chains in the sea. in (R.S. Russell, ed) Radioactivity and human diet Oxford: Pergamon Press, 421-453

Chisholm, B.S., Nelson, D.E. & Schwarcz, H.P., 1983a. Dietary information from delta 13C and delta 15N measurements on bone collagen. in (W.G. Mook & H.T. Waterbolk, eds) Proceedings of the first international symposium 14C and Archaeology, Groningen 1981. PACT 8. Strasbourg: Council of Europe, 391-395

Chisholm, B.S., Nelson, D.E. & Schwarcz, H.P., 1983b. Marine and terrestrial protein in prehistoric diets on the British Columbia coast. Current Anthropology 24, 396-398

Clark, C. & Haswell, M., 1964. The economics of subsistence agriculture. London: MacMillan

Clason, A.T., 1961. De beenderen van tumulus XIII bij 'De Ark', gem. Wervershoof. WFON 28, 91-96

Clason, A.T., 1964. The animal bones from the Bronze Age settlement of Zwaagdijk, gemeente Wervershoof, Prov. North Holland. BROB 14, 44-52

Clason, A.T., 1967. Animal and man in Holland's past. Palaeohistoria 13

Clason, A.T., 1983. A.E. van Giffen as archaeozoologist. Palaeohistoria 25, 1-6

Coles, J.M. & Harding, A.F., 1979. The Bronze Age of Europe. London: Methuen

Collander, R., 1941. Selective absorption of cations by higher plants. Plant Physiology 16, 691-720
Comar, C.L., 1963. Some Over-all Aspects of Strontium-Calcium Discrimination. in (R.H. Wasserman, ed) The Transfer of Calcium and Strontium Across Biological Membranes. New York: Academic Press, 405-417
Comar, C.L., 1967. Some principles of strontium metabolism: implications, applications, limitations. in (J.M.A. Lenihan, J.F. Loutit & J.H. Martin, eds) Strontium metabolism. London: Academic Press, 17-31
Comar, C.L., Russell, R.S. & Wasserman, R.H., 1957. Strontium-calcium movement from soil to man. Science 126, 485-492
Comar, C.L., & Wasserman, R.H., 1958. Strontium-calcium metabolism in man and animals as studied by radioisotope methods. in (R.C. Extermann, ed) Radioisotopes in Scientific Research Vol IV. London: Pergamon Press, 192-206
Comar, C.L., Wasserman, R.H., & Twardock, A.R., 1961. Secretion of calcium and strontium into milk. Health Physics 7, 69-80
Connor, M. & Slaughter, D., 1984. Diachronic study of Inuit diets utilizing trace element analysis. Arctic Anthropology 21, 123-134
Cordfunke, E.H.P. & Diederik, F., 1984. Schagen: ijzerwinning in de Romeinse tijd met behulp van steenkool. Westerheem 33, 5-10
DeNiro, M.J., 1985. Postmortem preservation and alteration of in vivo bone collagen isotope ratios in relation to palaeodietary reconstruction. Nature 317, 806-809
DeNiro, M.J. & Hastorf, C.A., 1985. Alteration of 15N/14N and 13C/12C ratios of plant matter during the initial stages of diagenesis: Studies utilizing archaeological specimens from Peru. Geochimica et Cosmochimica Acta 49, 97-115
Dennell, R.W., 1978. Early farming in South Bulgaria from the sixth to the third millenia BC BAR International Series 45
Dennell, R.W., 1979. Prehistoric diet and nutrition: some food for thought. World Archaeology 11, 121-135
Drasch, G.A., 1982. Lead burden in prehistorical, historical and modern human bones. The Science of the Total Environment 24, 199-231
Dupuis, Y. & Fournier, P., 1963. Lactose and the absorption of calcium and strontium. in (R.H. Wasserman, ed) The Transfer of Calcium and Strontium Across Biological Membranes. New York: Academic Press, 277-293
Eaton, S.B. & Konner, M., 1985. Paleolithic nutrition. A consideration of its nature and current implications. New England Journal of Medicine 312, 283-289
Ente, P.J., 1963. Een bodemkartering van het tuinbouwcentrum "De Streek". Verslagen Landbouwkundig Onderzoek 68-16. Wageningen.
Es, W.A. van, 1981. De Romeinen in Nederland. Haarlem: Fibula-Van Dishoeck (2nd edition)
Frissel, M.J., Jakubick, A.T., Klugt, N. van der, Penders, R.M.J., Poelstra, P. & Zwemmer, E.T.A., 1981. Modeling of the transport and accumulation of radionuclides of strontium, cesium and plutonium in soil. Experimental verification. Association Euratom-ITAL Technical Preliminary Research Report 101
Geel, B. van, Hallewas, D.P. & Pals, J.P., 1982-83. A Late Holocene deposit under the Westfriese Zeedijk near Enkhuizen (Prov. of Noord-Holland, the Netherlands): Palaeooecological and archaeological aspects. Review of Palaeobotany and Palynology 38, 269-335
Giffen, A.E. van, 1913. Die Fauna der Wurten. thesis Groningen
Giffen, A.E. van, 1930. Die Bauart der Einzelgräber. Mannus Bibliothek 44-45
Giffen, A.E. van, 1944. Grafheuvels te Zwaagdijk, gem. Wervershoof, N.-H. WFON XVII, 121-221

Giffen, A.E. van, 1953. Onderzoek van drie Bronstijdgrafheuvels bij Grootebroek, gem. Grootebroek, Noord-Holland. verbeterde en vermeerderde overdruk uit WFON XX, 1-32
Giffen, A.E. van, 1962. Grafheuvels uit de Midden-Bronstijd met nederzettingssporen van de Klokbekercultuur bij Oostwoud. WFON 29, 199-209
Giffen, A.E. van, 1966. Nederzetingssporen van de Vroege Klokbekercultuur bij Oostwoud (NH). in (W. Glasbergen & W. Groenman-van Waateringe, eds) In het voetspoor van A.E. van Giffen, tweede, vermeerderde druk. Groningen: Wolters, 66-71
Gilbert, R.I., 1975. Trace element analyses of three skeletal Amerindian populations at Dickson Mounds. unpublished Ph.D. dissertation, University of Massachusetts, Amherst
Gilbert, R.I., 1977. Application of trace element research to problems in archaeology. in (RL Blakely, ed) Biocultural adaptation in prehistoric America. Athens: Univ. Georgia Press, 85-100
Gilbert, R.I. jr., 1985. Stress, paleonutrition and trace elements. in (R.I. Gilbert jr. & J.H. Mielke, eds) The analysis of prehistoric diets. Orlando: Academic Press, 339-358
Gilbert, R.I. jr. & Mielke, J.H. (eds), 1985. The analysis of prehistoric diets. Orlando: Academic Press
Gilfillan, S.C., 1965. Lead poisoning and the fall of Rome. Journal of Occupational Medicine 7, 53-60
Gould, P.R. & Sparks, J.S., 1969. The geographical context of human diets in southern Guatemala. The Geographical Review LIX, 58-82
Groenman-van Waateringe, W., 1986. Grazing possibilities in the Neolithic of the Netherlands based on palynological data. in (K-E. Behre, ed.) Anthropogenic indicators in pollen diagrams. Rotterdam: Balkema, 187-202
Groot Bruinderink, G., 1976. Wilde zwijnen op de Veluwe. de Jager 80, 606-609
Grupe, G., 1986a. Multielementanalyse: Ein neuer Weg für die Paläodemographie. Materialien zur Bevölkerungswissenschaft, Sonderheft 7. Wiesbaden: Bundesinstitut für Bevölkerungsforschung
Grupe, G., 1986b. Rekonstruktion bevölkerungsbiologischer Parameter aus dem Elementgehalt bodengelagerte Knochen. in (B. Herrmann, ed) Innovative Trends in der prähistorischen Anthropologie Mitteilungen der Berliner Gesellschaft für Anthropologie, Ethnologie und Urgeschichte 7, 39-44
Haaff, G. van, 1973. Archeologie, een nevenaspekt van de ruilverkaveling Het Grootslag. Het Grootslag, december 1973
Haan, F.A.M. de & Zwerman, P.J., 1976. Pollution of soil. in (G.H. Bolt & M.G.M. Bruggenwert, eds) Soil Chemistry A. Basic Elements. Amsterdam: Elsevier. 192-271
Haaster, H. van, 1985. Schagen-Muggenburg. Een bijdrage aan de reconstructie van milieu en agrarische activiteiten rond een nederzetting uit de 2e/3e eeuw. Internal Report IPP, Amsterdam
Hallam, A. & Price, N.B., 1968. Environmental and biochemical control of strontium in shells of Cardium edule. Geochimica et Cosmochimica Acta 32, 319-328
Hallewas, D.P., 1981. Archaeological cartography between Marsdiep and IJ. BROB 31, 219-272
Hallewas, D.P., 1986. Archeologische kroniek van Zuid-Holland over 1985. Holland 18, 304-330
Harding, R.S.O. & Teleki, G., eds. 1981. Omnivorous primates. Gathering and hunting in human evolution. New York: Columbia University Press.
Hart Hansen, J.P., 1985. De mummies van Qilakitsoq. Natuur & Techniek 53 (12), 888-907

Hartog, C. den, 1976. De behoefte aan dierlijk eiwit. Voeding 37, 354-366

Hartog, C. den, Hautvast, J.G.A.J. & Hartog, A.P. den, 1978. Nieuwe Voedingsleer. Utrecht: Het Spectrum

Hassan, F.A., 1981. Demographic Archeology. New York: Academic Press

Hastorf, C.A. & DeNiro, M.J., 1985. Reconstruction of prehistoric plant production and cooking practices by a new isotopic method. Nature 315, 489-491

Hatch, J.W. & Geidel, R.A., 1985. Status-specific dietary variation in two (new?) world cultures. Journal of Human Evolution 14, 469-476

Hawkes, J.G., 1969. The ecological background of plant domestication. in (P.J. Ucko & G.W. Dimbleby, eds) The domestication and exploitation of plants and animals. London: Duckworth, 17-30

Hayden, B. 1981. Subsistence and ecological adaptations of modern hunter/gatherers. in (Harding, R.S.O. & Teleki, G., eds) Omnivorous primates. New York: Columbia University Press, 344-421

Heidinga, H.A., 1984. Indications of severe drought during the 10th century AD from an inland dune area in the central Netherlands. in (H.J.A. Berendsen & W.H. Zagwijn, eds) Geological changes in the western Netherlands during the period 1000-1300 AD. Geologie & Mijnbouw 63, 241-248

Helbaek, H., 1952. Early crops in Southern England. Proceedings of the Prehistoric Society XVIII, 194-233

Herrmann, B. 1972. Das Combe Chapelle Skelett. Ausgrabungen in Berlin 3, 7-69

Hobson, K.A. & Schwarcz, H.P., 1986. The variation in delta 13C values in bone collagen for two wild herbivore populations: implications for palaeodiet studies. JAS 13, 101-106

Hodge, A.T., 1981. Vitruvius, lead pipes and lead poisoning. American Journal of Archaeology 85, 486-491

Holdgate, M.W., 1979. A Perspective of Environmental Pollution. Cambridge: Cambridge University Press

Huizinga, J., 1964. Preliminary physical anthropological investigations. BROB 14, 35-36

Hulshof, K.F.A.M., 1985. Spoorzoeken in voedingsmiddelen. Voeding 46, 227-232

IJzereef, G.F., 1981, Bronze Age animal bones from Bovenkarspel. Nederlandse Oudheden 10. Amersfoort

IJzereef, G.F., 1983. Boeren in de Bronstijd bij Bovenkarspel. Spiegel Historiael 18, 635-643

Isermann, K., 1981. Uptake of Stable Strontium by Plants and Effects on Plant Growth. in (S.C. Skoryna, ed) Handbook of Stable Strontium New York: Plenum Press, 65-86

Jaarverslag ROB 1974

Jelgersma, S., de Jong, J., Zagwijn, W.H. & Regteren Altena, J.F. van, 1970. The coastal dunes of the Western Netherlands; geology, vegetational history and archeology. Mededelingen Rijks Geologische Dienst Nieuwe Serie 21, 93-167

Johansen, O.S., Gulliksen, S. & Nydal., R, 1986. Delta 13C and diet: analysis of norwegian human skeletons. Radiocarbon 28, 754-761

Jones, M. (ed), 1983, Integrating the subsistence economy. BAR International Series 181

Jonxis, J.H.P., 1983, Sporenelementen. Voeding 44, 266-273

Jørgensen, G., 1977. Acorns as food-source in the Later Stone Age. Acta Archaeologica 48, 233-238

Jowsey, J., 1977. Metabolic diseases of bone. Philadelphia: WB Saunders

Kahn, B., Jones, I.R., Porter, C.R., Straub, C.P., 1965. Transfer of radiostrontium from cows' feed to milk. *Journal of Dairy Science* 48, 1023-1030

Keeley, H.C.M., Hudson, G.E. & Evans, J., 1977. Trace element contents of human bones in various states of preservation. *JAS* 4, 19-24

Keene, A.S., 1981. *Prehistoric foraging in a temperate forest*. New York: Academic Press

Keene, A.S., 1985. Nutrition and economy: Models for the study of prehistoric diet. in (R.I. Gilbert jr. & J.H. Mielke, eds) *The analysis of prehistoric diets*. Orlando: Academic Press, 155-190

Klechkovsky, V.M. & Guliakin, I.V., 1958. Behaviour of tracer amounts of strontium, calcium, ruthenium and zirconium in soils and plants according to the data of investigations with radioactive isotopes of these elements. in (R.C. Extermann, ed) *Radioisotopes in Scientific Research* Vol IV. London: Pergamon Press, 150-172

Knizhnikov, V.A. & Marei, A.N., 1967. Strontium metabolism in man. in (J.M.A. Lenihan, J.F. Loutit & J.H. Martin, eds) *Strontium metabolism*. London: Academic Press, 71-82

Kobert, R., 1906-9. Chronische Bleivergiftung im klassischen Altertum. in (P. Diergart, ed) *Beiträge aus der Geschichte der Chemie*, 103-119

Kornberg, H.A. & Davis, J.J., 1966. Food chains in fresh water. in (R.S. Russell, ed) *Radioactivity and human diet*. Oxford: Pergamon Press, 385-418

Kyle, J.H., 1986. Effect of post-burial contamination on the concentrations of major and minor elements in human bones and teeth-the implications for palaeodietary research. *JAS* 13, 403-416

Kuyper, W.J., 1977. Molluscs. in (Bakker, J.A., Brandt, R.W., Geel, B. van, Jansma, M.J., Kuijper, W.J., Mensch, P.J.A. van, Pals, J.P. & IJzereef, G.F.) Hoogkarspel-Watertoren: towards a reconstruction of ecology and archaeology of an agrarian settlement of 1000 BC. in (B.L. van Beek, R.W. Brandt & W. Groenman- van Waateringe, eds) *Ex Horreo*. Cingula IV. Amsterdam: IPP, 198-200

Lambert, J.B., Szpunar, C.B. & Buikstra, J.E., 1979. Chemical analysis of excavated human bones from Middle and Late Woodland sites. *Archaeometry* 21, 115-129

Lambert, J.B., Vlasak, S.M., Thometz, A.C. & Buikstra, J.E., 1982. A comparative study of the chemical analysis of ribs and femurs in Woodland populations. *American Journal of Physical Anthropology* 59, 289-294

Lambert, J.B., Simpson, S.V., Buikstra, J.E., & Charles, D.K., 1984. Analysis of soil associated with Woodland burials. in (J.B. Lambert, ed) *Archaeological Chemistry* III, Advances in Chemistry Series No. 205. Washington: American Chemical Society, 97-116

Lambert, J.B., Vlasak Simpson, S., Gorell Weiner, S., & Buikstra, J.E., 1985. Induced metal-ion exchange in excavated human bone. *JAS* 12, 85-92

Lambert, J.B., Simpson, S.V., Szpunar, C.B. & Buikstra, J.E., 1984. Copper and barium as dietary discriminants: the effect of diagenesis. *Archaeometry* 26, 131-138

Lanting, J,N., 1979. Medemblik: Oostwoud. in (P.J. Woltering) Archeologische kroniek van Noord-Holland over 1978. *Holland* 11, 250-251

Lanting, J.N. & Mook, W.G., 1977. *The pre- and protohistory of the Netherlands in terms of radiocarbon dates*. Groningen

Lehmann, L.Th., 1963. Het partiele onderzoek van tumulus I in de gemeente Enkhuizen. *WFON* 30, 234-242

Lengemann, F.W., 1963. Over-all aspects of calcium and strontium absorption. in (R.H. Wasserman, ed) *The Transfer of Calcium and Strontium Across Biological Membranes*. New York: Academic Press, 85-96

Létolle, R., 1980. Nitrogen-15 in the natural environment. in (Fritz, P. & Fontes, J.Ch., eds) Handbook of environmental isotope geochemistry Vol.1. Amsterdam: Elsevier, 407-433

Lindsay, W.L., & Vlek, P.L.G., 1977. Phosphate minerals. in (J.B. Dixon & S.B. Weed, eds) Minerals in soil environments. 639-672

Longin, R., 1971. New method of collagen extraction for radiocarbon dating. Nature 230, 240-242

Louwe Kooijmans, L.P., 1974. The Rhine/Meuse delta; Four studies on its prehistoric occupation and Holocene geology. Analecta Praehistorica Leidensia 7 and Oudheidkundige Mededelingen Rijksmuseum Oudheden Leiden 53-4

Luten, J.B., 1983. Spoorelementen in voor de consumptie bestemde zeewieren. Voeding 44, 232-236

Maat, G.J.R., 1986. Features of malnutrition, their significance and epidemiology in prehistoric anthropology. in (B. Herrmann, ed) Innovative Trends in der prähistorischen Anthropologie Mitteilungen der Berliner Gesellschaft für Anthropologie, Ethnologie und Urgeschichte 7, 157-164

Maat, G.J.R., in press a. (Physical-anthropological report on a Bronze Age skeleton from Bovenkarspel). to be published in BROB

Maat, G.J.R., in press b. Human remains from a native settlement at Schagen-Muggenburg (2nd-3rd century AD). to be published in Cingula

Mackie, A., Townshend, A. & Waldron, H.A., 1975. Lead concentrations in bones from Roman York. JAS 2, 235-237

Mahanti, H.S. & Barnes, R.M., 1983. Determination of major, minor and trace elements in bone by Inductively Coupled Plasma Emission Spectrometry. Analytica Chimica Acta 151, 409-417

Mann, A.E., 1981. Diet and human evolution. in (Harding, R.S.O. & Teleki, G., eds) Omnivorous primates. New York: Columbia University Press, 10-36

Marschner, H., 1983. General introduction to the mineral nutrition of plants. in (A. Lauchli & R.L. Bieleski, eds) Inorganic plant nutrition Vol. 15A. Berlin: Springer Verlag, 5-60

Martin, R.P., Newbould, P. & Russell, R.S., 1958. Discrimination between strontium and calcium in plants and soils. in (R.C. Extermann, ed) Radioisotopes in Scientific Research Vol IV. London: Pergamon Press, 173-190

McConnell, D., 1973. Apatite. Its chrystal chemistry, mineralogy, utilization, and geologic and biologic occurences. Wien: Springer Verlag

Mensch, P.J.A. van & IJzereef, G.F., 1975. Animal remains from a Bronze Age settlement near Andijk, Prov. of North Holland. BROB 25, 55-68

Mensch, P.J.A. van & IJzereef, G.F., 1977. Animal and human remains. in (Bakker, J.A., Brandt, R.W., Geel, B. van, Jansma, M.J., Kuijper, W.J., Mensch, P.J.A. van, Pals, J.P. & IJzereef, G.F.) Hoogkarspel-Watertoren: towards a reconstruction of ecology and archaeology of an agrarian settlement of 1000 BC. in (B.L. van Beek, R.W. Brandt & W. Groenman- van Waateringe, eds) Ex Horreo. Cingula IV. Amsterdam: IPP, 204-208

Menzel, R.G. & Heald, W.R., 1955. Distribution of potassium, rubidium, cesium, calcium and strontium within plants grown in nutrient solutions. Soil Science 80, 287-293

Menzel, R.G. & Heald, W.R., 1959. Strontium and calcium contents of crop plants in relation to exchangeable strontium and calcium in the soil. Soil Science Society America Proceedings 23, 110-112

Mercer, R., 1981. Appendix. in (R. Mercer, ed) Farming practice in British prehistory. Edinburgh: University Press, 231-237

Modderman, P.J.R., 1964. Middle Bronze Age graves and settlement traces at Zwaagdijk, Gemeente Wervershoof, Prov. North Holland. BROB 14, 27-35

Modderman, P.J.R., 1974. Een drieperiodenheuvel uit de Midden Bronstijd op het Bullenland te Hoogkarspel. *WFON* 41, 251-258

Mook, W.G., 1968. Geochemistry of the stable carbon and oxygen isotopes of natural waters in the Netherlands. thesis Groningen

Moritz, L.A., 1958. *Grain-mills and flour in classical antiquity*. Oxford: Clarendon Press

Mraz, F.R., Wright, P.L. & Ferguson, T.M., 1967. Effect of dietary strontium on reproductive performance of the laying hen. in (J.M.A. Lenihan, J.F. Loutit & J.H. Martin, eds) *Strontium Metabolism*. London: Academic Press, 247-253

Mulder, E.F.J. de, & Bosch, J.H.A., 1982. Holocene stratigraphy, radiocarbon datings and paleogeography of the central and northern North-Holland (the Netherlands). *Mededelingen Rijks Geologische Dienst* 36-3, 111-160

Nelson, D.A., & Sauer, N.J., 1984. An evaluation of postdepositional changes in the trace element content of human bone. *American Antiquity* 49, 141-147

NVT, 1983. *Nederlandse Voedingsmiddelentabel* 34th edition. Den Haag: Voorlichtingsbureau voor de voeding.

Nriagu, J.O., 1983a. *Lead and lead poisoning in antiquity*. New York: John Wiley

Nriagu, J.O., 1983b. Saturnine gout among Roman aristocrats. *New England Journal of Medicine* 308, 660-663

O'Dell, B.L., 1976. Biochemistry and physiology of copper in vertebrates. in (A.S. Prasad, ed) *Trace elements in human health and disease*, Vol I: Zinc and copper. New York: Academic Press, 391-413

Ophel, I.L. & Judd, J.M., 1967. Skeletal distribution of strontium and calcium and strontium-calcium ratios in several species of fish. in (J.M.A. Lenihan, J.F. Loutit & J.H. Martin, eds) *Strontium metabolism*. London: Academic Press, 103-109

Pals, J.P., in press. Ecological and economic aspects of the medieval settlement at Kootwijk, as elucidated by archaebotanical research.

Pals, J.P., Geel, B. van & Delfos, A., 1980. Paleooecological studies in the Klokkeweel bog near Hoogkarspel (Prov. of Noord-Holland) *Review of palaeobotany and palynology* 30, 317-418

Panne, C. van de, 1976. *Linear Programming and related techniques*. Amsterdam: North Holland

Pate, D. & Brown, K.A., 1985. The stability of bone strontium in the geochemical environment. *Journal of Human Evolution* 14, 483-491

Parker, R.B., & Toots, H., 1980. Trace elements in bones as palaebiological indicators. in (A.K. Behrensmeyer & A. Hill, eds) *Fossils in the making*. Chicago: University of Chicago Press

Paul, A.A. & Southgate, D.A.T., 1978. *McCance and Widdowson's The composition of foods* 4th edition. London:HMSO; Amsterdam: Elsevier/North-Holland

Perizonius, W.R.K., & Pot, Tj., 1981. Diachronic dental research on human skeletal remains excavated in the Netherlands, I: Dorestad's cemetary on 'the Heul'. *BROB* 31, 369-413

Piepenbrink, H. 1986. Two examples of biogenous dead bone decomposition and their consequences for taphonomic interpretation. *JAS* 13, 417-430

Pories, W.J., Mansour, E.G., Plecha, F.R., Flynn, A. & Strain, W.H., 1976. Metabolic factors affecting zinc metabolism in the surgical patient. in (A.S. Prasad, ed) *Trace elements in human health and disease*, Vol.I: Zinc and copper. New York: Academic Press, 115-141

Posner, A.S., 1969, Chrystal chemistry of bone mineral. *Physiological Review* 49, 760-792

Prasad, A.S., 1976. Deficiency of zinc in man and its toxicity. in (A.S. Prasad, ed) Trace elements in human health and disease, Vol I: Zinc and Copper. New York: Academic Press, 1-20

Price, T.D., 1985. Late Archaic subsistence in the Midwestern United States. Journal of Human Evolution 14, 449-459

Price, T.D., 1986. Conference Report: Bone chemistry and past behaviour. Santa Fe, New Mexico, March 1986. SAS Newsletter 9(3), 8-9

Price, T.D., Connor, M. & Parsen, J.D., 1985a. Bone chemistry and the reconstruction of diet: strontium discrimination in White-Tailed Deer. JAS 12, 419-442

Price, T.D., Schoeninger, M.J. & Armelagos, G.J., 1985b. Bone chemistry and past behaviour: an overview. Journal of Human Evolution 14, 419-447

Prummel, W., 1979. Environment and stock-raising in Dutch settlements of the Bronze Age and Middle Ages. Palaeohistoria XXI, 91-107

Randsborg, K., 1985. Subsistence and settlement in Northern temperate Europe in the First millenium A.D. in (G. Barker & C. Gamble, eds) Beyond domestication in prehistoric Europe. London: Academic Press, 233-265

Regteren Altena, H.H. van & Bakker, J.A., 1968. Opgravingen bij Medemblik. WFON 35, 201-210

Regteren Altena, J.F. van, Bakker, J.A., Clason, A.T., Glasbergen, W., Groenman-van Waateringe, W. & Pons, L.J., 1962. The Vlaardingen Culture (I). Helinium 2, 3-35

Regteren Altena, J.F. van, Mensch, P.J.A. van & IJzereef, G.F., 1976. Bronze Age clay animals from Grootebroek. in (B.L. van Beek, R.W. Brandt & W. Groenman-van Waateringe, eds) Ex Horreo Cingula IV. Amsterdam: IPP, 241-254

Renfrew, J.M., 1973. Palaeoethnobotany. The prehistoric food plants of the Near East and Europe. London: Methuen

Reynolds, P., 1981. Deadstock and livestock. in (R. Mercer, ed) Farming practice in British prehistory. Edinburgh: University Press, 97-122

Rheingold, A.L., Hues, S. & Cohen, M.N., 1983. Strontium and zinc content in bones as an indication of diet. Journal of Chemical Education 60, 233-234

Riordan, J.F. & Vallee, B.L., 1976. Structure and function of zinc metalloenzymes. in (A.S. Prasad, ed) Trace elements in human health and disease, Vol I: Zinc and copper. New York: Academic Press, 227-256

Roberts, H.J., 1983. Potential toxicity due to dolomite and bonemeal. Southern Medical Journal 5, 556-559

Rogers, J. & Waldron, T., 1985. Lead concentrations in bones from a Neolithic long barrow. JAS 12, 93-96

Rosenblatt, M., 1906. Beiträge zur Kenntnis der chronischen Bleivergiftung.

Rosenthal, H.L., 1957. Uptake of calcium-45 and strontium-90 from water by fresh-water fishes. Science 126, 699-700

Rosenthal, H.L., Cochran, O.A. & Eves, M.M., 1972. Strontium content of mammalian bone, diet and excreta. Environmental Research 5, 182-191

Rosenthal, H.L., Eves, M.M. & Cochran, O.A., 1970. Common strontium concentration of mineralized tissues from marine and sweet water animals. Comparative Biochemistry and Physiology 32, 445-450

Rowley-Conwy, P., 1981. Slash and burn in the temperate European Neolithic. in (R. Mercer, ed) Farming practice in British Prehistory. Edinburgh: University Press, 85-96

Runia, L.T., 1985. Gebruik van strontium, andere spoorelementen en stabiele isotopen als voedingsindicatoren in de archeologie. Voeding 46, 368-375

Runia, L.T., 1986. Noord-Holland: Zwaagdijk. Bulletin KNOB 85, 137-138

Runia, L.T., 1987a. Analysis of bone from the Bronze Age site Bovenkarspel-Het Valkje, the Netherlands: a preliminary report. Archaeometry 29
Runia, L.T., 1987b. Strontium and calcium distribution in plants: effect on palaeodietary studies. JAS 14
Runia, L.T., in prep. Discrimination factors on different trophic levels in relation to the trace element content in human bones. in (G. Grupe & B. Herrmann, eds) Proceedings of the symposium 'Trace elements in environmetal history', Göttingen, June 1987. Berlin: Springer
Russell, R.S., 1966a. Nature of food chains and the nuclides of major concern. in (R.S. Russell, ed) Radioactivity and Human Diet Oxford: Pergamon Press, 45-62
Russell, R.S., 1966b. Radioactive strontium in food chains: general review. in (R.S. Russell, ed) Radioactivity and Human Diet (Oxford: Pergamon Press, 173-187
Russell, R.S. & Newbould, P., 1966. Entry of strontium-90 into plants from the soil. in (R.S. Russell,ed) Radioactivity and Human Diet Oxford: Pergamon Press, 213-245
Sandstead, H.H., Vo-Khactu, K.P. & Solomons, N., 1976. Conditioned zinc deficiencies. in (A.S. Prasad, ed) Trace elements in human health and disease, Vol 1: Zinc and copper. New York: Academic Press, 33-49
Sanzharova, N.I., 1978. Change in the ratio of strontium-90 to calcium during uptake from soil by herbaceous plants. Moscow University Soil Science Bulletin 33, 42-43
Scheinberg, I.H. & Sternlieb, S., 1976. Copper toxicity and Wilson's disease. in (A.S. Prasad, ed) Trace elements in human health and disease, Vol. I: Zinc and copper. New York: Academic Press. 415-438
Schoeninger, M.J., 1979. Diet and status at Chalcatzingo: some empirical and technical aspects of strontium analysis. American Journal of Physical Anthropology 51, 295-310
Schoeninger, M.J., 1981. The agricultural "revolution": its effect on human diet in prehistoric Iran and Israel. Paleorient 7, 73-91
Schoeninger, M.J., 1982. Diet and the evolution of modern human form in the Middle East. American Journal of Physical Anthropology 58, 37-52
Schoeninger, M.J., 1985. Trophic level effects on 15N/14N and 13C/12C ratios in bone collagen and strontium levels in bone mineral. Journal of Human Evolution 14, 515-525
Schoeninger, M.J., in manuscript. Dutch whalers
Schoeninger, M.J., & DeNiro, M.J., 1984. Nitrogen and carbon isotopic composition of bone collagen from marine and terrestrial animals. Geochimica Cosmochimica Acta 48, 625-639
Schoeninger, M.J., DeNiro, M.J. & Tauber, H., 1983. Stable nitrogen isotope ratios of bone collagen reflect marine and terrestrial components of prehistoric human diet. Science 220, 1381-1383
Schoeninger, M.J., & Peebles, C.S., 1981. Effect of mollusc eating on human bone strontium levels. JAS 8, 391-397
Schroeder, H.A. & Balassa, J.J., 1966. Abnormal trace metals in man: arsenic. Journal of Chronical Diseases 19, 85-106
Schroeder, H.A., Nason, A.P., Tipton, I.H., & Balassa, J.J., 1966. Essential trace elements in man: Copper. Journal of Chronical Diseases 19, 1007-1034
Sealy, J.C., & Van der Merwe, N.J., 1985. Isotope assessment of Holocene human diets in the southwestern Cape, South Africa. Nature, 138-140
Sherratt, A.G., 1981. Plough and pastoralism: aspects of the secondary products revolution. in (I. Hodder, G. Isaac & N. Hammond, eds) Pattern of the past. Studies in honour of David Clarke. Cambridge: Cambridge Univ. Press, 261-306

Shipman, P., Foster, G. & Schoeninger, M.J., 1984. Burnt bones and teeth: an experimental study of color, morphology, crystal structure and shrinkage. JAS 11, 307-326

Sillen, A., 1981. Strontium and diet at Hayonim cave, Israel: an evalution of the strontium/calcium technique for investigating prehistoric diets. Ph.D. dissertation, Univ. of Pennsylvania

Sillen, A. & Kavanagh, M., 1982. Strontium and paleodietary research: a review. Yearbook of Physical Anthropology 25, 67-90

Sillen, A. & Smith, P., 1984. Weaning patterns are reflected in strontium-calcium ratios of juvenile skeletons. JAS 11, 237-245

Slicher van Bath, B.H., 1960. De agrarische geschiedenis van West-Europa 500-1850. Utrecht: Het Spectrum

Slicher van Bath, B.H., 1962. Accounts and dairies of farmers before 1800 as sources for agricultural history. AAG bijdragen 8, 5-33

Slicher van Bath, B.H., 1963a. De oogstopbrengsten van verschillende gewassen, voornamelijk granen, in verhouding tot het zaaizaad, ca. 810-1820. AAG bijdragen 9, 9-28

Slicher van Bath, B.H., 1963b. Yield ratios, 810-1820. AAG bijdragen 10, 3-264

Smith, J.L., 1976. Metabolism and toxicity of lead. in (A.S. Prasad, ed) Trace elements in human health and disease, Vol II: Essential and toxic elements. New York: Academic Press, 443-452

Smith, K.A., 1971a. The comparative uptake and translocation by plants of calcium, strontium, barium and radium. I Bertholettia excelsa (Brazil Nut Tree). Plant and Soil 34, 369-379

Smith, K.A., 1971b. The comparative uptake and translocation by plants of calcium, strontium, barium and radium. II Triticum vulgare (wheat). Plant and Soil 34, 643-651

Smith, L.H., Rasmussen, D.C. & Myers, W.M., 1963. Influence of genotype upon realtionship of strontium-89 to calcium in grain of barley and wheat. Crop Science 3, 386-389

Spencer, H., Osis, D., Kramer, L. & Norris, C., 1976. Intake, excretion and retention of zinc in man. in (A.S. Prasad, ed) Trace elements in human health and disease, Vol 1: Zinc and copper. New York: Academic Press, 345-361

Staarink, T. & Hakkenbrak, P., 1984. Het contaminantenboekje. 's Gravenhage: Staatsuitgeverij

Tanaka, G-I., Kawamura, H. & Nomura, E., 1981. Reference Japanese man-II. Distribution of strontium in the skeleton and in the mass of mineralized bone. Health Physics 40, 601-614

Tauber, H., 1981. 13C evidence for dietary habits of prehistoric man in Denmark. Nature 292, 332-333

Tauber, H., 1983. 14C Dating of human beings in relation to dietary habits. in (W.G. Mook & H.T. Waterbolk, eds) Proceedings of the first international symposium 14C and Archaeology, Groningen 1981. PACT 8. Strasbourg: Council of Europe. 365-375

Tauber, H., 1986. Analysis of stable isotopes in prehistoric populations. in (B. Herrmann, ed) Innovative Trends in der prähistorischen Anthropologie Mitteilungen der Berliner Gesellschaft für Anthropologie, Ethnologie und Urgeschichte 7, 31-38

Therkorn, L.L., 1984. Schagen: Muggenburg. in (P.J. Woltering) Archeologische kroniek van Holland over 1983. I Noord-Holland. Holland 16, 215-216

Therkorn, L.L., Brandt, R.W., Pals, J.P., & Taylor, M., 1984. An Early Iron Age farmstead: Site Q of the Assendelver Polders Project. Proceedings of the Prehistoric Society 50, 351-373

Therkorn, L.L., & Runia, L.T., in prep. Stock raising and cattle trade in a native Roman settlement. Cingula

Tipton, I.H., Stewart, P.L. & Martin, P.G., 1966. Trace elements in diets and excreta. Health Physics 12, 1683-1689
Toots, H. & Voorhies, M.R., 1965. Strontium in fossil bones and the reconstruction of food chains. Science 149, 854-855
Tylecote, R.F., 1976. A history of metallurgy. London: The Metals Society
Ubelaker, D.H., 1978. Human skeletal remains; excavation, analysis, interpretation. Chicago: Aldine
Underwood, E.J., 1977. Trace elements in human and animal nutrition. New York: Academic Press
Van der Merwe, N.J., 1982. Carbon isotopes, photosynthesis and archaeology. American Scientist 70, 596-606
Van der Merwe, N.J. & Vogel, J.C., 1978. 13C Content of human collagen as a measure of prehistoric diet in Woodland North America. Nature 276, 815-816
Veen, H.E. van de, 1979. Food selection and habitat use in the red deer (Cervus elaphus L.). thesis Rijksuniversiteit Groningen
Veen, H.E. van de, & Wieren, S.E. van, 1980. Van grote grazers, kieskeurige fijnproevers en opportunistische gelegenheidsvreters. Internal report, IVM, Amsterdam
Vons-Comis, S.Y., 1978. Excavation report Hoogkarspel-Watertoren 1978. Internal report, IPP, Amsterdam
Waals, J.D. van der, 1961. De zool van tumulus XIII bij 'De Ark', gemeente Wervershoof. WFON XXVIII, 52-96
Wahl, J., 1982. Leichenbranduntersuchungen. Ein Uberblick über die Bearbeitungs und Aussagemöglichkeiten von Brandgräben. Prähistoriches Zeitschrift 57, 1-125
Waldron, H.A., 1982. Human bone lead concentrations. in (A. McWhirr, L. Viner and C. Wells) Romano-British cemetaries at Cirencester. Cirencester excavations II Cirencester: Cirencester Excavation Committee, 203-204
Waldron, H.A., 1983. On the post-mortem accumulation of lead by skeletal tissues. JAS 10, 35-40
Waldron, H.A., Khera, H., Walker, G., Wibberley, G. & Green, C.J.S., 1979. Lead concentrations in bones and soil. JAS 6, 295-298
Waldron, H.A., Mackie, A. & Townshend, A., 1976. The lead content of some Romano-British bones. Archaeometry 18, 221-227
Wallace, A. & Romney, E.M., 1971. Some interactions of Ca, Sr and Ba in plants. Agronomy Journal 63, 245-248
Wasserman, R.H., Comar, C.L. & Papadopoulou, D., 1957. Dietary calcium levels and retention of radiostrontium in the growing rat. Science 126, 1180-1182
Waterbolk, H.T., 1973. A.E. van Giffen, 1884-1973. Palaeohistoria XV, 7-12
Waterbolk, H.T., 1977. Walled enclosures of the Iron Age in the North of the Netherlands. Palaeohistoria XIX, 97-172
Weast, R.C. (ed), 1973. Handbook of chemistry and physics. Cleveland: CRC (54th edition)
Weerd, M.D. de, 1966. Nederzettingssporen van de vroege klokbekercultuur bij Oostwoud (N.H.). Voortgezet onderzoek 1964. in (W. Glasbergen & W. Groenman-van Waateringe, eds) In het voetspoor van A.E. van Giffen, tweede, vermeerderde druk. Groningen: Wolters, 174-175
White, E.M. & Hannus, L.A., 1983. Chemical weathering of bone in archaeological soils. American Antiquity 48, 316-322
Wijn, J.F. de & Staveren, W.A. van, 1980. De voeding van elke dag. Utrecht: Bohn, Scheltema & Holkema
Wijngaarden- Bakker, L.H. van, 1986. Trace elements in prehistoric environment and food chains. in (B. Herrmann, ed) Innovative Trends in

der prähistorischen Anthropologie Mitteilungen der Berliner Gesellschaft für Anthropologie, Ethnologie und Urgeschichte 7, 25-29

Wing, E.S., & Brown, A.B., 1979. Paleonutrition. Method and theory in prehistoric foodways. New York: Academic Press

Woltering, P.J., 1979. Archeologische kroniek van Noord-Holland over 1978. Holland 11, 242-273

Woltering, P.J., 1985. Prehistorie en Romeinse tijd in West-Friesland. WFON 52, 199-232

Woltering, P.J., 1986. Archeologische kroniek van Noord-Holland over 1985. Holland 18, 273-303

Zeuner, F.E., 1963. A history of domesticated animals. New York: Harper & Row

APPENDIX 1
CATALOGUE OF HUMAN REMAINS FROM WEST-FRIESLAND

Introduction

The human remains from West-Friesland are catalogued on the basis of year of excavation and publication. The basis for the present catalogue is the preliminary list by J.A. Bakker (1974). The catalogue numbers 1-53 are present in Bakker's list, the higher numbers are newly added.

The catalogue contains the following information per entry:

General information: Number, site, year of excavation and publication, place where the material is stored.
A: Anthropological data
1. General data: which elements are present/absent, state of conservation
2. Measurements, body height
3. Estimation of sex
4. Estimation of age
5. Special features such as pathology
6. If more than one individual is present, the number of individuals

B. Archeological data: position of the body in the grave, date.

Sexing according to the morphological method of AeA (1979), score -2 (feminine) to +2 (masculine).
Age determination according to Brothwell (1981, tooth wear) and Ubelaker (1978, tooth eruption) and AeA (1979, fusing of epiphyses).
Body lengths estimates according to Trotter & Gleser (in Brothwell 1981).

Abbreviations:
L: left
R: right
Dentition:
M1: first molar, M3: third molar
C: canine teeth
P1: first premolar, P2 second premolar

Sex characteristics on pelvis (AeA 1979):
- P1 Sulcus praeauricularis
- P2 Incisura ischiadica major
- P3 Angulus pubis
- P4 Arc compose
- P5 Os coxae
- P6 Foramen obturatem
- P7 Corpus ossis ischii
- P8 Crista iliaca
- P9 Fossa iliaca
- P10 Pelvis major

Sex characteristics on cranium (AeA 1979):

S1 Glabella
S2 Arcus superciliarus
S3 Tubera frontalia & parietalia
S4 Inclinatio frontale
S5 Processus mastoideus
S6 relief planum nuchale
S7 Protuberantia occipitalis externa
S8 Processus zygomaticus
S9 Os zygomaticum
S10 Crista supramastoidea
S11 Margo supraorbitale & Forma orbitae

Sex characteristics on mandibula (AeA 1979):

S12 general impression
S13 Mentum
S14 Angulus
S15 Margo

CATALOGUE

1–10 A series of burials from a group of barrows near Zwaagdijk, excavated 1942 (Van Giffen 1944). Stored at the BAI.

1–2
Cremations.

3 Zwaagdijk I, no.16
A 1. Very incomplete, only parts of long bones and two pelvis fragments preserved.
3. Incisura ischiadice major appears rather wide: female?
4. Proximal epiphysis of ulna fused, indicating age >18.
B. On back extended E-W in upper part of centre of barrow.

4 Zwaagdijk I, no. 17
A 1. Incomplete skeleton. Large parts of hands, feet and axial bones missing.
3. Probably female, characteristics S1, S2, S4, S5, S12, S13 and S14 score -1 - -2, but sexing somewhat ambiguous due to relatively low age.
4. Third molars in mandibula not yet erupted, very little wear on first and second molars. Age c. 15.
5. Excavation and storage of skeleton was not done very carefully. Bones with numbers 15 and 16 fit to bones of skeleton 17.
B. On back extended E-W in upper part of centre of barrow.

5 Zwaagdijk IV, no. 10
A 1. Very incomplete skeleton; only fragments of skull, lower arms and lower limbs present.
3. Female? Lower jaw somewhat less gracile than **4**, but female in appearance. Skull rather weathered, clear masculine features are lacking.

4. No third molars have erupted in mandibula. L maxillar M3 lost ante-mortem. Molar wear suggests age of 25-35, probably <30.
5. M3 in maxilla L lost ante-mortem in connection with periapical abscess.
B. On back extended E-W in top of barrow.

6 Zwaagdijk IV, no. 11
A 1. Very incomplete skeleton, only fragments of skull, pelvis and limbs present.
3. Distinct sulcus praeauricularis (Pl): female.
4. Epiphyses of present metacarpalia and radius (proximal) have fused, pointing to an age > c. 20.
5. Poor state of preservation.
B. On back extended E-W in top of barrow.

7 Zwaagdijk IV, no. 12
A 1. Very incomplete skeleton. Fragment of pelvis, some skull and mandibula fragments, some rib fragments and parts of upper and lower limbs present.
2. Three more or less complete bones allow calculation of body length: c. 170-175 cm.
3. Male? Pelvis fragment too small for sexing. Caput femoris diameter 47 mm, mentum appears masculine.
4. Mandibular R M3 lost post-mortem. Molar wear suggests age of 25-35.
B. In top of barrow, extended on back, S-N or N-S.

8 Zwaagdijk IV, no. 13
A 1. Very incomplete, only incomplete skull, mandibula and some fragments of lower limbs present.
3. Sex ambiguous; on mandibula, female characteristics dominant, on skull male characteristics dominate.
4. Mandibular R M3 lost post-mortem. Molar wear indicates age of 25-35.
B. In top of barrow, extended on back E-W.

9 Zwaagdijk IV, no. 14
A 1. Very incomplete, besides incomplete skull only small fragments of postcranial bones present.
3. Pelvis absent. Skull surface rather weathered. Glabella and arcus superciliarus masculine rather than feminine.
4. Mandibular L M3 lost post-mortem. Age of 25-35 suggested by wear of M1 and M2.
B. In top of barrow, extended on back N-S or S-N.

10 Zwaagdijk IV, no. 15
A 1. Very incomplete, only some small skull fragments and small fragments of postcranial skeleton preserved.
3. Sexing not possible due to low age.
4. Age can only be guessed because no fragments of skull, dentition or epiphyses are present. Dimensions of long bones suggest age <10
B. In top of barrow, N-S or S-N.

11-20 A series of cremations and skeletons from two barrows near Grootebroek, excavated 1949. (Van Giffen 1953) The material is stored at the IPP

11 Grootebroek I, no. 1
Cremation.

12 Grootebroek I, no. 2
Cremation.

13 Grootebroek I no. 3
Cremated woman (?).

14 Grootebroek I no. 3 (2)
A 1. Incomplete skeleton of young child.
3. Sexing not possible due to age.
4. Child.
B. Buried together with cremated individual **13.**

15 Grootebroek I, no. 7
A 1. Incomplete skeleton. Hand, feet, axial bones and large part of cranium missing.
2. Length of femur R and humerus R indicate body length of about 173 cm.
3. Pelvis characteristics P1 and P2 score +1; also on the mandibula male characteristics are predominant.
4. Both M3's in the mandibula are present. Molar wear indicates age of 20-25.
B. Skeleton placed on back in extended S-N position.

16 Grootebroek I, no. 4
A 1. Very incomplete skeleton, only parts of arms, legs and pelvis present.
3. Sulcus praeauricularis and incisura ischiadica major suggest female sex.
4. Adult.
B. Body was placed on R side legs contracted, arms folded in front of chest. NW-SE, facing SW.

17 Grootebroek III, no. 1
Cremation.

18/20 From Grootebroek III only one skeleton present, though two skeletons were found (Van Giffen 1953).

18 Grootebroek III, no. 12
This skeleton was probably not excavated carefully because Van Giffen assigned it to a relatively recent period. Skeleton on back, extended NNE-SSW position. Bones could not be traced.

19 Grootebroek III, no. 13
A 1. Very incomplete skeleton. Incomplete skull and parts of lower limbs present.
2. Trochanteric oblique length of L femur c. 45 cm.
3. Glabella and arcus superciliarus masculine, mandibula too weathered for sexing.
4. Mandibular R M3 not yet erupted, L M3 lost post-mortem. Together with wear of present molars (M1 R, M2 L), this suggests an age of 15-20.
5. There is some doubt if skull and limb bones belong to same skeleton.
B. Rectangular grave pit suggests extended position. Orientation of pit is approximately NNE-SSW, position of head and feet not indicated.

20
(empty number)

21-22 Hoogkarspel-Watertoren I
Bakker (1959) mentions find of a cremation and some human bone fragments. These fragments have not (yet) been traced.

23-24 Zwaagdijk XIII
Human bones mentioned by Clason (1961) could not be traced. No. 23 represents disturbed central grave, and consists of fragment of L humerus, R and L femur. No. 24 comprises finds from ring ditch: R femur (fragment?) and three non-determinable fragments. Fig. 10 in Clason (1961) shows no. 23; fragments appear too small to allow any sex, age or stature estimate.

25-36 A series of skeletons from two barrows near Oostwoud, excavated 1956-57 (Van Giffen 1962, Lanting 1979). Stored at the University of Amsterdam.

25 Oostwoud I, no. 230
A 1. Incomplete skeleton, hands, feet and major part of ribs and vertebrae are missing. Large part of cranium and mandible present.
2. Most of long bones damaged. Only one bone present in full length: L humerus, length c. 36 cm, indicating body length of c. 182 cm.
3. Pelvis and skull suitable for sexing; both have male characteristics
4. Mandibula and maxilla present. L M3 in mandibula not yet erupted, wear suggests age of 25-35.
5. Bone surface weathered.
B. Body on back, arms alongside chest, extended E-W position in centre of barrow.

26 Oostwoud I, no. 231
A 1. Incomplete skeleton. Hands, feet, vertebrae and ribs missing. Skull partly present but deformed.
2. No complete long bones present.
3. P1 and P2 are clearly female, characteristics on skull less clear, sex most probably female.
4. Mandibular M3 not yet erupted. Maxilla fragment too small to observe state of M3. Molar wear suggests age of 25-35.
5. Bones in poor state of conservation due to cracking after excavation. Periapical abscess cavities are present in the L half of the mandibular C and M1. In connection, M1 lost ante-mortem.
B. The body was laid on back in flank of barrow, extended E-W, arms alongside chest.

27 Oostwoud II, no. 127
A 1. Incomplete skeleton; hands, feet and axial skelton missing.
2. Femora and tibia present. Epiphyses not fused, so measuring length problematical. With this restriction, body length can be estimated at 155-165 cm.
3. Sex?
4. Age estimation difficult. Epiphyses of long bones not fused, suggesting age below c. 19 years. All M3 however erupted. All molars show very little wear (maximum 2+ on M1). All teeth rather small. In sum, age at death probably was 15-20.

B. Secondary grave; body crouched on L side, E-W, facing S.

28 Oostwoud II, no. 228

A 1. Incomplete skeleton, feet and large part of axial bones missing.

2. Body length can be extrapolated from lengths of three long bones: c. 172 cm.

3. Skull and part of pelvis present, both suggesting male sex.

4. Dentition suggests age of c.20. Part of the M3 erupted, M1 and M2 show little wear, stage 2 - 2+.

B. Crouched on L side, arms in front of chest, E-W, facing S. R hand and distal parts of R ulna and radius found together with manubrium sterni 'onder de voeten' (below the feet). Exact position unknown due to ambiguous word 'below' the meaning of which depends on reference (body, i.e. 'caudal', or the soil surface). 'Caudal' position resulting of post-burial displacement is suggested by presence of part of sternum.

29 Oostwoud II, no. 229

A 1. Incomplete skeleton, hands and axial bones not present. Mandible and large part of L half of skull missing.

2. Four long bones more or less complete; extrapolated body length c. 173 cm.

3. Sex characteristics on skull and pelvis indicate male sex.

4. Mandible absent, maxilla partly present. R M3 in maxilla post-mortem lost. Molar wear suggests age of ca. 25-30.

5. Tibiae very flat, platycnemic index 51.

B. Excavation plan (Van Giffen 1962) shows location of 229, but position of body unclear.

30 Oostwoud II, no. 232

A 1. Incomplete skeleton, removed in a block in fixed position. Individual bones cannot be taken out. Ribs, sternum and almost all hand- and foot bones missing. Skull fractured and pressed together. Pelvis broken and only partly visible. Most of long bones broken.

2. Exact measurements cannot be made due to fixation and fractures. Length of femur c. 43 cm, tibia c. 37 cm, suggesting body length of 160 and 169 cm, respectively.

3. Skull not suitable for sex determination. Pelvis broken and partly covered by soil. L half of pelvis visible from behind. Incisura ischiadica major not easily visible, but probably rather wide. Sulcus praeauricularis appears present. Both characteristics suggest female sex.

4. Age estimation difficult. M1, M2 and M3 in upper and lower jaw L appear to be present. Occlusal surfaces not visible. Molar wear probably not very extreme, so an age of 25-35 is suggested.

5. Left femur and tibia used for 14C dating (GrN 8801: 3530 ± 25 BP) and replaced by casts.

B. Crouched on R side, hands in front of face. N-S, facing W. For further comments, see **33**.

31 Oostwoud II, no. 233

A 1. Very incomplete skeleton. Only skull, mandibula, part of L arm and R half of pelvis present.

3. Sex characteristics on skull and pelvis not very clear but probably this was a female.

4. All molars present. Molar wear on M3 stage 2+ - 3+, on M1 5+. Age c. 33-45.

5. Caries in P2 and M1 in mandibula L, periapical abscess cavities below both second premolars in mandibula.
B. Position of body unknown.

32 Oostwoud II, no. 235
A 1. Incomplete skeleton, skull, hands, feet and most axial bones missing.
2. Six bones can be used for body length estimation. Stature was c. 165 cm.
3. Pelvis shows clear male characteristics.
4. Adult.
B. Though mentioned in finds list of excavation documents of Van Giffen, position of skeleton was not drawn on excavation plans.

33 Oostwoud II, no. 236
A 1. Almost complete skeleton, lower L arm, R hand and both feet missing. Skull almost complete but deformed.
2. Femora and tibiae damaged at proximal and distal ends. Only R humerus complete, suggesting body length of c. 171 cm.
3. Sexing of pelvis is problematical: P1 scores -1, P2 +1. Skull and mandibula, however, clearly male.
4. M3 in mandibula R not erupted. Heavily worn M1 and M2 suggest fairly advanced age (>40).
5. A number of pathological features can be observed:
   - dentition in very poor state. Premolars from mandibula lost ante-mortem in connection with periapical abscesses; M1 R and M2 L lost ante-mortem, other molars very heavily and unequally worn,
   - vertebra of neck show clear traces of osteoarthritis,
   - R ulna broken and healed, R distal ends of ulna and radius show osteoarthritis,
   - joint of humerus and scapula R shows eburnation.
B. Crouched on L side, arms folded in front of chest, E-W, facing S. Together with the skeleton, bones (skull, mandibula, long bones) of a marten (Marter sp.) were found. According to Van Giffen, grave 232 (**30**) was primary grave of barrow. Lanting (1979), on the contrary, is of the opinion that skeleton 236 is primary burial. The latter opinion may be corroborated by the anthropological data, as it would mean that the barrow was raised for a relatively old male rather than for a younger female.

34 Oostwoud II, no. 239
A 1. Incomplete skeleton, only lower limbs, part of pelvis, part of L arm and parts of mandibula and maxilla present.
2. Length of tibia and femora suggest body length of c. 180 cm.
3. Pelvis shows clear male characteristics.
4. M3 in manibula R probably lost post-mortem, three molars present in R maxilla. Wear of molars suggests age of 20-25.
B. Crouched on L side, arms in front of chest. E-W, facing S.

35 Oostwoud II, no. 242
A 1. Incomplete skeleton, only skull, mandibula, part of upper limbs, L femur and some vertebra present (fig. 1.1).
2. Length of L femur suggests body length of c. 181 cm.
3. Skull shows clear male characteristics; diameter of caput femoris 51 mm, both suggesting male sex.

4. All molars present except for not yet erupted M3 in mandibula R. Molars show little wear (stage 3 on first molars) suggesting age of 17-25.
B. Excavation plan of Van Giffen suggests crouched position on L side, E-W, facing S (see also **38**).

36 (1) Oostwoud II, no. 243
A 1. Incomplete skeleton, ribs and vertebrae for large part absent.
2. Body length can be estimated on basis of lengths of three long bones: c. 165 cm.
3. Both pelvis and skull show female characteristics.
4. Dentition in very poor state. M3 in mandibula R shows wear stage 4+, M1 have wear stage 5, suggesting age of 35-50.
5. L tibia and fibia bowed. Dentition in very poor state, with caries in present molars. Several elements lost ante-mortem in connection with periapical abscesses. Radiographs of tibiae show number of Harris' lines.
B. Crouched on R side, hands in front of face. E-W, facing N.

36 (2) Oostwoud II, no. 247
A 1. Incomplete skeleton. Only skull and mandibula, and parts of upper and lower limbs present.
3. Incisura ischiadica major rather wide, skull too shows female characteristics.
4. M3 probably all erupted. Molar wear suggests age of 25-35.
B. Probable position of body: crouched on R side, NWN-SES, facing W.

37 - 39 Oostwoud II, excavation 1963 (De Weerd 1966). Material stored at the IPP (**38**) and WestFriesch Museum (Hoorn).

37 Oostwoud II
A. 1. Almost complete skeleton, except for complete and reconstructed skull in-situ embedded and fixed in soil. State of preservation good, some long bones broken.
2. Exact measurements not possible due to fixation of bones. Length of femur c. 47.5 cm, tibia c. 38.0 cm, humerus c. 33.0 cm, suggesting stature of c. 175 cm.
3. Sex characteristics on skull and pelvis suggest male sex.
4. All dental elements completely erupted. Molar wear suggests age of 25-35 year.
5. The skull is asymmetric to medial plane, possibly due to deformation in soil. In this aspect, it can be compared to the Molenaarsgraaf II skull (Louwe Kooymans, 1974, Plate XV). Both skeletons were lying on L side. R processus mastoideus larger than L. Medial part of linea nuchalis superior forms a crest. In lambdoid suture some five Wormian bones.
B. Crouched on L side, arms folded in front of chest. E-W, facing S.

38 Oostwoud II, no. 533
A. 1. Bones from lower half of body (fig. 1.1).
2. L tibia measures c. 41 cm, suggesting body length of c. 181 cm.
3. Pelvis fragments show clear male characteristics. Body length also suggests male sex.
4. Adult.
6. Though bones were not found in anatomical position, they probably are from one individual.

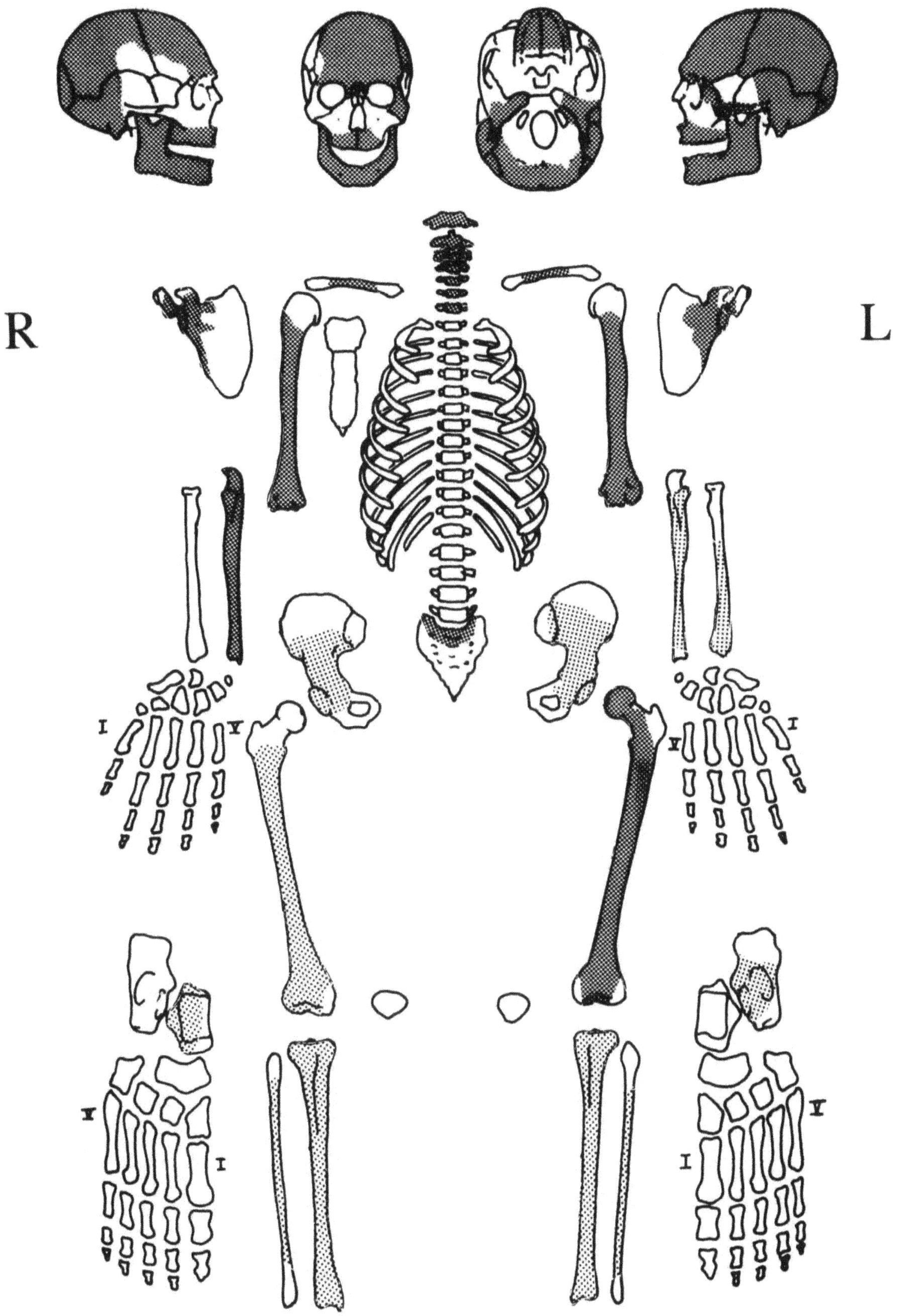

figure 1.1 Scheme showing the recovered skeletal elements of 35 (dark shading) and 38 (light shading).

B. Bones were found above and next to **37**, and may represent a disturbed grave. The bones of **35** and **38** most likely represent one individual as suggested by fig.1.1, the dimensions of the bones and chemical analysis. In the cluster of bones some bones of fox (Vulpes vulpes) were found.

39 Oostwoud II
A.1. According to De Weerd, another incomplete human skeleton was found.
2-6. No further information can be given because the bones could not be traced.

40 Barrow 'De Tent' near Enkhuizen, excavated 1960 (Lehmann 1963). Material stored at the IPP.
A 1+2. five bones:
27. fragment of clavicula R, sternial part and acromial facet missing,
37. neck and parts of acromion and coracoid process of scapula R,
50. fragment of os temporale R, squamous part and zygotomatic process missing,
56. fragment of clavicula L, medial part and acromial facet missing,
58. cervical vertebra, spine missing.

3. Sexing not possible, 50 may be female (S5:-1, S10:-1).
4. Adult .
5. 58: osteoporosis?
6. These bones were found in SW quadrant of barrow, 56 and 58 close to each other in second period ring ditch, 27 and 37 in th flank of barrow, 50 possibly in first period ring ditch. Distance between 56/58 and 27 some 10 m. All fragments stem from the upper part of the body, possibly from one individual. Claviculae are almost perfect counterparts. An old grave may have been disturbed during construction of the barrow. Lehmann (1963, p.240) writes (my translation) that "two fragments of what may have been a human mandible" were found in the first period ringditch. No human mandible fragments were, however, found in the storage box containing the mobilia of the excavation neither does the finds list mention a human mandible. During the excavation, only 37 and 50 were recognized as being human.
B. Fragments were found in the ditches from a two-period Bronze Age barrow.

41 - 45 Flat graves near Zwaagdijk, excavated 1961 (Modderman 1964) and preliminary described by Huizinga (1964). Material at present at IPP, but owned by the ROB.

41 Zwaagdijk, flat grave 1, storage box no. 636
A 1+2. Incomplete skeleton, only part of skull, upper arms and legs present.
3. Eight sex characteristics on the skull could be scored, suggesting female sex.
4. Only right half of mandible present. M1 lost post-mortem, M2 and M3 show little wear, indicating age of c. 20-25 years.
B. Bones were collected after the grave had been disturbed, so no information on burial position is available.

42 Zwaagdijk, flat grave 2, storage box no. 637

A 1+2. Almost complete skeleton. Part of sacrum, patellae and proximal parts of R fibula and of L tibia and fibula missing. L and R femur and R tibia indicate stature of c. 169 cm.

3. Pelvis and skull have clear male characteristics.
4. M3 present in mandibula and lost in maxilla. Wear indicates age of 30-40.
5. Some pathological features can be observed:
   - L ulna broken and healed,
   - M2 and M3 in maxilla L show severe caries; more than half of M3 has disappeared,
   - R apex capitis fibulae is surrounded by bone exostotes, unfortunately R caput fibulae absent,
   - lower lumbar vertebrae and basis ossis sacri show bone exostoses around the articulation facets. The lower part of the vertebral column shows scoliosis.

B. On back extended E-W, R arm straight alongside body, L arm in front of chest, hand on neck.

43 Zwaagdijk, flat grave 3, storage box no. 638

A 1+2. Incomplete skeleton, hand, feet, lower arms and axial bones missing. Complete L femur suggests stature of c. 185 cm.

3. Pelvis and skull show clear male characteristics. Robustness of bones and diameter of the caput femoris (51 mm) also suggest male sex.
4. M3 present in maxilla and mandibula, tooth wear suggests age of 20-25.
5. On the place of incisura radialis of R ulna some bone exostoses are present. M3 in R maxilla has caries.

B. On back extended ESE-WNW, arms alongside body. A recent drain trench had been dug through middle of body. In this grave, a bronze sword, amber beads, a piece of worked flint, a piece of sandstone and a small animal bone were found.

44 Zwaagdijk, flat grave 4, storage box no. 639A

A 1+2. Very incomplete skeleton in poor state of preservation. Only fragments of skull, mandibula, vertebrae, ulnae and radii, and diaphyses of both femurs and tibiae and of R humerus present.

3. Though Huizinga (1964) suggests female sex, in my view male sex is also possible.
4. Small part of R half of mandibula with M1 and M2 preserved. Both show very little wear. Though not certain because mandible is incomplete, M3 had probably not yet erupted. Age estimated c. 15-20.

B. On back extended W-E.

45 Zwaagdijk, flat grave 5, storage box no. 639B

A 1+2 Almost complete skeleton of child.

4. Dentition suggests age of c. 6.

B. Position of body reconstructed by Huizinga (1964). Child buried on back, legs above chest and arms around legs. Orientation ?

46 - 47 Secondary grave in barrow II of Hoogkarspel-Tolhek, excavated 1965 (Bakker & Brandt 1966). Material stored at the IPP and WestFriesch Museum (Hoorn).

46

A 1+2. Fragments of cremated bone and some fragments of incompletely burnt bones. Present are incompletely burned parts of pelvis, sacrum and femora. Skull fragments were also found, but are now missing. Large part of skeleton in-situ fixed and kept in the WestFriesch Museum at Hoorn.

3. Dr. de Boer, who examined the skeletal remains in 1966, concluded that the person was female (letter of Dr. W de Boer to director of IPP, May 26, 1966). Of remaining bones, pelvis fragments show distinct sulcus praeauricularis and suggest a rather wide incisura ischiadica major, which suggest female sex. Diameter of caput femoris rather large (c. 47 mm).

4. No age estimation can be given on basis of the now present material. De Boer estimated age of about 30-40, probably 35 or older.

B. see **47**.

47

A 1. Incomplete skeleton of child. Lower legs, hands and skull not present. Studied by Dr. de Boer in 1966 (see **46**).

2. Both femora present, but proximal epiphyses missing. Length of diaphyses 18.5-19 cm.

4. Skull missing, so no exact age estimation can be given. On basis of femur diaphyses length, age can be estimated at 4-5. This is somewhat lower than de Boer's estimate of 7.

5. Some small fragments (of ribs, hands ?) are charred .

B. Found together with **46**, who was deposited in a secundary, tangential grave and incompletely burnt in grave pit, crouched on R side, E-W, facing N. Small pieces of charred bone of **47** suggest that the child was deposited near the woman shortly after she had been cremated. The child was on its R side, arms and legs folded in front of body, in front of **46**.

48 Hoogkarspel-Tolhek

In a series of excavations near Hoogkarspel (section II.C.2.7) a number of isolated human bones were found in occupation features, as were animal bones, stones and pottery fragments. Bones from a maximum number of 31 individuals is present. Estimation of sex and age in most cases not possible. Material at present stored at the IPP.

HKL 18

A 1. Fragment of L clavicula.

4. Adult.

HKL 65

A 1+2. Part of R half of mandibula. C, P1 and P2 lost post-mortem, M1 and M2 present, M3 not yet erupted. Part of ramus present, but angulus mandibulae absent.

3. Fragment too small to allow for sex determination.

4. Molar wear (M1:5, M2:2) and absence of M3 suggest age of 15-20.

HKL 83

A 1+2. Part of distal half of L femur, parts of condyles present. Length c. 20 cm.

4. Adult.

HKL 173

A 1+2. Phalanx.

4. Adult.

HKL 177
A 1. Small skull fragment.
4. Adult.

HKL 194
A 1. Small skull fragment.
4. Adult.

HKL 207
A 1+2. Fragment of humerus shaft, length 9 cm.
4. Adult.

HKL 217
A 1+2. (1) Distal part of R humerus, length c. 15 cm,
(2) fragments of two vertebrae bodies.
4. Adult.

HKL 242
A 1+2. Calcined, deformed, whitish skull fragment.

HKL 257
A 1+2. Proximal end and shaft of R radius, length c. 17 cm.
4. Adult.

HKL 258
A 1+2. (1) Distal end of R radius, length c. 11 cm,
(2) small fragment of proximal end and caput of L radius.
4. Adult.

HKL 269
A 1+2. (1) Proximal part of small R femur,
(2) M1 with small part of mandibula.
4. (1) child (< 10), epiphysis not fused.
(2) wear stage 5, adult: 25-35?
6. Obviously, these are fragments of two individuals.

HKL 278
A 1+2. Fragment of diaphysis of fibula.
4. Adult.

HKL 320
A 1+2. Fragment of L os parietale with part of margo sagittalis and margo occipitales.
4. Adult ?
5. Osteoporosis.

HKL 322
A 1+2. Small skull fragment.

HKL 323
A 1+2 Skull fragment.

HKL 352
A 1+2. Diaphysis of R femur, clearly marked linea aspera.
3. Male ?
4. Adult.

HKL 370
A 1+2. Small, calcined, whitish skull fragment.

HKL 425
A 1+2. Diaphysis of tibia, length 19 cm.
4. Adult.

HKL 475
A 1+2. Small skull fragment.

HKL 479
A 1+2. Diaphysis and proximal part of L ulna, olecranon missing, length c. 20 cm.
4. Adult.

HKL 482
A 1+2. Small part of a humerus diaphysis, length 7.5 cm.
4. Adult.

HKL 485
A 1+2. Shaft of femur, length c. 22 cm, clearly marked linea aspera.
3. Male?
4. Adult.

HKL 494
A 1+2. Small fragment of fibula shaft, length 9 cm.
4. Adult.

HKL 496
A 1+2. (1) Shaft of femur, length c. 13 cm,
(2) Shaft of L humerus, length c. 22 cm.
4. (1) and (2) : adult.
6. Probably from two individuals.

HKL 528
A 1+2. Shaft of femur, length c. 20 cm.
4. Adult.

HKL 543
A 1+2. Shaft of tibia, length c. 14 cm.
4. Adult.

49 Medemblik, barrow II (Van Regteren Altena & Bakker 1968)
Cremation.

50–53 An incomplete skeleton and some cremated human bones from a barrow Ia at Hoogkarspel-Watertoren, excavated in 1972. (Modderman 1974). Material stored at the WestFriesch Museum (Hoorn).

50 Hoogkarspel Ia, no. 207
Cremation. In the storage bag containing this cremation, a few fragments of non cremated bones of a very young child were present.

51 Hoogkarspel Ia, no. 228

A. 1. Incomplete skeleton. State of preservation rather poor, only diaphyses of long bones are preserved. Pelvis and large part of skull missing.

3. Sexing problematical due to absence of pelvis and large part of skull. Some characteristics are male: heavy mandibula, rough surface of planum nuchale, clearly marked linea aspera.

4. Adult. R M3 in mandibula erupted but does not show much wear, L M3 not present, pathological features and wear of M1 suggest age >35.

5. Pathological features present in mandibula and upper in cervical vertebrae. R M1 caries and periapical abscess cavity.

B. Extended E-W. A kitten tibia might represent a grave gift.

52 Hoogkarspel Ia, no. 227

Cremation.

53 Hoogkarspel-Watertoren

A human bone fragment was found in the occupation traces of Hoogkarspel-Watertoren (Bakker et al. 1977). Stored at the IPP.

A 1+2. Fragment of R part maxilla, C1, P1, P2, M1, M2, M3 present.

4. Tooth wear suggests 17-25 year.

54 Andijk

A number of human bones from settlement traces near Andijk, excavated by the ROB in 1973-74 (Van Mensch & IJzereef 1975). Stored at the ROB.

II-64

A 1+2. R femur, length 51 cm.

3. Diameter caput femoris 53 mm, suggesting male sex.

4. Adult, epiphysis fused.

II-117

A 1+2. Diaphysis of L humerus, length 23.7 cm.

4. Adult.

III-3

A 1+2. Almost complete L os temporale.

3. Sex? Processus mastoideus not very large.

4. Adult.

III-30

A 1+2. Small skull fragment, probably of os temporale.

4. Adult.

III-36

A 1. Fragment of os frontale.

4. Adult.

III-37, III/IV-37

A 1+2.

(1) L pelvis, os pubis missing,

(2) R femur, length 45.2 cm, suggesting body length of c. 166 cm,

(3) diaphysis fragment of R radius, length 16.0 cm, marked tuberosity,

(4) fragment of L os temporale, squamous part and processus zygomaticus missing,

(5) fragment of L half of os frontale,

(6) fragments of os frontale and os parietale.
3.
(1) P1 and P2 indicate female sex,
(2) diameter caput femoris 45 mm suggests female sex,
(4) S1 and S10 suggest female sex,
(5) S2 indicates male sex.
4. All fragments probably adult.
6. (5) and (6) of two individuals. L counterpart of (2) would probably fit in (1). Fragments are therefore of at least two, at most six individuals.

III-38
A 1+2.
(1) R femur, length 46.5 cm suggesting body length of 169 cm, proximal epiphysis not fused,
(2) fragment of diaphysis R femur, length 25.5 cm, well developed linea aspera,
(3) fragment of diaphysis R tibia, length 22.5 cm,
(4) part of R os parietale, margo occipitalis partly present. In this margo a small wormian bone,
(5) humerus fragment, length 7.6 cm.
3.
(1) Female sex suggested by caput diameter, 43 mm.
4.
(1) Epiphysis suggests age under 16-19.
(2)-(5) Adult.
6. At least two individuals.

III-39
A 1+2. Diaphysis and proximal part of L femur, length 36.5 cm, diameter caput 45 mm.
3. Diameter of caput femoris may suggest female sex.
4. Adult.

III-44
A 1. Complete L ulna.
2. Length 28.2 cm, suggesting body length of c. 180 cm.
3. Body length may suggest male sex.
4. Adult.

III/IV-45
A 1+2. Diaphysis and proximal part of L femur, length 37 cm. Caput not present.
4. Epiphysis not fused, suggesting age < 20.

III-46
A 1+2.
(1) Complete mandible, C2 L lost post mortem, L P2 damaged post mortem,
(2) fragment of L pelvis,
(3) small skull fragment.
3. Mandible probably female; incisura ischiadica major of pelvis wide suggesting female sex.
4. In mandible all elements erupted, wear suggests age of 17-25. Pelvis probably adult.
5. L and R M1 and M2 have caries.
6. Number of individuals ?

III-48
A 1+2. Fragment of os frontale, posterior part missing.
3. Glabella and arcus supraciliaris suggest male sex.
4. Adult.

III-49/5
A 1. Almost complete R radius, only caput missing.
2. Length of probably about 27 cm, suggesting body length of about 180 cm.
3. Body length suggests male sex.
4. Adult.

III-50A
A 1+2. Part of L os parietale, parts of margo occipitalis and margo squamosus present.
4. Adult.

III-62
A 1+2.
(1) Two skull fragments and fragment R os temporale,
(2) fragment of small mandibula, no elements preserved,
(3) fragment of corpus ossis ischii,
(4) diaphysis of R femur, length c. 30 cm,
(5) diaphysis of R tibia, length c. 28 cm,
(6) diaphysis of fibula, length c. 25 cm,
(7) fragment of distal part of radius, length c. 20 cm,
(8) R humerus, proximal part missing, length c. 35 cm,
(9) diaphysis of small child's L femur,
(10) three diaphysis fragments.
4. Except (2) and (9), adult.
5. Exostosis at locus tuberositas deltoidea on (8).
6. At least two individuals.

55 Bovenkarspel-Het Valkje
During 1974-1975, the ROB excavated a large settlement site near the small lake Het Valkje near Bovenkarspel. Human bones were found mixed with other finds in ditches and pits. IJzereef (1981) has listed the finds. After re-examination, a list is also given here. Find nos. 40-1-40, 101-2-15 and 173-0-1, all long bone diaphysis fragments listed by IJzereef, could not be studied. Bones stored at the ROB.

1-2-45
A 1+2.
(1) Incomplete skeleton, skull, mandibula, femur and feet bones preserved.
(2) Incomplete skeleton, skull, mandibula, femur and feet bones preserved.
3.
(1) Characteristics of skull and mandibula suggest female sex,
(2) According to IJzereef (1981, 1983) male individual. Mandibula less gracile than (1) but S12-S14 score not feminine. S5 suggests male, but S1 and S2 female. Conclusion: probably female, but uncertain due to age.
4.
(1) M3s not yet erupted, wear on other molars suggest age of c. 15.
(2) M3 in maxilla erupted, in mandibula erupting, suggesting age of c. 17-19.
B. Extended alongside each other in grave in ditch.

8-1-4/24
A 1+2. Small fragment of os occipitale.
4. Adult.

17-1-1
A 1+2. Mandible fragment, all elements erupted but post-mortem lost.
3. S12 and S13 suggest female sex.
4. Adult.

30-1-4/1
A 1+2. Shaft and distal end of L humerus, length c. 20 cm.
3. Clearly marked tuberositas deltoidea: male?
4. Adult.

31-1-3
A 1+2. Incomplete skeleton of infant.

38-2-1
A 1. Three skull fragments: two small fragments of the cranium and a complete R os zygomaticum.
2. Cranium fragments both measure about 8 square cm.
3. The os zygomaticum has a somewhat rough surface and the edge of the orbit is rather rounded. Both suggest male sex.
4. Adult.
6. One or two individuals.

40-1-35
A 1+2. Diaphysis of R femur, length c. 27 cm.
3. Linea aspera might suggest male sex.
4. Adult.

44-1-15
A 1. Complete phalanx.
4. Adult.

45-1-9
A 1+2. Diaphysis of L femur, length 34 cm.
4. Adult.

48-1-1/23
A 1+2. L femur, length 45 cm suggests body length of c. 170 cm.
3. Diameter caput 51 mm suggests male sex.
4. Adult.

97-2-16
A 1. Complete phalanx.
4. Adult.

98-1-3
A 1+2. Proximal part of R femur.
3. Female sex suggested by diameter caput, 42 mm.
4. Adult.

99-2-26
A 1+2. Fragment diaphysis femur, length 18.5 cm.
4. Adult.

102-2-2
A 1+2. Proximal and distal fragment of R femur, diaphysis not present
3. Diameter of caput 45.5 mm might suggest female sex.
4. Adult.

103-1-11
A 1+2. Fragment of L os parietale, part of margo frontalis and parietalis present.
4. Adult.

103-2-21
A 1+2. Diaphysis of L femur, length 26 cm.
4. Adult.

117-2-8
A 1+2. Fragment of os frontale and R os parietale.
3. S1 and S2 suggest male sex.
4. Adult.

117-2-12
A 1+2. Complete slightly damaged skull, all elements in maxilla erupted but except L M1 post mortem lost.
3. Clear male characteristics.
4. Adult. Wear of L M1 suggests age 17-25.

117-1-15
A 1+2. Small skull fragment.

117-2-24
A 1+2. Diaphysis of R tibia, length 29.5 cm.
4. Adult.

150-3-8
A 1+2. Small fragment of femur diaphysis, length 9 cm.
4. Adult.

150-3-17
A 1+2. Large part of R half of cranium, almost complete os frontale.
3. Probably female.
4. Adult.

157-2-1
A 1. Part of R calcaneus.
4. Adult.

185-2-2
A 1+2. Small fragment of proximal part of L femur of young child.
4. Dimension of femur suggests age under c. 7.

197-2-1
A 1+2. Almost complete mandibula, all elements erupted.
3. S12-S14 suggest male sex.
4. Wear of molars suggests age of 17-25.

201-1-3
A 1+2. L os temporale, squamous part missing, and fragment of R os zygomaticum.

3. S 5, S10 suggest male sex.
4. Adult.

56 Hoogkarspel-Watertoren
Excavation of an area N of Hoogkarspel in 1978 (Bakker 1979). A skeleton from a barrow and some small human bone fragments. Stored at the IPP.

Hw 71
A 1. Incomplete skeleton, skull and mandibula almost complete, major parts of arms and legs present. Ribs and vertebra partly present, but in small fragments.
2. No complete long bones are present.
3. In the pelvis, both P1 and P2 score -2, on skull female characteristics present. Female.
4. Dentition suggests rather advanced age. A number of elements lost ante-mortem, alveolar bone resorption is considerable. Both M1 in mandibula present, but heavily worn (stage 5++) and with considerable calculus. Age probably over 45.
5. Dentition is poor state, elements heavily worn, alveolar bone resorption and periapical abcesses (at both P2's in the mandibula). L ulna broken some 3 cm above distal end, callus present but bone not fused.
B. In small grave pit in small barrow, crouched on back, S-N.

Hw 78
A 1+2. Fragment of skull and fragment of condyle(?).

57 Bovenkarspel-Monument terrein Visser
Almost complete skeleton of and old woman, nicknamed 'the witch of Bovenkarspel' because of advanced age and a number of pathological features. Described by G.J.R. Maat (in press a). Stored at the ROB.

58 Andijk 1982
During a small excavation (de Vries-Metz 1983, IPP, pers. comm..) some human bone fragments were found:

An 82-3
A 1+2. Fragment of cranium, c. 10 cm2, with part of margo.
4. Fragment relatively thin which suggests sub-adult age.

An 82-39
A 1+2. Part of fractured L os parietale, part of margo sagittalis and occipitalis present.
4. Thin bones, suggesting low age.

59 Schagen-Muggenburg
At Schagen-Muggenburg, remains of five human individuals were found. The material was studied and described by G.J.R. Maat. Here, they are numbered Mug 1-5. Description based on Maat (in press b). Bones stored at the IPP.

Mug 1. Isolated human bone from feature 27
A 1. Incomplete R os coxae.
3. Characteristics P1, P2, P4 and P7 indicate male sex.
4. Adult (epiphyses fused).

Mug 2. Skeleton from feature 77
A 1. Almost complete child's skeleton, bones fragmented.
4. A number of characteristics indicate this was a perinatal child with gestational age of 9 months.

Mug 3. Skeleton from feature 150
A 1. Almost complete skeleton, bones fragmented.
2. Stature of 149 cm measured in situ.
3. Pelvis characteristics indicate female sex.
4. Age of 17-24 is suggested by molar wear and internal bone remodelling.
B. On back extended, orientation? face turned R, R hand on R hip.

Mug 4. Skeleton from feature 321
A 1. Almost complete skeleton, bones fragmented.
2. Insitu length 160-165 cm, length of R femur indicates body length of c. 165 cm.
3. Complete pelvis indicates male sex.
4. Age 50-56, based on state of dentition and on AeA complex method.
5. Caries in R M3s, abscess at apex M3 mandibula.
B. On back, extended orientation?, L hand on R pelvis, face turned R.

Mug 5. Skeleton from feature 322
A 1. Almost complete skeleton, bones fragmented.
2. In situ length not measurable, long bones too fragmented to allow measuring.
3. Pelvis indicates this was a male.
4. Age of 23-25 suggested by dentition, fused proximal epiphysis of clavicula, and obliteration of sutures of tabula interna.
B. Crouched on L side, arms in front of chest.

60 Venhuizen-Kestelo

Mr. Kestelo of Venhuizen on his land found some human bone fragments in addition to pot sherds and flint artifacts.

(1)
A 1+2. Part of os frontale, width c. 7 cm, squama frontalis absent.
3. Arcus superciliaris not very pronounced, suggesting female sex.
4. Adult.

(2)
A 1+2. Small cranium fragment, c. 6 square cm, part of margo present.

(3)
A 1+2. Small cranium fragment, c. 25 square cm, part of margo present.

(4)
A 1+2. Fragment of os frontale, R processus zygomaticus and part of margo orbitalis, c. 2x4 cm.
3. Rather sharp margo orbitalis suggests female sex.
4. Adult.
5. Colour whitish, suggesting it was (incompletely) burnt.

APPENDIX 2

Abbreviations

AAS	Atomic Absorption Spectrometry
APM	Average Plant Material, i.e. young, green shoots and plant parts (section IX.D.4)
BAI	Biologisch-Archeologisch Instituut, State University at Groningen
CV	Coefficient of variation: mean/standard deviation x 100%
delta 13C	((13C/12C sample)/(13C/12C standard)-1)x1000 per mil, standard is PDB (section I.B)
delta 15N	((15N/14N sample)/(15N/14N standard)-1)x1000 per mil, standard is atmospheric nitrogen (AIR) (section I.B)
DR	Distribution Ratio = (Sr/Ca ratio in item x) / (Sr/Ca ratio in item y); (Runia 1987b, section IX.C)
ECN	Netherlands Energy Research Foundation, Petten (N-H)
ICP-AES	Inductively Coupled Plasma Atomic Emision Spectrometry
IDMS	Isotope Dilution Mass Spectrometry
IPP	Albert Egges van Giffen Instituut voor Prae- en Protohistorie, University of Amsterdam
IPL	Instituut voor Praehistorie, State University at Leiden
L	left
OR	Observed Ratio = (Sr/Ca ratio in sample)/(Sr/Ca ratio in precursor); (Comar et al. 1957, section V.A)
R	right
Rc	mg Sr/g Ca in cattle bones (section V.C.4.3)
Rd	mg Sr/g Ca in human diet (section XI.C.2)
Rh	mg Sr/g Ca in human bones (section V.C.4.3)
ROB	Rijksdienst voor het Oudheidkundig Bodemonderzoek, Amersfoort

www.ingramcontent.com/pod-product-compliance
Lightning Source LLC
LaVergne TN
LVHW071206210926
848482LV00015B/737
* 9 7 8 0 8 6 0 5 4 4 7 1 5 *